Developing
Retirement
Facilities

Developing Retirement Facilities

PAUL A. GORDON, J.D.
Hanson, Bridgett, Marcus, Vlahos & Rudy
San Francisco, California

JOHN WILEY & SONS
New York • Chichester • Brisbane • Toronto • Singapore

This publication is designed to provide accurate and
authoritative information in regard to the subject
matter covered. It is sold with the understanding that
the publisher is not engaged in rendering legal, accounting,
or other professional service. If legal advice or other
expert assistance is required, the services of a competent
professional person should be sought. *From a Declaration
of Principles jointly adopted by a Committee of the
American Bar Association and a Committee of Publishers.*

Library of Congress Cataloging in Publication Data:

Gordon, Paul A. (Paul Anthony), 1950–
    Developing retirement facilities / Paul A. Gordon.
       p.   cm.
    Bibliography: p.
    ISBN 0-471-85799-8
    1. Life care communities—United States—Planning. 2. Retirement
communities—United States—Planning. 3. Old age homes—United
States—Planning. I. Title.
HV1454.2.U6G67 1988   87-22475
362.1'6'068—dc19   CIP

Printed in the United States of America
10 9 8 7 6 5

To Robin, Keith,
and my parents

Preface

The burgeoning growth of the elderly population, and its increasing preeminence as a bastion of wealth and influence, now and well into the next century, have helped draw many newcomers into the field of retirement facility development.

Once considered a last resort for the old, retirement facilities are now being designed as resorts for active seniors, with a full panoply of services, amenities, and care available when needed, or as a mere convenience. Many entrepreneurs and major corporate concerns have recently entered the field, traditionally dominated by church and fraternal groups. Novices and experienced providers alike have never had a complete business guide to formulation and development of the retirement facility product.

This book is designed to address comprehensively all the major business, legal, and tax issues facing any person contemplating or involved in the development of a retirement facility. Developers, lenders and investors; financial and marketing consultants; attorneys; and others involved in the process need to be aware of important issues, discussed in this book, that go far beyond those presented by conventional housing. The provision of hospitality services, health care, insurance programs, and other features can require licensing, unique service contracts, unusual fee payment mechanisms, consideration of special tax issues, and business and program structures designed to maximize developer and resident advantages.

While presenting the many divergent, sometimes opposing, views on the components of successful retirement facility development, this book attempts also to maintain a pragmatic, useful, how-to-do-it approach. Extensive contract forms, lists, and tables explaining applicable laws, facility features, development processes, and joint venture options; brief summaries of business structure options; state property tax laws, federal and private health insurance programs; and other topics are presented in an organized fashion intended to bring numerous complex issues into sharp focus, and to make reader access to specific information as easy as possible. In addition, however, most chapters include detailed analyses of the issues and options faced by development teams, and are heavily referenced with authoritative citations from legal, statistical, or industry expert sources.

Many of the topics discussed relatively briefly in this book (e.g., Medicare), have been the subject of volumes elsewhere. Others (e.g., retirement facility tax exemptions) are probably nowhere covered as thoroughly as here. The relative weights given to these subjects have been based on their importance in the product design and development processes, and the extent to which they are uniquely a part of the retirement facility domain.

It is my sincere hope that this book will prove to be a valuable and timely reference work both for persons first seriously exploring the field, as well as those who are already familiar with it.

PAUL A. GORDON

San Francisco, California
November 1987

Acknowledgments

My partners and associates at Hanson, Bridgett, Marcus, Vlahos & Rudy deserve first acknowledgment for making it possible for me to devote the necessary time and make use of the firm's ample resources to undertake this work. Steve Taber's authorship of the tax exempt and conventional finance sections of Part VI was indispensable to a complete survey of the subject. John Hays also deserves particular credit for his extensive work on the HUD financing and operations sections, and excellent research assistance with many other portions of the book. My partners Allan Jergesen and Joel Goldman are also responsible for the content of many of the forms in Part IX.

A debt of gratitude is owed to the American Association of Homes for the Aging and the California Association of Homes for the Aging, where my foundations in the industry stand. Andy Leon of the National Real Estate Development Center has also made it possible for me to greatly expand my knowledge by involving me in the Center's excellent series of retirement facility conferences. Many other friends, clients, and colleagues, too numerous to mention, have educated and guided me in this field for over a decade, but Raymond Hanson and Judge Thomas Jenkins—two of my firm's founding partners and pioneers in the industry—really paved the way for my involvement.

Several people have provided very helpful insights and commentaries on the text, including John Panetta, whose extensive review of tax issues is greatly appreciated, and Denice Spangler, on development and marketing issues. Thanks also to Mary Webb, Ralph Knight, Bob MacKenzie, Rob Wexler, Deborah Harris, Lydia Freeman, and Kathy Cheatum.

One of the greatest efforts is typing the seemingly endless drafts of the manuscript. A superb, and sometimes superhuman, job was done by Hilde Nivens, Bondy Pastorino, and Mark Borrowman. And, of course, none of this could have been done without Jeanne Littas and the staff at John Wiley & Sons.

Finally, I want to thank my family for its patience and support for the better part of a year while I was distracted with this work.

Contents

1   2

One

Elderly Markets and Development Responses

§ 1 AMERICAN ELDERLY PROFILE

§ 1.1 RETIREMENT FACILITY FEVER

"Real estate developers, large and small, are falling all over each other as they scramble to get into this market. Only a few seem to really know what they are doing."

(Anonymous lender)

In the latter half of this decade, the development of retirement facilities has emerged as one of the most sought after real estate investments. What has engendered this rather sudden surge of interest is the recent recognition of factors that have been evolving for many years. These include the greatly increasing numbers of elderly people in the United States and their growing wealth, the spiraling proportion of the population consisting of the very old and their soaring demand for health care, and the arrival of seniors as a consumer force with which the business world must reckon.

A 1985 study estimates that approximately one million to 1.3 million people over age 75 can afford the relatively costly life care services now being enjoyed by only about 200,000.[1] It has been predicted that by the year 2000,

[1]ICF, Inc. "Private Financing of Long Term Care: Current Methods and Resources," Phase I Final Report, U.S. Department of Health and Human Resources (1985), 74.

approximately one million new nursing beds, 812,000 new conventional retirement facility units, and 116,000 new continuing care units will be needed to meet this demand.[2] One observer expects that $33 billion will be raised between 1985 and 1990 alone to develop over 1800 retirement communities with a care component.[3] Another expects 4400 life care and congregate developments to be created by 1995, resulting in a $46 billion industry.[4]

But it is not only the burgeoning masses of the nation's elderly that have attracted devotees to the retirement facility cause. Developers who are having trouble filling office buildings, selling condominium units, or finding another good shopping center site are driven to explore new territories and markets. Hospitals and other health providers, stinging from cuts and restrictions in government reimbursement programs, are looking for ways to diversify their portfolios and to find more customers who can pay their charges in full. Insurance companies are seeking alternatives to writing liability insurance. Nonprofit groups and others already established in the field are positioning themselves to beat the others to the finish line. Hoteliers, universities, pension funds . . . it seems everyone is getting into the act.

Retirement facilities are neither simple nor homogenous products. A thorough understanding of the ranges of options available and their business and legal implications is necessary for developers, lenders, market analysts, lawyers, financial advisors, managers, marketing specialists, and others connected with the project. Eventually, retirement facility residents, with the help of their advisors, will gain a complete comprehension of these matters, for they may be embarking upon one of the most important transitions of their lives. Public awareness of the importance of careful selection among retirement community options is also heightened by the increasing interest of the press in the industry. The project development team needs to know what it is doing, what options are not being pursued, and why.

To meet the needs of the elderly, those entering the industry may have to create specialized programs and packages, beyond mere housing, that combine elements of the amenities and services of a hotel, the care available at a nursing facility, the social and recreational activities of a private club, the benefits of insurance coverage, and the shops, bank, post office, chapel, and other conveniences of a small town. The presence of many of these elements, and the way in which they are structured financially and legally can

[2]American Association of Homes for the Aging. *Market and Economic Feasibility Studies—Guidelines for Continuing Care Retirement Facilities*, 2, citing *Healthcare Financial Management*, Vol. 38, No. 4 (April 1984).

[3]K. Harney, "Facilities for the Elderly Booming" *Washington Post*, March 9, 1985, quoting Aaron Rose, then of Laventhol & Horwath.

[4]J. Lublin, "Costly Retirement-Home Market Booms, Raising Concern for Aged," *Wall Street Journal*, Oct. 22, 1986, 35, col. 4. *See also*, J. Graham, "Demand Should Foster Rapid Growth in Retirement Center Industry," *Modern Healthcare*, April 24, 1987.

have a profound impact on facility financing, income and taxation of income, marketability, control over operations, exposure to liability, government regulation, obligations to residents, and other factors that can spell success or failure for any project.

Similarly, lenders, lawyers, financial and marketing advisors, architects, and others involved in the development process should have a comprehensive knowledge extending beyond the particular project at hand. Often, the hybrid character of many retirement facilities can create discomfort among lenders and others familiar with more conventional real estate developments. While a healthy dose of caution is prudent in any undertaking as complex and expensive as these, a blanket, reflexive reaction against sophisticated or innovative retirement projects may result in a triumph of simplicity over success, and peace of mind instead of a piece of the market. Whether a complicated or straightforward program is chosen, it should be because a full spectrum of alternative structures has been considered, and the needs and wants of the consumer identified and targeted. It is therefore important first to know something about who the elderly are.

§ 1.2   THE NUMBERS OF OLDER PEOPLE

The number of people age 65 and over in the United States is increasing at a dramatic rate.[5] Census Bureau figures indicate that the number of Americans in that category will increase from 25.5 million in 1980, to 35.1 million in 2000, to 64.3 million in the year 2030. In the same time span, they will grow from 11 percent of the total population to over 18 percent.[6] Some observers have noted the increasing evidence of national interest in older people in all aspects of our culture, which will culminate with the maturation of the baby boom generation (the "pig in the python") early in the next century.[7]

The aging of America is not only due to more people reaching maturity, but also to their remaining there longer. The old are getting older, and staying healthier, so that four- and even five-generation families are becoming more commonplace (see § 1.3).[8] Especially in the upper age groups, most of the elderly are women. These facts about the *ways* in which the elderly are multiplying may have a significant bearing on how developers respond, or at least should respond, to this explosive growth.

[5]Elderly growth is even greater in countries such as Japan (three times the U.S. rate). Japan is rapidly developing senior centers, and encouraging development of facilities in other countries for Japanese elderly use. *See*, "Elderly Japanese May Be Encouraged to Retire Abroad," San Francisco *Chronicle* (UPI), Aug. 8, 1986, "Japan Is Turning Gray Fast," San Francisco *Examiner*, Sept. 14, 1986, A-16; "Japan to Export Seniors," San Francisco *Examiner*, Oct. 26, 1986, A-23.

[6]*See* Warner, "Demographics and Housing," *Housing For A Maturing Population*, Urban Land Institute (1983).

[7]*See* K. Dychtwald, ed. *Wellness and Health Promotion for the Elderly.* (Rockville, MD: Aspen Publications, 1986) 1–17.

[8]*See* A. Otten, "The Oldest Old," *Wall Street Journal*, July 30, 1984.

It is the sheer numbers of people who can be categorized as elderly that constitute the major impetus for the surge in the development of retirement housing. However, several other factors point to the need for additional development of retirement facilities, and for the development of particular types or styles of facilities to suit the needs of the consumer.

§ 1.3 AGES OF THE ELDERLY

Because of the great strides made in this century in extending the life spans and life quality of Americans, the elderly can no longer be lumped together as a uniform group. When Prussia's Bismarck decreed in the 19th century that citizens over age 65 would receive state pensions, the average life expectancy was so low that the promise amounted to little more than a political stratagem. Since 1900, when the average age at death was 49 years, life spans have climbed 50 percent to an average of about 75 years.[9] This is a leap in longevity probably unparalleled in our evolution.

Remarkable advances in medical science, and perhaps the increasing health consciousness of the population, have helped make the fastest growing age group in the country, for both men and women, the 85-and-over population.[10] At present, there are about 29.9 million people over the age of 65, 2.9 million of whom (9.7 percent) are over the age of 85. By the year 2040, approximately 66.6 million will be over 65, and about 13 million of these (19.5 percent) will be over 85.[11] Thus, while the fast-growing over-65 population will slightly more than double in roughly the next 50 years, the number of persons over the age of 85 is expected to multiply by nearly five times.

According to Census Bureau predictions, the number of persons aged 85 or more will about double as we approach the millennium, and then grow startlingly as post-World War II baby boomers reach old age.[12]

Year	Millions 85 and Over	Percent of Population
1982	2.5	1.1
2000	5.1	2.0
2050	16+	5.2

These oldest of the old consist overwhelmingly of women. In a 1982 federal government study of nursing and related care (personal care) facilities, it was found that the approximate ratio of resident women to men varied according to age as follows:

[9]*Id.*

[10]*Id. See also Aging America: Trends and Projections,* 1985–86 ed. U.S. Senate Special Committee on Aging, at 15.

[11]*Older American Reports,* June 26, 1987, 6; and "Who's Taking Care of Our Parents?," *Newsweek,* May 6, 1985, 61.

[12]*See* Otten, note 8, above.

Under 65 years	1 to 1
65–74 years	1.5 to 1
75–84 years	3 to 1
85 and over	4 to 1[13]

Women outlive men, and as a consequence, older women often live alone. In 1980, about three out of five women over 65 were single, divorced, or widowed, compared with slightly over one out of four males in the same age group.[14] At the same time, female life expectancy at age 65 was 18.7 years, whereas men could expect to have only about 14.3 more years.[15]

Of course, age frequently has a bearing upon functional ability. For ease of reference, some commentators have divided seniors into subcategories based upon their levels of independence and energy:

Go-Go
Slow-Go
No-Go[16]

These generalizations do not necessarily correlate directly to age however. Some of the very old (e.g., George Burns and Bob Hope) may still be considered Go-Gos, while some 65-year-olds unfortunately have become No-Gos due to disease or disability.

Other approaches link age broadly with general functional independence:[17]

"Empty nesters" (preretirement)	55–64	active
Young old	65–74	independent
Old	75–83	semi-independent
Very old	84+	dependent

Despite the prolonged life spans of persons over age 65, older people continue to retire from employment long before they are forced to do so by reason of functional impairment. A 1978 survey found that nearly two-thirds of retirees left work before age 65.[18] By 1980, the average male spent 20 percent of his lifetime in retirement.[19]

---

[13]Sirrocco, A., "An Overview of the 1982 National Master Facility Inventory Survey of Nursing and Related Care Homes," *Advancedata*, National Center for Health Statistics, Sept. 20, 1985.

[14]Feldblum, C., "Home Health Care for the Elderly: Programs, Problems, and Potentials," *Harvard Journal on Legislation*, 22:193 (1985, 193).

[15]*Id.*

[16]Attributed to Herb Shore, Dallas Home for Jewish Aged.

[17]This is a composite of approaches used by such commentators as Gerald Glaser of Oxford Development, and James Sherman of Laventhol & Horwath.

[18]*Aging America*, note 10 above, at 74, citing Harris, Louis & Associates, *A Nationwide Survey of Employees, Retirees and Business Leaders*, 1979.

[19]*Id.*, at 71.

The age and functional ability of a given segment of the senior population often dictates the particular type of retirement facility in which they live, and the kinds of services they want or need. One recent survey reports that although only 12.6 percent of the 65 through 74 age group required assistance with daily activities, such help was needed by 25 percent of those between the ages of 75 and 84, and by nearly 46 percent of those 85 and over.[20] On the other hand, the younger old—aged 50 to 65—have been credited with buying more warm up suits per capita than any other age category.[21] This younger, and probably more affluent, group has been affectionately labeled Grumpies (Gray-haired Urban Mature Professionals). (See § 1.6 for further discussion of the need for care.)

The character of retirement facilities can vary widely, from retirement villages offering essentially only age-restricted housing, to nursing homes, where the housing element is really incidental to health care (see § 2.2). One estimate has placed the average entry age for residents at the various types of retirement facilities as follows:

Retirement village	58
Congregate housing	62
Lifecare/continuing care	77
Nursing facility	83[22]

Much of the focus of this book will be upon the middle ranges of this spectrum, where combinations of independent housing, convenience services, personal care, or health care may exist in a single community.

§ 1.4   WHERE THE AGING LIVE

The elderly reflect society in general, with all its diversity and many of its shared attributes. Accordingly, nearly half of all Americans 65 or older live in the otherwise populous states of California, New York, Florida, Illinois, Ohio, Michigan, Pennsylvania, and Texas.[23] On the other hand, the highest concentrations of elderly are overwhelmingly in many of the less populated midwestern states, where they remain after younger people have left (see Figure 1.1).[24] For the first time, more elderly now live in suburbs than in major cities.[25]

[20] See Aging America, note 10 above, at 87.

[21] P. Petre, "Marketers Mine for Gold in the Old," Fortune, March 31, 1986, 70.

[22] See Allen, Grubb & Ellis, Investor Outlook, 6, No. 2, (2d quarter 1986), 4. Note however, that opinions vary considerably on this topic. See Todd, note 111 below, indicating that rental units attract more older persons than life care, and The Senior Living Industry 1986, Laventhol & Horwath, showing an average age of 79 years for both rental and entrance fee facilities.

[23] See Aging America, note 10, above, at 30.

[24] Id., at 34.

[25] Id., at 33.

FIGURE 1.1

**PERCENTAGE OF POPULATION 65 YEARS AND OLDER
COUNTIES WITH 15 PERCENT OR MORE, 1980**

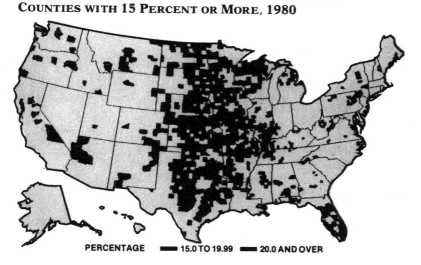

PERCENTAGE ▬ 15.0 TO 19.99 ▬ 20.0 AND OVER

Source: U.S. Bureau of the Census, Decennial Census of the Population, 1980. Prepared by Michael Callahan, U.S. Senate Computer Center.

While there are many seniors in the sunbelt states such as Florida, Arizona, and California, most industry sources seem to agree that the retirement housing market is nationwide. In fact, some elderly countermigration from sunbelt states back to states of origin has been noted in recent years.[26] Less than one in 10 of all retired persons is reported to move more than 200 miles from the area where he or she lived prior to retirement.[27] In continuing care facilities, the primary market area, from which 60 to 75 percent of the residents are expected to be drawn, may have a radius of only 25 to 50 miles.[28] In some urban areas, an even smaller radius may be applicable. For the most part, therefore, retirement communities must appeal to people who already live in the vicinity.

The vast majority of the elderly remain in their own homes rather than make a planned transition to a retirement facility.[29] However, many of them hold out for so long in their homes that when they are forced to move to a supportive environment, the transition can be abrupt and traumatic (see § 1.6). While only about five percent of the elderly live in nursing facilities, approximately one in four eventually will need long-term care.[30]

[26]*Id.,* at 37.

[27]*See* Allen, note 22, above.

[28]*Market and Economic Feasibility Studies,* note 2, above.

[29]*See* Allen, note 22, above.

[30]*Aging America,* note 10, above, at 97.

Table 1.1   Expected Additional Nursing Home and Personal Care Beds: Selected States

State	1980	Additional Beds by Year 2000	Percent Increase
Arizona	9,308	45,002	483
California	163,481	191,043	117
Florida	36,121	94,990	263
Georgia	30,040	50,294	167
Illinois	88,382	61,338	69
Louisiana	21,671	34,168	158
Maryland	20,725	37,903	183
Nevada	2,021	19,378	959
New York	103,951	76,577	74
North Carolina	32,172	69,238	215
Ohio	76,279	81,036	106
Pennsylvania	75,906	93,541	123
South Carolina	11,989	29,556	247
Texas	101,327	96,018	95
Virginia	27,376	44,363	162

Tremendous growth is expected in nonhospital facilities offering long-term care and services to the aging. The U.S. Department of Health and Human Services has predicted that the number of nursing home and personal care beds will increase by over 100 percent from the year 1980 to 2000, for a total of over three million beds.[31] Among the most significant increases projected are in the states depicted in Table 1.1.

§ 1.5   SENIOR WEALTH

The older population of the United States is arguably becoming one of the wealthiest segments of our society. About 70 percent of the net worth of all American households ($7 trillion) is controlled by people over 50, and they are spending more and saving less than ever before.[32] The elderly are doing increasingly well when compared with the rest of the populace. In 1985, households with heads aged 65 or older constituted only eight percent of the $25,000-and-over income bracket, but that share is expected to increase to 16 percent by 1995, 29 percent by 2005, and 34 percent by the year 2015.[33] One survey found that approximately 35 percent of families headed by a person at least 65 years of age earned incomes of over

[31] See Sirrocco, A., note 13, above.

[32] See Petre, note 21, above.

[33] Calculated in 1980 dollars and not including income from assets, such as interest or dividends. See ICF, Inc., note 1 above, at 78.

$25,000.[34] And the net worth of the general populace ($32,700) is well below that of elderly households ($60,300), even where the head is 75 years or older ($55,200).[35] In fact, nearly a quarter of elderly households are estimated to have a net worth of between $100,000 and $250,000.[36] Seven percent had net worths in excess of $250,000.[37] Although once considered an economically disadvantaged group, the elderly have been declared to have achieved, on the whole, financial parity with the rest of the population.[38]

Americans age 65 and over had fewer of the poor among their numbers in 1985 (12.6 percent) than those under 65 (14.1 percent).[39] Nevertheless, while the elderly make up 21 percent of the nation's households, they represent about 30 percent of those receiving government housing subsidies and Medicaid payments.[40] Many large pockets of poverty exist among the elderly. Poverty statistics from 1983 indicate that while the elderly in general compared favorably with others, minority group elderly fared poorly.[41]

Group	Percent at Poverty Level
All under 65	15.3%
All 65 and over	14.1
Blacks 65 and over	36.3
Hispanics 65 and over	23.1
Whites 65 and over	12

Women, who make up the bulk of the very old population (see § 1.3) bear a disproportionate share of the burden of poverty. While constituting only 59.1 percent of the total elderly population, women represented 71.1 percent of the elderly poor.[42] This phenomenon is probably because women generally outlive men and, as single persons, have fewer sources of income.[43]

---

[34]*A Profile of Older Americans*, American Association of Retired Persons and Administration on Aging, U.S. Department of Health and Human Services (1986).

[35]*Id.*

[36]"Insurance for the Twilight Years: Life Care Takes the Uncertainty Out of Retirement," *Time*, April 6, 1987, 53.

[37]*A Profile of Older Americans*, note 34, above.

[38]*See* J. Seaberry, "CEA Says Aged Have Attained Economic Parity," *Washington Post*, February 6, 1985, citing President's Council of Economic Advisors Annual Report. Note, however, that elderly cash income is substantially less than that of nonelderly persons, and that some observers argue that, even taking noncash resources into account, elderly persons are economically disadvantaged as a group. *See Aging America*, note 10, above, at 40–68.

[39]*A Profile of Older Americans*, note 34, above.

[40]*See* Seaberry, note 38, above.

[41]*Id.*

[42]*Id.*

[43]Average cash income for elderly couples in 1980 was $16,600, but for elderly single persons was only $8500. *See* ICF, Inc., note 1, above, at 54.

Perhaps even more significant than cash income is the increasing hold that the elderly population has upon this country's assets. Close to 80 percent of the deposits in banks and savings and loan institutions belong to people aged 55 or older.[44] Indeed, much of the income of senior citizens is generated from assets, as opposed to earnings. According to a nationwide survey, elderly income comes from the following sources:

Source	Percent
Social Security	40%
Assets	25
Earnings	15
Private Pensions	15
Miscellaneous	5[45]

In addition, the elderly, perhaps more than any other segment of the population, have benefited from the dramatic upswing in real estate values that took place during the double-digit inflation years of the 1970s and early 1980s. For many seniors, their homes have undergone astonishing appreciation in value over the past 30 or more years of ownership. When they sell their homes to move into a retirement facility or some other form of group living arrangement, release of the locked up equity, $125,000 of which is tax free (see § 7.1(d)(1)), may make their often modest incomes pale by comparison.

The sale by a retired person of his or her principal residence creates perhaps the greatest single financial investment opportunity in that person's lifetime. In 1980, almost 75 percent of elderly households owned their own homes, and 80 percent of these were owned free of any mortgage.[46] In 1984, the median value of older Americans' homes was $55,000.[47] Even among the elderly poor, 65 percent are homeowners, and 22 percent have over $50,000 in net home equity.[48] According to one estimate, the value of locked up home equity controlled by people over 65 is approximately $700 billion.[49] In most instances, there is no other time in life when so much asset value can be liquidated and be available for future investment or use.

---

[44]*See* Allen, note 22, above.

[45]*See* Seaberry, note 38, above.

[46]*Aging America*, note 10, above, at 67.

[47]U.S. Bureau of the Census, Current Population Reports, July 1986, cited in O'Shaughnessy et al., note 49, below.

[48]Jacobs & Weissart, "Long Term Care Financing and Delivery Systems," Conference Proceedings, Health Care Financing Administration, Washington, DC, Jan. 1984, p. 83, cited in O'Shaughnessy et al., note 49, below.

[49]U.S. Department of Health and Human Services, "Catastrophic Illness Expenses," Report to the President, Nov. 1986, cited by O'Shaughnessy, Price, & Griffith, "Financing and Delivery of Long-Term Care Services for the Elderly," Congressional Research Service, Feb. 24, 1987, 69.

There are doubtless many entrepreneurs and others in the marketplace who want the opportunity to assist retired persons in deciding what to do with their new-found liquid wealth, and investment in a retirement facility or lifestyle can be one of the most important and attractive options facing the elderly person. One imaginative observer, describing the recent "old rush," which seems to have possessed many in and out of the real estate development field, mused:

> Like Europeans stumbling across the New World, mass marketers are belatedly realizing that 'mature' households—the vogue term for households headed by people over 50—control a disproportionate share of the nation's buying power and most of its wealth, and are becoming more prone than ever to spend their formidable resources.[50]

Some developers eager to mine the wealth of the elderly are expecting a return on investment of 20 percent or more, largely from providing services to residents.[51] Because of the potential for unscrupulous, or well meaning but incompetent, developers to get their hands on these large amounts of dollars without giving full value in return, many states have adopted statutes that extensively regulate retirement facility transactions in which large sums of money are received from elderly persons in exchange for promises to provide housing, services, and health care in the future. (See § 21 for a detailed discussion of these laws.)

§ 1.6   THE NEED FOR SERVICES, CARE, AND FINANCIAL SECURITY

Popular misconceptions about the elderly include that they are poor, frail, sick, or bordering on mental incompetence. While older people certainly have a greater need for care than other population segments,[52] the aged in fact comprise a cross section of the entire spectrum of American life and culture. Therefore, a given facility model cannot serve and satisfy all needs, and there is a market for projects ranging from pure independent housing to intensive custodial and health care. Nevertheless, many elderly are moving through a phase in their lives that gives them some common desires and needs. In general, these common needs point to the provision of varying levels of services and activities beyond mere housing.

Because many older people have retired from their employment, with children long since grown and out of the household, most have a good deal of unoccupied time, and retirement facilities may serve as a focal point for social and recreational activities. As a further consequence of retirement, elderly persons are often living on fixed incomes earned from financial

---

[50] *See*, Petre, note 21, above.

[51] *See*, W. Swallow, "Elderly Seen As Giant New Market," Washington *Post*, Sept. 15, 1984.

[52] People over 65 comprise 12 percent of the population, but account for 31 percent of total personal health care expenditures. *A Profile of Older Americans*, note 34, above.

holdings, pensions, annuities, or other investments. Accordingly, retirees are often looking for a stable living situation with predictable or controlled costs for future contingencies. To some, housekeeping, dining, and other similar services may be a convenience that adds to the enjoyment of retired living. For others, such services may be necessary because of physical limitations caused by advancing age.

Not all seniors need health care or personal care, but all face the growing possibility that an illness or disability will deplete their assets and disrupt their lives. Only about five percent of the elderly live in nursing facilities. However, 23 percent of those over the age of 85 live in one.[53] Nearly 50 percent of people 75 or older have significant limitations walking, climbing, or bending (see also § 1.3).[54]

In a nationwide random survey of the elderly's preferences for retirement facility services, approximately 50 percent believed that they must have access to nursing home care, even though over 80 percent of those with incomes over $25,000 believed they were presently in excellent health.[55] Sixty-six percent of survey respondents indicated they felt a retirement facility with a nurse on call 24 hours per day was a "must," and 47 percent stated they would want health services delivered in their residences.[56]

The absence of services, personal assistance, and health care can also create problems of transition for retirement housing operators. Retirement communities built according to the Sun City model, which have few or no personal services to supplement housing, may face major obstacles when their populations age and begin to need or want more assistance with daily tasks or require health care.[57] Both facility owners and residents may unwittingly conspire in a scenario where the resident deteriorates to a crisis point (see below). In addition, a housing development with a population of increasingly dependent people eventually may find itself operating illegally as an unlicensed board and care facility (see § 20.3). Even if the facility faces up to the problem of dependent residents, it may be difficult to place residents in care facilities, or forcibly transfer those who resist. Some experts believe that continuing care facilities, which bring in residents while they are independent, and then provide varying levels of services and care, as needed, offer an ideal model for elderly housing in that they can serve all the person's progressive needs in a single setting.[58]

One of the greatest wild cards in the future of a retired person is the potential cost of health care. Although government programs such as Medicare

[53] "Who's Taking Care of Our Parents?," *Newsweek*, May 6, 1985, 61.

[54] Feldblum, note 14, above, citing U.S. General Accounting Office, Report No. PAD-80-12, Nov. 26, 1979.

[55] M. Dwight, "Affluent Elderly Want To Live Where Quality Care's Readily Available," *Modern Healthcare*, Apr. 26, 1985.

[56] *Id.*

[57] A. Mariano, "As Old Grow Older, Housing Needs Change," Washington *Post*, Sept. 15, 1984.

[58] *Id.*

and Medicaid provide a safety net for certain kinds of catastrophic medical needs (see discussion in § 26.1), the expenses associated with medical care remain one of the greatest threats to an elderly person's long-term financial security. On the average, nursing home care costs range from $20,000 to $25,000 per year.[59] However, costs may vary widely depending on location; for example, nursing care may cost well over $100 per day in New York. Older people may sometimes require months or even years of sustained nursing care, virtually none of which is covered by the Medicare program. To lessen the resident's risk of financial adversity, retirement facilities can offer health plans, insurance programs, or the availability of health care on a fixed cost basis, or for a prepayment or some other predictable method of payment. (See §§ 21, 27, 28.4 and 28.6 for a full discussion of financial security plans.)

Although many elderly people do not wish to face the prospect of dependence or a long-term illness, or the possibility of debilitating feebleness or mental impairment, all people share a substantial risk that such an affliction will befall them. Many seniors in single family homes—often widows or widowers living alone—will hold out against advancing disability until a crisis takes place, such as a fall from which they cannot get up. An all-too-typical pattern at that point is that the older person's children must hurriedly find a nursing home or convalescent hospital, which is sometimes many miles from the person's residence, where they can place their dependent parent. Often, these decisions made in haste do not result in the best placement for the elderly person.

Sometimes, the nursing facility is geared toward a type of patient who is in need of a more intense and sustained level of medical care than that required by the elderly person. In 1977, the Congressional Budget Office determined that inappropriately high levels of care were being received by 10 to 20 percent of skilled nursing patients and 20 to 40 percent of intermediate care patients.[60] More recent estimates conclude that between 10 and 30 percent of nursing home patients are there because they could not obtain adequate outpatient services.[61]

The nursing facility can be cold and institutional in character, and may look more like a hospital than a place to live. Because of bed shortages, available facilities may be too far away to make visiting convenient for relatives. Facilities with immediate vacancies also may have less desirable services and amenities, or even quality of care problems, when compared with projects

[59]Doty, Liu, & Wiener, "An Overview of Long Term Care," *Health Care Financing Review*, 6, no. 3, (Spring 1985) 74.

[60]Feldblum, note 14 above, referencing Baltay, M., "Long-Term Care for the Elderly and Disabled," Congressional Budget Office (1977).

[61]*See*, "Special Report: The Future of Medicare," *New England Journal of Medicine*, 314, no. 11, (March 13, 1986) 725, citing Morris, R. & Youket, P., "The Long Term Care Issues: Identifying the Problems and Potential Solutions," in *Reforming the Long Term Care System*, Callahan, J. & Wallack, S., eds., (Lexington, Mass: Lexington Books, 1981), 11–28.

that have waiting lists. It is difficult enough for the elderly person to cope suddenly with the physical and emotional burdens of dependence, but to have to endure at the same time a move away from home, family, and friends into an unfamiliar environment inhabited by strangers seems, and is, an unnecessary torment.

A retirement facility that integrates housing, personal care, health care, and assistance with activities that may be difficult for a feeble person to perform, can accommodate a person in the transition from independent to dependent status without giving rise to the trauma that so often accompanies a move from a private residence to a nursing facility. However, a well planned facility designed to take a person through this transition will emphasize the independent aspects of the program to encourage a positive outlook among residents and an atmosphere that attracts new prospects.[62] One commentator[63] has observed that the elderly consumer feels the same about having long-term nursing facilities in his retirement home as he does about automobile airbags: You would prefer that they're kept out of sight, but when you need them, they should pop into place instantly.

Retirement facilities can offer a broad latitude of amenities, services, and payment mechanisms in varying combinations. While some facilities may not serve all the needs of the older person, all are designed to respond to the common interests and desires of a particular segment of the elderly population to whom they are marketed. The key in developing retirement facilities is first to identify the market segment to which the program will be directed and then to create a package of physical facilities, services, and payment structures to attract and satisfy the needs of the consumer.

§ 2 HOW RETIREMENT FACILITIES HAVE EVOLVED TO MEET SENIOR NEEDS

§ 2.1 THE ESSENCE OF A RETIREMENT FACILITY

The numerous housing options[64] available to elderly persons have been grouped as follows:[65]

Independent Elderly

Homeownership

Rental housing

Condominiums or cooperatives

---

[62]Of course, it can be beneficial to have dependent and independent residents commingle in various group activities, as this fosters a sense of community.

[63]Gerald Glaser, Oxford Development Enterprises, Inc.

[64]For a general discussion of elderly housing options, *see* Hancock, J., ed., *Housing the Elderly*, (New Brunswick, NJ: Center for Urban Policy Research, 1987).

[65]L. Elrod, "Housing Alternatives for the Elderly," *Journal of Family Law*, 18 (1979–1980), 723.

Retirement communities
Mobile homes

Semi-independent Elderly

Living with family
House sharing with another senior
Residential hotels
Life care communities

Dependent Elderly

Nursing homes

This listing is probably too much of a generalization, and leaves out certain prevalent retirement facility types. For example, life care facilities usually house people spanning the full range of independence to dependence. Congregate housing facilities may offer meals and services to independent elderly, while board and care homes offer, in addition, personal assistance for the semi-independent and dependent.

People in the business surely will disagree about what a retirement facility is. Yet it seems clear that certain forms of elderly housing, such as a self-owned or shared home, or an apartment, condominium, or hotel room, standing alone, do not deserve the title. Groups of single-family homes, apartments, or condos in which seniors live, by accident or design, are not qualitatively different by reason of their numbers, without something more. That something else is services and amenities specially designed for the center's older inhabitants.

Accordingly, an emphasis in this book is placed upon facilities that offer some form of specialized elderly services and amenities in addition to housing. Age restricted housing, or even large residential communities designed for retirees, do not raise as vast an array of business and legal issues as is present in a service oriented facility. Nevertheless, service oriented facilities can use all of the devices of housing development to serve the elderly, from condos to rentals, and from multifamily high rises, to single-family residential communities, to mobile home parks.

On the other hand, some facilities, such as hospitals, which may offer extensive services to the elderly, and provide food and shelter as well, should not be grouped with retirement facilities. It is not just the short-term stay usually associated with a hospital that puts it outside the bounds of the retirement facility definition, but also the extreme dominance of the medical services element over the housing component. Retirement facilities have, in addition to a service element, the characteristic that they serve at least some people who are not totally dependent, and who have voluntarily chosen the placement as their home. Accordingly, this book does not deal extensively with the business and law of nursing home and other health facility operations, except as part of retirement facility programs.

By narrowing the scope to exclude housing and health care, it may seem that there is nothing left to discuss. In fact, however, only "pure" housing and "pure" health facilities are treated in passing. This leaves *everything* to discuss, because retirement facilities can include independent housing, health care for the dependent, and every gradation of services in between.

§ 2.2   THE FOUR BUSINESSES OF FULL SERVICE RETIREMENT FACILITIES

Retirement facilities can consist of one or more of essentially four businesses: housing, convenience services, health care or personal care, and financial security/insurance. These disparate businesses may converge to provide, in a single setting, all of the basic needs of the older person. Facility developers must draw on resources from each field and bring them together in an integrated product.

An individual facility may provide all, or only some mixture, of these four basic components. Those that provide all elements are sometimes referred to as "continuing care" or "life care facilities," but these terms may have different meanings and implications, both legally and in the marketplace, depending upon the jurisdiction or the local terminology of choice. Because many of the newer providers of these services do not necessarily fit the traditional model of continuing care or life care facilities, the term "full service retirement facility" is used here as a generic description for those facilities providing all four of the elements described below. Those that provide less than all the elements may be called congregate living facilities, nursing homes, board and care homes, or simply elderly housing.

(a) Housing

Retirement housing is more than simply housing in which elderly people live. While it may take on many of the physical attributes of family housing, such as high-rise construction, planned communities of single family residences, or campus-type environments of multiunit low-rise dwellings with common use recreation centers, elderly housing in addition caters to the particular physical and emotional needs and desires of its clientele.[66]

There are certain basic guidelines and rules of thumb regarding design criteria for elderly housing of which everyone involved in development of a facility should be aware. As with other types of real estate, location is of paramount importance. Facilities should be close to shopping, transportation, health care and other community services and amenities. Facilities should be planned taking into account the physical needs or potential physical needs of the elderly market segment for whom the facility is being built. In addition to curb appeal, interior design is of great importance so that the facility is functional, but retains homelike qualities.

---

[66]For discussions of various facility models and architectural and amenities options, *see, generally, Professional Builder*, Sept. 1985 and Apr. 1986.

If units are designed to accommodate residents both when they are independent and later when they may become in need of personal assistance, certain design features can be incorporated into every residence. These may include such features as skid-proof floors, elevated switches and electrical outlets that do not require the user to bend or crouch, grab bars (when needed) at bathtubs and toilets, doors wide enough to accommodate wheelchairs, emergency call buttons, and similar conveniences. In addition, living quarters that are at ground level or can be reached by elevator are generally preferable to those that may require a resident to climb stairs. Design considerations for the elderly may also include special soundproofing measures, extra lighting without glare, avoidance of certain colors, automatic doors, particular corridor dimensions, specially positioned sinks and mirrors, care in the selection of chair designs, and numerous other factors related to the visual, auditory, ambulatory, and other impairments that may accompany old age (see also Exhibit 2.1).[67]

EXHIBIT 2.1
PREFERRED RETIREMENT CENTER AMENITIES

Interiors

The affluent elderly make up a very small percentage of the market. If the project is designed to attract them it should be luxurious and loaded with recreational amenities. The wealthy buy downsized versions of their former homes. Units of 2,000 to 2,500 square feet sell well and two bedrooms are a must.

The majority of the market is middle income. This is what they want:

- Privacy within the living unit is essential whether it is a for-sale or for-rent unit. The ability to have an area to oneself is very important to older couples. The privacy issue extends to the congregate living format where the number one issue is a private toilet area (shared baths are acceptable). Even common areas both indoors and out ought to provide for some measure of privacy while also maximizing the opportunity for residents to meet face-to-face. This issue may explain why efficiency units are far less popular than one bedroom plans and why nursing homes are so disliked by the overwhelming majority of people.

- Security inside and outside the living unit. An emergency call system and smoke alarms are virtually essential.

- A liberal use of natural light in the individual living units and in all common areas. All corridors, lobbies, etc. ought to offer views to the outside.

Source: Reprinted with permission from Allen, John B. "Housing for the Elderly," *Investor Outlook*, Vol. 6, No. 2, Grubb & Ellis, Second Quarter 1986.

[67]Testimony of Jack L. Bowersox, House Committee on Aging, May 22, 1984.

EXHIBIT 2.1 *(Continued)*

- Careful attention to artificial light levels. As people age they need access to more light.
- Low cost occupancy features such as:

   Cross ventilation in all rooms rather than air conditioning except in those climates where air conditioning is an absolute must.

   Individually controlled heating. The aged vary greatly in how they perceive heat and cold.

   Well-insulated structures to keep fuel costs down and assist in noise control.

   Liberal use of stained woodwork rather than high maintenance painted surfaces.

- Large areas of unbroken wall space to make furniture placement easy. An open space plan that also maximizes ease of movement with or without a wheelchair is usually very successful. Small, walled-in areas should be avoided.
- Very careful attention to avoiding barriers such as high door steps, multiple living levels, uneven walking surfaces, thick carpet (which is very hard to walk on as people get older), hard to open doors (use lever handles) and difficult to operate plumbing fixtures.
- Unobtrusive safety features such as large bathrooms, seats in all showers, non-slip floors, wide doors and halls sell well. Grab rails and railings do not sell and, in fact, are a hindrance to sales or rentals for the pre-retired or first generation elderly. Installing the bracing for them is a good idea, but it doesn't sell or rent many units. Electrical outlets and plugs that are accessible without bending over also help the unit to sell or rent.
- Storage space. It is almost impossible to provide too much closet or display space. The elderly have a lot of prized possessions. Built-in bookcases are very popular.
- Flexibility. The ability to adjust shelving, closet rod and even bath and kitchen counter heights is a saleable feature that adds very little cost to a project.
- Kitchens. A kitchen is a powerful amenity. In all product types except nursing homes, compact kitchens with at least thirty inches of counter space useable while seated and which are visible to the dining and living room area are the most popular. You can avoid installing most kitchen gadgets including, in many cases, dishwashers as many of the elderly have few dishes to wash and quite a few don't want the expense of operating one. Top-mounted freezers should be avoided. All appliances should have front-mounted, easy-to-read dials and gauges. In projects without kitchens, the residents respond well to a snack bar or to some area where they can buy snacks whenever they feel like it.

EXHIBIT 2.1 *(Continued)*

- Laundry facilities should be located on the main living level, not in a basement.
- Mail. Provide easy access to mail delivery areas. Large graphics on housing units and mailboxes make it easy for residents to identify their units and mail slots.
- Elevators are wanted in any multi-story project but you can get by without them in two-story projects. Elevators must be large enough for wheelchairs and must have slow-operating doors.
- Bathrooms. Most people want only one bathroom, however, the affluent elderly will want at least two. Separating the toilet area from the tub or shower is very desirable. Bathrooms should have wide doors and be large enough to allow a wheelchair to maneuver. Mirrors should start at 40-inch level and there should be a dressing table and basin which allow a seated person to use them. Showers are more desired than bathtubs.
- Entry doors which are recessed to give protection against weather and to give a sense of "ownership," even in a high-rise project, are popular. Peepholes at two levels, one accessible to a seated person, are appreciated. All entries must be well lit.
- Bedrooms. One bedroom units are the most popular, no bedroom units are least popular. Bedrooms ought to be large enough to allow a wheelchair to move around the bed.
- Unit size. Median size is 600 to 650 square feet. The trend is toward a larger size. Typical unit sizes are:
  Efficiency:
  Median—415; Range—325 to 450
  1 bedroom:
  Median—600; Range—520 to 740
  2 bedroom:
  Median—900; Range—750 to 1,100
- Housing Preference. The single-family residence is number one. Duplexes sell and rent well and cluster housing with buildings up to four units are very saleable or rentable. Least desired housing is multistory, especially high-rise.

Those projects that feature a health care facility generally have one of about 21,000 square feet; the size range is 13,000 to 30,000 feet. The facility is typically a 60-bed center divided into a short-term stay area and a long-term care area.

Activity centers such as are found in congregate and lifecare facilities average 30,000 square feet; the range is 15,000 to 50,000 square feet. An allocation of 125 feet per resident is a good rule of thumb.

EXHIBIT 2.1 *(Continued)*

Exteriors

Site sizes range from one to two acres for a small, in-town congregate project to hundreds or thousands of acres for a destination retirement village. The median lot size for an in-city lifecare project is six acres; those located in rural areas have a median size of 29 acres.

Density, the number of units per acre, varies widely. It ranges from 6.5 units per acre for rural projects to up to 50 units per acre for metropolitan developments. High density projects are, of course, generally the most profitable. It is possible to design pleasant environments at 35 to 50 units per acre but it can't be done without using a mid-rise or high-rise format. High-rises are the least popular with elderly residents.

Project size varies from 50 to 200 units; a 150-unit project seems most manageable. Absorption time ranges between 18 and 24 months. Rental or sale of four to six units per month is normal.

It is not necessary to provide a lot of parking especially as the entry age of the customer group increases. Even in congregate projects that appeal to the 65+ segment, a parking ratio of one space for every three units is satisfactory. Most projects that have tried one parking space for every four units have found they are eventually short of parking. Vehicle access to entries is quite important; covered access is desirable, but not essential. All walkways leading to the parking area should be smooth surfaces without any steps.

Because the elderly are either on limited budgets or have better things to do with their time, it is wise to provide low-maintenance exteriors. Brick construction or stucco finishes are good; stained, rather than painted, exterior wood trim is excellent.

A small yard or access to a garden plot will help to sell or rent the units. The cluster format lends itself to small backyards.

Open areas that are accessible but offer some areas for privacy are very popular. Golf courses are very much overdone. Few people play golf and those who do so seldom play championship golf. Courses are valuable as open spaces and will be used for walking if paths are provided. In many cases, however, projects could succeed without a golf course if the money normally spent on this amenity was put into the living units and interior common areas. A number of surveys designed to uncover what the elderly really want have shown that golf courses are never ranked among the first ten most desired features. Indoor swimming pools usually rank ahead of golf courses and even they are well down on the list. A lot more people play cards, listen to concerts, dance and socialize than play golf.

When judging the overall desirability of a project don't be taken in by the scope of the outdoor common areas. The best designed common areas won't make up for a lack of adequate size or privacy in the living units.

The old are not very different from the young in their housing needs. There are enough differences to justify developing projects especially for the elderly, but few plans will succeed if they are designed merely to serve the old.

It is a common experience that larger units tend to be preferred by the elderly over smaller units. Some developers are finding that it is difficult to sell studio units, whereas there is significant demand for one- and two-bedroom units. Residents wish to use their own furnishings and frequently desire large amounts of space to store the possessions they have accumulated over a lifetime. Often, residents wish to be able to accommodate overnight guests, such as visiting family members. Even though a facility may provide one or more meals in a common dining area, at least rudimentary kitchen facilities in the unit are desirable to enable the resident to prepare simpler meals, such as breakfast or lunch, and to promote an atmosphere of independence and self-direction, rather than that of dependence and institutionalization. In addition, retirement centers should be designed to provide for security, recreational facilities, gardening areas, group meeting rooms, art and craft rooms, cable television, and other amenities that will promote a homelike, community atmosphere.

Where a retirement facility includes a health care center or personal care center, the conventional wisdom is that such facilities should be separated from high visibility areas such as entranceways, lobbies, and common dining areas, and instead should be equipped with separate dining facilities and located in a place where it is convenient for other residents to visit their friends who are in need of health services or personal care. Entrance areas and highly visible portions of the building should be devoted to activity centers, shops, attractive dining facilities, or other areas that will promote a sense of independent living, luxury, or homelike qualities.

The housing element of a retirement facility may be offered to the resident on a rental basis, as a life lease, as a membership privilege, or on an ownership basis, among others. Provision of services or care as part of the same arrangement can have an impact upon the form of property interest the developer transfers to residents. Generally, where it is expected that care or services are to be available to residents for extended periods, facility operators may want to retain control over the disposition of property and avoid transfer of an unrestricted fee interest.

(b) Convenience Services

Services are that aspect of retirement housing that most distinguish it from any other form of housing. The kinds of services offered by many retirement facilities may be likened to those provided in the hotel or hospitality industries. They may include restaurants or group dining facilities, weekly or other periodic housekeeping and flat laundry services, game rooms, fitness centers, tennis and golf facilities, barber shops and beauty salons, on-site banks, convenience stores and gift shops, concierge or activity director services, local minibus transportation, and a host of other programs and features (see Exhibit 2.2). In addition to the quality of the physical surroundings, it is the extent and scope of these services and amenities that

EXHIBIT 2.2
TYPICAL CONTINUING CARE SERVICES AND FEATURES

Included General Services

Meals
Activities Director
Apartment Cleaning
Apartment Maintenance
Carports/Garages
Flat Linens Supplied
Flat Linens Laundered
Guest Accommodations
Kitchen Appliances
Personal Laundry Facilities
Prescribed Diet
Scheduled Transportation by Facility
Storage (outside of living unit)
Telephone Service (generally local only)
Tray Service When Ordered By Physician
Utilities

Health Related Services

Annual or Routine Physical Exams
Community's Physician (services of)
Dental Care
Emergency Call System
Home Health Care (in apartment)
Hospitalization in Acute Care Hospital
Illness or Accident Away from Facility
Occupational Therapy
Optician
Physical Therapy
Podiatry
Prescription Drugs
Recreational Therapy
Referred Specialists

Source: Reprinted with permission from *National Continuing Care Directory* by Ann Trueblood Raper, American Association of Homes for the Aging, American Association of Retired Persons, 1984.

EXHIBIT 2.2 *(Continued)*

Health Related Services

Resident's Own Physician
Social Service
Therapy for Psychiatric Disorders
Treatment for Pre-existing Condition

Special Features

Bank (this sometimes means a check cashing service)
Barber Shop (may be part of Beauty Salon)
Beauty Salon
Cable TV
Chapel
Coffee Shop
Craft Areas
Exercise Program
Financial Aid Available
Fireplaces
Garden Plots
Greenhouse
Hiking/Walking Trails
Library
Master TV Antenna
Pharmacy
Private Dining Room (for small parties)
Religious/Vesper Services
Resident Association
Sauna/Spa Whirlpool
Security Gate/System (many communities have security guards)
Store/Gift Shop
Swimming Pool (outdoor)
Woodworking Shop

will differentiate the luxury facilities from those directed to the lower-
and middle-income population. The very top of the line in luxury retirement facilities can be modeled after a resort or cruise ship lifestyle. Such
facilities are helping change the image of retirement centers as desirable
places to live, rather than refuges of last resort, for those who can afford
such amenities.

One small survey published in 1986 showed that food service, social programs, common rooms, housekeeping, laundry, transportation, and an on-call attendant ranked high in terms of the number of facilities offering them.[68] Allowance of pets, security services, swimming pools, libraries, guest rooms, and beauty shops were less frequently encountered.[69]

Payment for these services is often included in a monthly fee charged to the resident, which also covers rent, or which supplements the entrance fee or the purchase price of the residential unit. Many developers are finding that, if financially feasible, it is desirable to make many of the services available on an à la carte basis to enable individual residents to customize a service package that meets their individual wants and needs. Oftentimes, however, economies of scale and the developer's capital investment in particular portions of the facility require that all residents purchase certain basic services, for example, a minimum of one meal per day to cover the cost of kitchen and dining room construction and staffing. However, making use of certain services a mandatory condition of occupancy can create regulatory problems or even give rise to antitrust issues (see § 22.5(d)).

Services should be carefully distinguished from care, which usually involves hands-on personal assistance, and may be a licensable activity. Gray areas can exist when services that may be a convenience to some persons amount to a necessity for others who are dependent. In such circumstances, it is important to consider the possible licensing implications of facility activities and resident mix.

(c) Health Care or Personal Care

A sharp dividing line exists between many facilities that offer only the two elements of housing and services, and those that venture into the business of providing health care or related forms of care and physical assistance to the residents. There is a wide divergence of opinion among developers and marketers of facilities regarding the desirability of offering health services in a retirement facility. Some older people would rather postpone thinking about the probabilities of their eventually needing assistance, rather than plan for them. However, the reasons for this debate may not be so much a lack of consumer interest in these services as a reluctance of many developers to venture into a field that is so foreign to them (see § 11.1(a)).

Facilities that offer only health care or personal care as part of a single program that does not include housing for, or services to, independent residents generally are not considered to be retirement facilities, but are more

---

[68]A. Jeck and Carlson, J., "Retirement Housing: Exploring the Gray Area of Housing's Gray Market," *Real Estate Finance* (Winter 1986).

[69]*Id.* Note, however, that such amenities may be very popular where they are installed. See "Continuing Care Retirement Communities: An Industry in Action," American Association of Homes for the Aging, Ernst & Whinney (Washington, DC 1987) 20.

properly characterized as health care facilities, nursing facilities, inter-mediate care facilities, convalescent hospitals, or similar titles (see § 2.1). Retirement facilities usually offer health care and personal care as a sup-plement to housing and services in a homelike environment.

Retirement facilities with health care or personal care services offer them in a wide variety of ways and combinations. Generally speaking, facil-ities identify and provide these services at various points along a continuum of care, which may range from minimal assistance with daily tasks for resi-dents who are slightly enfeebled, to long-term, 24-hour skilled nursing care for those with chronic debilitating conditions, to acute hospitalization for the seriously ill.

Personal care[70] may include assistance with such activities as bathing, grooming, dressing, transferring from bed to a walker or wheelchair, and related tasks. Assistance with such activities as letter writing, shopping, maintaining a checkbook, and similar activities that do not involve care of the body may not rise to the level of licensable care in most states (see § 20.3(b)). The presence of care and the type and level of care being offered will have a significant impact on the kinds of regulations imposed on the facility operator and can often have an impact on construction standards and physical plant amenities required by law, as well as the numbers and kinds of staff required to operate the facility.

Unlike the concept of personal care, which may vary from state to state, the notion of skilled nursing facility services is more broadly and consist-ently recognized across the country as a level of care that requires the availability of trained nursing personnel on a full time basis. Almost all states have extensive regulatory requirements that apply to such facilities (see § 20.2). Retirement facilities may offer skilled nursing services in a unit attached to or adjacent to the residential portion of the facility, and usually require a resident to give up his or her unit whenever the facility's medical director determines that a permanent transfer to nursing services is required. (See § 28.9 concerning alternative transfer options for resident agreements.)

The emergence of home health care as a distinct type of health care or personal care service, when applied to the full service retirement facility, blurs the distinction between programs requiring a facility license and unli-censed services contracted for privately by an individual. An elderly person contracting for delivery of home health services in a private residence does not result in the home becoming a retirement facility. On the other hand, substantial utilization of home health by a significant number of dependent elderly in a multiunit housing project could be viewed by state inspectors as circumstances warranting licensure of the facility, especially where the facility helps arrange or provide the service (see § 20.3(b)).

---

[70]There are many other names for this level of care, depending on state or local usage. *See* § 20.3, below.

Few retirement facilities in the nation offer general acute care hospital services on the retirement facility site. However, many will assure that hospital services are available by making special arrangements with nearby facilities, and may pay for some or all of the expenses related to the hospitalization[71] as part of the retirement facility's overall fee structure. For the most part, retirement facilities that agree to cover the costs of health care services rendered in-house or at another facility as part of a prepaid or fixed fee arrangement are entering into a fourth business, that of insurance or provision for residents' financial security.

(d) Financial Security/Insurance

Because most retired persons are living on fixed incomes, they are concerned about preserving their life-styles for the rest of their days. They may wish to minimize the risk that a catastrophic event, such as a sudden serious illness, or a long and gradual one, will force them to become dependent upon government aid, to move to undesirable housing, or to become a burden upon their families. Consequently, many retirement facilities have established financial mechanisms, which are akin to insurance programs, to help ensure that the costs of living for the remainder of a person's lifetime will be predictable and stable.

One method of ensuring stability in terms of health care costs is to require residents upon admission to a facility to pay a large, lump sum entrance fee, which is then invested by the facility and reserved for payment of future health care costs and other needs of the resident. In return for the entrance fee, the facility will guarantee coverage for the costs of certain of the resident's health care needs in the future. The money to pay such an entrance fee is often available because the resident has sold his or her home just prior to moving into the retirement facility.

This method of self-insurance by the retirement facility has been prevalent among not-for-profit continuing care facilities. An emerging development is that facilities increasingly may, as employers have in the past, purchase group health insurance, which is available exclusively to occupants of the particular retirement facility in return for a fixed monthly premium. Although relatively scarce at present, insurance policies are being offered that cover those medical and health services (for example, long-term skilled nursing care) that are not covered by government programs such as Medicare (see § 27.2).

§ 2.3 TRADITIONAL RETIREMENT FACILITY MODELS

(a) Overview

Centers for the elderly have evolved along two separate paths, with housing at the genesis of one, and health and custodial care at the source of the

---

[71]In excess of Medicare payments.

other. With time, these two branches have intertwined so much that retirement centers currently are thought of as places that are neither pure housing nor pure care, but a little of each, and a lot of added services and amenities that form the middle ground. Accordingly, freestanding nursing facilities, where there is no independent housing, and age restricted housing, where there is no service or care element, are distinguished here from true retirement facilities.

Over the years, many different models of retirement facilities have developed that incorporate some mixture of housing, convenience services, care, or insurance. Principally, these fall into three basic patterns: congregate housing, board and care,[72] and continuing care or life care. However, even these traditional points of departure are rapidly becoming arbitrary stereotypes that do not fit the marketplace.

Figure 2.1 places the traditional retirement facility models of congregate housing, board and care, and life care, plus retirement villages and skilled nursing facilities, along a spectrum of basic amenity/service types: housing, convenience services, personal care, and health care.[73] These service/amenity types can be loosely associated with independence or dependence of the facility's elderly residents. While facilities may offer several of the service/amenity types, only one or two features may characterize the facility, and other attributes will be incidental to the primary features. For example, nursing facilities are characterized principally as health care providers. Housing is provided, but not to independent residents, and more as a necessary incident of full time health care, rather than as a primary objective. On the other hand, independent housing and some provision for health care or personal care are more coequal attributes of a life care community. As more and more developers with a diversity of backgrounds and experience enter this growing field, one can expect to see distinctions between the traditional types of retirement facility product blur, and new products evolve from various combinations of physical facilities, services, delivery systems, and payment mechanisms. With that, we will probably also see a whole new lexicon develop to help us describe what is going on.

In some respects, the retirement facility field is presently at a stage where ice cream making was many years ago: there were just a few available flavors, selected by the manufacturer. As the elderly population grows, becomes more affluent, and discovers itself to be a powerful segment of the consumer public that can generate innovation and demand variety and custom tailored quality in the marketplace, we can expect to see rapid diversification and creativity of the type that took vanilla, chocolate, and strawberry to 31 flavors, and ice cream to frozen yogurt, gelato, and sorbet.

---

[72]Also known as personal care, assisted living, and by other names. *See* § 20.3, below.

[73]Financial security is not considered in the analysis represented in Figure 2.1, in that it reflects a payment system usually associated with life care, but potentially applicable to any facility type.

FIGURE 2.1
TYPICAL RETIREMENT FACILITY MODELS

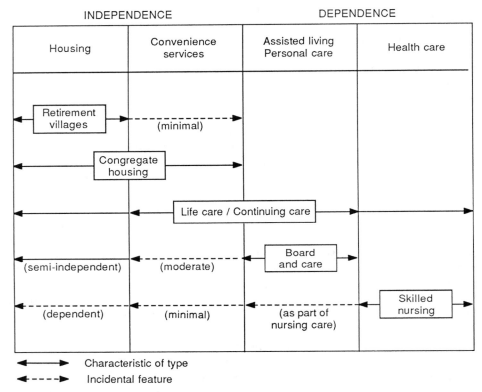

(b) **Congregate Housing**

Congregate housing was defined, in its formative years, as:

> An assisted independent group living environment that offers the elderly who are functionally impaired or socially deprived, but otherwise in good health, the residential accommodations and supporting services they need to maintain or return to a semiindependent lifestyle and prevent premature or unnecessary institutionalization as they grow older.[74]

However, today congregate housing has come to mean more universally a multiunit housing facility that provides, often to independent elderly, a rental program that includes supportive services (predominantly meals), but generally not the personal assistance or health care needed by the functionally impaired. Unlike board and care, it generally does not

[74]See Elrod, note 65 above, quoting the 1976 National Conference on Congregate Housing for Older People.

require institutional licensure, and is made up of self contained, single family occupancy units.[75]

Congregate housing is a concept that was fostered largely by the creation in 1978 of the Congregate Housing Services Act,[76] which provides funding for meals and other services to be provided in low income or otherwise federally subsidized housing (see § 22.3(c)). Over the last decade, the congregate housing concept has been greatly expanded in the marketplace to include market rate multiunit facilities that offer meals, housekeeping, laundry, transportation, recreational programs, and other convenience services, in settings that can range from modest to luxurious.[77]

Although one often hears reference to congregate care facilities, this is sometimes a misnomer in that, technically, care of the sort that is usually licensed by state regulatory agencies is not commonly offered in such facilities, although the facility may assist residents in obtaining access to care in the community. Due in part to the confusing terminology associated with assisted living facilities (see below), some writers have equated congregate facilities with life care endowment programs.[78] Although congregate living is an element of life care and other retirement housing options, standing alone it constitutes a distinct and growing option.

Congregate housing facilities traditionally do not exact any lump sum payment or entrance fee from residents, but are made available on a monthly rental basis. The parties are in the relationship of landlord and tenant. Both the nonprofit and for profit sectors are well represented in the field of congregate housing.

(c) Board and Care/Assisted Living

Facilities where residents need assistance with daily activities such as bathing, grooming, and dressing, but are otherwise independent and not in need of full time nursing care, have been variously described as assisted living, residential care, board and care, personal care, congregate care, or sheltered living facilities, among numerous other names.[79] The House Select Committee on Aging estimated, in 1981, that there were 100,000 boarding homes in the country (five times the number of nursing facilities), that they served a million people, and generated $12 billion to $20 billion of revenue per year.[80]

---

[75]See Thompson, M., and Donahue, W., *Planning and Implementing Management of Congregate Housing for Older People* (Washington, DC: International Center for Social Gerontology, 1980), 5–6.

[76]42 U.S.C. § 1437e (1978).

[77]See, generally, Chellis, R., Seagle, J., & Seagle, B., eds. *Congregate Housing for Older People* (Lexington, Mass: Lexington Books, 1982).

[78]Caulfield, L., and Carlucci, J., "The Adult Congregate Living Facility—A Comparison and Critical Discussion of Assistance-Oriented Facilities and an Alternative Concept for the Marketplace," *The Real Estate Appraiser and Analyst* (Fall 1985), 43.

[79]See § 20.3, below..

[80]House Select Committee on Aging, "Fraud and Abuse in Boarding Homes" June 25, 1981.

Such facilities have been broadly defined to include any "publicly or privately operated residence that provides personal assistance, lodging, and meals to two (2) or more adults who are unrelated to the licensee or administrator."[81] The kind of assistance that may be received by residents in such facilities, on an as-needed basis, has been broadly construed to include help with:

Walking
Bathing, shaving, brushing teeth, combing hair
Dressing
Eating
Getting in and out of bed
Laundry
Cleaning room
Managing money
Shopping
Using public transportation
Writing letters
Making telephone calls
Obtaining appointments
Self-administration of medication
Recreational and leisure activities
Other similar activities[82]

In addition, facility staff monitor residents' activities on the premises, and are generally aware of their whereabouts when outside of the facility.[83]

Assisted living facilities should be distinguished, however, from facilities, such as congregate housing, that may offer housekeeping, recreational programs, or similar services, as a convenience for truly independent residents. Assisted living involves dependent people who, because of physical or mental infirmity, require assistance with one or more essential daily tasks, and especially matters of personal physical care, such as grooming and hygiene.

Personal care facilities are also quite different from nursing facilities, where patients need full time, licensed nursing care or supervision. Personal care residents are usually ambulatory, and somewhat independent, in that they may leave the premises (perhaps in groups, with or without supervision). They may have no mental impairment whatsoever, but

---

[81] Beyer, Bulkley, & Hopkins, "A Model Act Regulating Board and Care Homes: Guidelines for States," *Mental and Physical Disability Law Reporter* 8 (March–Apr. 1984) 157, defining "Board and Care Home."

[82] *Id.*, at 159.

[83] *Id.*

simply need some physical help to get up and about, or to perform household tasks.

Board and care homes, some of which housed mentally handicapped, developmentally disabled, and other nonelderly dependent groups, were the subject of considerable criticism in the past decade due to serious problems of fraud and abuse, as well as a series of deadly fires in elderly facilities.[84] In response to these problems, Congress passed the Keys Amendment,[85] requiring states to enact minimum standards for facilities serving a significant number of recipients of federal Supplemental Security Income (SSI) payments.[86]

It has been more recently estimated that there are nationally approximately 300,000 unlicensed boarding homes (with room and meals) and about 30,000 licensed board and care facilities that include supportive services.[87] Taken together, these facilities are housing between 500,000 and 1.5 million people.[88] A 1983 study of licensing programs found that of 458,500 identified board and care beds, about 324,000 were occupied by elderly or handicapped adults.[89] The remainder were for mentally retarded or developmentally disabled persons.[90]

Board and care is a very attractive alternative to a nursing home placement for an elderly person who needs assistance and wants a homelike environment, but neither needs full time nursing care nor wants the more institutional, medical-model surroundings of many nursing facilities. Unfortunately, board and care has not received the kind of government financial support (Medicare and Medicaid) that health care facilities have enjoyed, and therefore many facilities rely on residents' rather meager SSI payments as a funding source.[91] Many facilities have been run by small mom and pop types of operators. Poor reimbursement may be a principal reason both for the extent of inferior quality existing in many board and care facilities, and the high rate of placements in nursing facilities of people requiring a lower level of care.

As the number of elderly who can pay their own way grows, and as government looks for less expensive and medically intensive ways to care for

---

[84] See House Select Committee on Aging, "Fraud and Abuse in Boarding Homes," June 25, 1981.

[85] Pub. L. 94-566, § 505(d) (1976).

[86] See "State Laws and Programs Serving Elderly Persons and Disabled Adults," (excerpting an American Bar Association Commission study), *Mental Disability Law Reporter*, 7 (March–Apr. 1983) 158, for a comprehensive survey of individual state board and care licensing laws. See also § 26.1(d)(1), below, regarding the SSI program.

[87] See Newcomer, R., and Stone, R., "Board and Care Housing: Expansion and Improvement Needed," *Generations* (Summer 1985), 38.

[88] Id.

[89] Id.

[90] Id.

[91] Id., at 39.

the elderly, we should expect a significant rise in the development of quality assisted living facilities as an alternative to skilled nursing care.

(d) Continuing Care Facilities

A hundred years ago, retirement homes arose in this country within church groups, fraternal organizations, and social welfare organizations as a means of caring for those who had served as missionaries, were abandoned by their families or had no families, or who were too poor to care for themselves.[92] In some cases, the elderly would be asked to turn over whatever meager assets they had to the nonprofit organization operating the facility, and in return would be assured of a place to live, a square meal, and care, when needed, for the rest of their lives. Such facilities came to be known as life care facilities.

Life care facilities evolved over the last century into what are perhaps more appropriately called continuing care facilities.[93] In the past decade, the number of continuing care retirement facilities has doubled, and it is expected to at least double again in the next 10 years.[94] Many have waiting lists of five to eight years, especially for larger units. Continuing care facilities, or continuing care retirement centers (CCRCs), continue to be designed to offer food, shelter, convenience services, personal assistance, and often medical care, to the extent needed by a resident for the rest of his or her life. However, instead of transferring all of one's assets, residents will usually pay a substantial entrance fee, sometimes called an endowment or founder's fee, and will, in addition, be charged a monthly fee ranging on the average from $500 to $1500, subject to adjustment to cover fluctuations in the cost of operating the facility. Deposits on entrance fees are sometimes collected prior to facility construction as a financing vehicle or to ensure sufficient demand for the project.

[92]A brief history of CCRCs is discussed in Winkelvoss and Powell, *Continuing Care Retirement Communities—An Empirical, Financial and Legal Analysis,* (Pension Research Council, Wharton School, University of Pennsylvania, Richard D. Irwin, 1984), 6–11. A more recent, general discussion of life care facilities is contained in "Sizing Up Life Care," *Changing Times,* May 1987, 65.

[93]There is some confusion over the distinctions of meaning and usage between the terms *life care* and *continuing care*. Sometimes, *life care* is used to distinguish the archaic fully prepaid programs from those that charge monthly fees in addition to an entrance fee. Others may use *life care* to refer to contracts that promise care and residence for life, and reserve *continuing care* as a more generic term covering contracts of any duration where a person can receive varying levels of health care or personal care along a continuum of benefits. At least one study has referred to *life care* facilities as those that offer care, when needed, without an increase in the regular monthly charge for residence, as distinguished from *continuing care*, where the facility merely arranges for health services to be available at fee for service rates. *See* ICF, Inc., note 1, above, at 36. In this book, the terms are used, more or less interchangeably, to refer to contracts offering long-term care and residence, usually with some form of prepayment for, or priority access to, health benefits. *See also* the statutory definitions set forth in Part VII, *below.*

[94]Raper, A., ed., *National Continuing Care Directory,* (Washington, DC: American Association of Homes for the Aging/American Association of Retired Persons, 1984), 5.

According to a 1986 study, the median one bedroom entrance fee for surveyed facilities was $45,000, and the median monthly fee was $739,[95] but entrance fees may range from as little as $10,000 to $400,000 or more, in some cases. Fees vary greatly depending upon location, unit size and luxury, the extent of prepaid services, the refund policy of the home, and similar factors. Although eligible for tax exemption (see § 9.2), these facilities often cater to middle and upper income elderly who can afford the expense of extensive service programs.[96]

The life care industry has been estimated to be $4 billion strong.[97] The field continues to be dominated by nonprofit church and fraternal groups, although for profit developers are entering the field in increasing numbers. In 1981, 97 percent of continuing care communities studied nationwide had nonprofit owners or sponsors.[98] It has been estimated that about 700 continuing care facilities exist in the United States,[99] with an average resident population, according to one study published in 1984, of 245.[100] However, the trade association for nonprofit retirement facilities, the American Association of Homes for the Aging, headquartered in Washington, D.C., has stated that only about 300 facilities fit the traditional definition of life care.[101]

In continuing care facilities, the facility operator has historically retained ownership of the premises and granted residents the right to occupy a residential unit for life or some other long-term period. If for life, the interest transferred may be considered a life lease, except that the right of occupancy is personal to the resident and may not be sublet or transferred in any fashion. A generally accepted rule of thumb for determining whether the term of the arrangement is considered to be continuing care is whether the promise to provide residents with care and services is for more than one year.[102]

Continuing care facilities usually accept as residents only those who are healthy and capable of independent living, and provide services, personal care, and health care, as needed, as the resident moves along the continuum of care from the status of complete independence to greater dependence

---

[95]*The Senior Living Industry 1986*, Laventhol & Horwath, 44, 46. See also the exhaustive study of continuing care facilities, note 69 above, published as this book was going to press.

[96]An exhaustive empirical study of continuing care retirement communities, their fees, services, amenities, resident mixes, and other characteristics, together with an analysis of actuarial projection methodologies, pricing theory, budgeting and general accounting and financial considerations appears in Winkelvoss and Powell, note 92, above.

[97]Fairchild, T., "Profit or Nonprofit Retirement Housing: Is There a Difference?" *Aging Network News* (July 1986), 6.

[98]Raper, A., note 94 above, at 11.

[99]"Insurance for the Twilight Years: Life Care Takes the Uncertainty Out of Retirement," *Time*, Apr. 6, 1987, 53.

[100]Mariano, A., "As Old Grow Older, Housing Needs Change," Washington *Post*, Sept. 15, 1984.

[101]Rosenblatt and Peterson, "Life Care: Insurance Against Age," Los Angeles *Times*, Aug. 5, 1986, 6.

[102]Raper, A., note 94 above, at 4.

and possibly long-term illness. Sometimes, health care or personal care is provided without any significant increase in monthly fees. Recently, facilities offering a broad range of services and assistance along the continuum of care have used alternative payment mechanisms, such as an entrance fee with fee-for-service payments for care and conveniences on an à la carte basis, or straight rental payments for shelter, food, and services. Though nontraditional in format, these may also be considered to be CCRCs.[103]

(e) Related Facilities

(1) Planned Residential Communities

Planned residential communities for seniors have been popularized since the late 1950s by such developments as Sun City, Arizona. Sometimes called retirement communities or retirement villages, these projects essentially provide only a housing component and, perhaps, a modicum of common area recreational facilities and maintenance services such as gardening. Except for age restrictions applicable to residents of such communities, they are essentially pure real estate developments that do not raise as many of the unusual business, marketing, and legal questions involved in the development of a retirement facility offering extensive services.

Generally, planned residential communities consist of single family residences, duplexes, or condominium or apartment units, which are sold or leased to residents. While there may be monthly association fees, these are generally used for such purposes as maintenance of common areas and facilities and not for provision of meals, convenience services, or care.

Although these communities were not designed to offer extensive services, personal assistance, or health care to their residents, some are finding that it may be necessary or advantageous to construct care facilities on the premises or nearby as their populations age in place. If the increasing age and dependence of such a population is ignored, significant problems can arise in dealing with transfers of residents out of the community, or caring for them on site.[104]

(2) Nursing Homes

Facilities in which elderly people receive or have available to them round-the-clock nursing care are generally referred to as skilled nursing facilities,

[103]However, some commentators have advised that an essential element of continuing care is that some form of below cost or prepaid health care be included [Raper, note 94 above, at 4, and Winkelvoss and Powell, note 92 above, at 23]. Under that definition, for example, facilities that charge full fee-for-service rates for nursing care but give priority health center admission status to independent living residents would not be considered continuing care, contrary to some state statutes, such as California Health and Safety Code §§ 1770 et seq.

[104]See "Who's Taking Care of Our Parents," Newsweek, May 6, 1985, for a discussion of health care needs at Sun City, 25 years after its opening.

nursing homes, or convalescent hospitals. While these facilities provide many of the elements of shelter, food services, and health care that are present in the retirement facilities discussed above, nursing homes are essentially health care facilities that are based upon a medical model and do not provide the homelike environment that typifies a retirement facility. Moreover, such facilities are not available to healthy persons who desire retirement living in a group setting, but are not in need of constant health care or personal attention. Most states recognize this distinction and separately group skilled nursing facilities with hospitals and other health facilities in their licensing laws and regulations, whereas retirement facilities, if regulated at all, are regulated by such government entities as departments of real estate, social services, or even insurance.

Nursing facilities have been the prevalent choice for placement of many dependent elderly who are not in need of the constant nursing attention such facilities are designed to provide (see § 1.6). Moreover, the institutional character of many such facilities is considered by some observers to be detrimental to many elderly persons who would adjust better to a more homelike setting. Many providers of nursing care are expanding into the true retirement field and offering board and care, independent living, or other levels of service below skilled nursing. In addition, life care or continuing care facilities often offer skilled nursing on site, or by special arrangement with a neighboring facility. Therefore, while a skilled nursing facility, standing alone, is not considered here as a true retirement facility, the subject is discussed throughout this book (see, e.g., § 20.2).

(3) Other Elderly Housing

Numerous other types of facilities that restrict admission to elderly persons may exist in communities across the United States. However, these are not properly characterized as retirement facilities unless they provide some significant measure of services designed to cater to the particular needs of independent or semidependent elderly persons. Examples of such facilities include adults only apartments or condominium units, or rent-assisted or other low income housing. In addition, an estimated 76,000 elderly live in urban residence hotels that rent rooms to urban elderly persons on a monthly or longer term basis.[105] As the populations of these essentially pure housing projects age, they can become excellent candidates for conversion into more traditional retirement programs by the addition of services or arrangement for care, on or off the premises.

---

[105]Elrod, note 65 above, referencing HUD, *How Well Are We Housed, The Elderly* 1979.

§ 2.4 EMERGING TRENDS IN RETIREMENT FACILITY DEVELOPMENT

(a) New Participants in the Marketplace

The new interest of for profit real estate developers in the retirement housing field is due in part to the demographics of the elderly population and its expected rapid growth. In addition, many real estate developers are finding it difficult to find a large measure of success in certain types of real estate developments that, in the past, had been lucrative, such as shopping centers, condominiums, and high-rise office buildings. Whatever their motivations, for profit entities have, since approximately 1984, made a concerted effort to capture a substantial segment of the retirement housing marketplace, particularly service oriented facilities. One can look to any of the four businesses that make up the retirement facility industry—housing, hospitality, health, insurance—and find a major for profit group that has actively explored the development of new facilities. Not only is there expanded interest from those real estate developers who have extensive experience in the development of housing, but also from those experienced in providing hospitality and convenience services, including hotel chains. Major hospital chains and insurance companies as well have expressed an interest and are taking steps toward significant involvement in the retirement facility field. Well known corporate names such as Marriott, Avon, Sears, and Hyatt have become associated with the field in recent years. A new, nationwide organization of largely for profit retirement facility developers, service providers, and consultants, the National Association of Senior Living Industries, was formed in 1985 and is very active and growing in membership.

Expanded interest has been witnessed not only in the for profit sector but also among nonprofit institutions. Most notable are hospitals, which, over the past several years, have been suffering under increasingly strict limitations upon government reimbursement for health care services. The emergence in the Medicare program of such cost-saving devices as diagnosis related groups (DRGs) has forced hospitals to look to other sources of revenue to help diversify and balance their financial pictures. Development of retirement facilities is a natural next step for hospitals, and many are exploring retirement facility development.[106] Many can develop retirement facilities on available land adjacent to the hospital site and can furnish health care, dining, housekeeping, and other services from a central location at the hospital itself. However, hospitals should be cautioned that the location may not be attractive to the well-elderly, and that the institutional style of dining, housekeeping, and other services provided by hospitals in their own facilities are likely to be inappropriate in a retirement facility, where home-style qualities are expected.

---

[106]See § 11.2(a), below.

(b) New Business Structures and Partnerships

The new found interest of real estate developers, and other for profit enterprises, in the retirement field will naturally bring about changes in the complexion of the industry. For example, in a field such as continuing care, nonprofit organizations have dominated the industry. Historically, nonprofit organizations, and particularly church groups, have been engaged in the operation of health facilities such as hospitals and nursing homes. It was a logical transition for them to move into the provision of health care in homes for the aging.

Many real estate developers, on the other hand, have experience almost exclusively in the development of housing, and are not generally familiar with the health care business, nor with the provision of basic services such as meals and housekeeping, which go routinely along with the provision of health care in facilities. Nevertheless, real estate developers may recognize consumer desires and needs for the provision of health care in a retirement facility, and are looking for ways to provide the full panoply of services available at many of the existing nonprofit centers, without being required to learn the new business of provision of health and hospitality services.

A natural consequence of the desire of real estate developers to provide services not normally associated with the real estate business is the development of joint ventures or of contractual relationships with management companies or health care service providers, or purchase of long-term care insurance to cover the risk of future health care costs. These and other methods help the real estate developer provide the full spectrum of services by tapping the resources and expertise of existing companies already in the health care, service, or financial security businesses (see § 11 regarding joint ventures).

Tax laws, and the desire to create new products that will be competitive with those offered by charitable organizations, have also led to the development of different ownership and operational structures (discussed below, in subsections (c) to (f), and more fully in Part III).

The influx of eager developers in the elderly marketplace has raised some controversy. Nonprofit providers have expressed concerns that many of the flood of new, profit oriented developers will not remain interested in keeping long-term commitments to residents and may sell off retirement facilities once they are depreciated, or overbuild and be forced to turn over unprofitable projects.[107]

For profit developers counter that many of the major retirement facility failures have been those of nonprofit operators, who, due to misguided altruism, inexperience, incompetence, or even criminally fraudulent business practices, have caused some elder people to be displaced or lose money (see § 5.1).

---

[107] See, e.g., "What's Putting New Life Into 'Life Care' Communities," *Business Week*, March 3, 1986, 108, quoting Sheldon Goldberg, Executive Vice President, American Association of Homes for the Aging.

To some extent, these exchanges between the for profit and nonprofit sectors are a byproduct of competitive pressures. On the other hand, non-profit retirement centers have, over the years, had to repeatedly distinguish themselves before the public, the press, and the lawmakers from the pre-dominantly for profit nursing homes where allegations of poor care seem to be regularly raised. Ironically, however, these for profit nursing facilities are largely responsible for caring for poor, Medicaid patients, while many nonprofits cater to a greater proportion of private pay patients who can afford a better standard of care. At present, both groups seem to be compet-ing most vigorously for the more affluent market segment.

Most thoughtful observers recognize that quality of care and commit-ment to service of the elderly is not the exclusive property of either group, and that nonprofits and for profits have much to offer the public and each other. Still, latent stereotypes and prejudices may have to be overcome to pursue a successful joint venture.

(c) Resident Ownership versus Rental

One of the greatest current debates in the retirement housing field is whether the trend will be toward development of rental housing or a resi-dent ownership structure. Until recently, most of the service oriented re-tirement housing market has been devoted to a rental type of format, even where facilities and services are offered on a lifetime or other long-term basis. Despite the existence of large retirement village developments where residents own their own homes, most congregate housing, board and care, continuing care, and HUD financed retirement housing has been made available on the basis that the premises are not owned by the resident, but are essentially leased, whether the term be on a month-to-month basis, re-newable annually, or for life.

More recently, a trend toward increasing development of ownership models of retirement facilities is detectible. Studies have shown that elderly persons overwhelmingly prefer home ownership to rentals or other ar-rangements.[108] The 1986 Tax Reform Act also creates some serious impedi-ments to investment in rental housing, which may hasten the trend (see § 8.2). Nevertheless, tax considerations may not predominate when com-pared with countervailing issues that affect operations, especially in facili-ties with substantial services.

An interesting example of the phenomenon of increased ownership in fa-cilities with services is the development of continuing care-styled communi-ties that are sold to residents as condominiums. Health care and service packages are made available through the residents' association, which can contract for services with a management company. Unfortunately, home-owner associations are not well suited to management of complex operations

---

[108]See Adams, E., "Meeting the Varied Market For The Graying of America," *Professional Builder,* April 1986, 68.

that may affect members' health and welfare in ways well beyond the usual housing and maintenance issues that face most such groups. While there are many advantages to ownership, especially tax advantages to the consumer (see § 7.1(d)(1)), the desire of the developer/operator to maintain control over the facility on a day-to-day basis will probably result in the continued preeminence of the rental format over true ownership in service oriented retirement housing. Nevertheless, the proportion of retirement communities with an ownership structure, or a related equity factor such as a membership, stock ownership, or refundable fee system, should continue to grow.

(d) Monthly or Annual Rental versus Continuing Care

A further division lies between traditional monthly rentals or annual leases, and life care or continuing care structures where (sometimes after an initial probation period) residents cannot be evicted except for cause.[109] Because continuing care promises are more complex and generally are accompanied by substantial entrance fees or endowment payments, sales can require more consumer education. In markets where there is little familiarity with a particular breed of retirement community, developers may face exceptional challenges in educating buyers. One consultant[110] tells the story of a developer who had created beautiful models of proposed life care units, but was having difficulty closing any but a few sales. When asked why they were not buying the units, prospects responded that they could not assess whether they would be getting their money's worth. The nearest life care facilities were in a neighboring state. After developing brochures comparing the project with other life care facilities, with little added success, the developer, to improve sales, eventually had to charter a bus to take prospects across state lines to visit the other communities.

In the opinion of an experienced marketing consultant, rental retirement facilities have advantages and disadvantages when compared with a traditional entrance fee model:[111]

Rental Pros

1. No major lump sum cost commitment.
2. Resident controls investment of the proceeds of sale of home.
3. If dissatisfied with the facility, resident can leave without a significant financial loss.

---

[109] See, generally, Carlson, J., "What The Experts Are Saying: New Developments in Retirement Housing," Retirement Housing Report, Sept. 1986, 16, for a discussion of rental versus life care trends.

[110] Remarks of James Sherman, Laventhol & Horwath, Philadelphia, PA, at Sandy & Babcock seminar on "Proprietary Lifecare," San Francisco, July 19, 1985.

[111] Linda Todd, Senior National Vice President, National Retirement Consultants, Inc., Fort Lauderdale, FL. Retirement rental rates average about $1,050 per month for a single person, one bedroom unit. "Rental Retirement Housing," The Stanger Report, Sept. 1986, 2.

4. Resident's children are generally more receptive.

5. Less education of the prospect may be required.

Rental Cons

1. Resident's perception that the facility has only a short-term commitment to them.

2. Any price increases are likely to have a greater impact than in an entrance fee structure.

3. Rental can be perceived as low income or lesser quality.

4. Age group responding is typically older.[112]

From a financing perspective, rentals and traditional endowment projects may have some of the following attributes and problems:[113]

Rentals

1. Less than full occupancy can jeopardize meeting of debt service.

2. Renters are more subject to rent increases to pay for construction debt due to interest fluctuations, vacancies, or other factors.

3. Residents are subject to displacement as a result of foreclosure action.

Endowment

1. Helps control fluctuations in monthly fees.

2. Helps retire construction debt, making residence more secure.

3. Public bond issues can greatly increase project costs.

4. Repayment of bonds can be dependent on turnover and resale of units many years after the facility opens.

5. The resident's position is always secondary to the bondholders.

However, consumer preferences may be guided not so much by the financial arrangement as by product image. In a recent survey by the American Association of Retired Persons, about half of the respondents reported that they would consider living in a continuing care facility. About the same number would consider moving into congregate housing. Yet only 26 percent would consider a cooperative, and only 17 percent a board and care home. [114]

Continuing care is an attractive, but not a simple, product. Experienced developers estimate that the creation of a life care facility can last an average four to five years: a year of planning before marketing, another year to reach the 50 to 60 percent presales level often required for financing, 18

---

[112]*But see* Allen, § 1.3, above, indicating congregate care residents are younger than life care residents.

[113]*See* Caulfield, & Carlucci, note 78, above. Note that this comparison assumes bond financing for the endowment project, but not for the rental.

[114]*See* L. Dobkin, "AARP Releases Nationwide Housing Survey of Older Consumers," *Aging Network News*, June 1987, 5.

months of construction, and six months or more to move in residents.[115] Marketing costs can reach $4000 to $6000 per unit in a life care facility, whereas in rental projects, such fees may be about half that amount.[116]

Despite the complexities of continuing care, it probably has attracted more attention during the recent retirement housing boom than any other form of facility. This is due in part to the growing ranks of the very old and the probabilities of their eventual need for care, in a financially secure environment, on a long-term basis (see §§ 1.3, 1.6). As a consequence, the number of life care communities is expected by some to triple over the next 10 years.[117] Because of the simplicity of straight rentals, and the familiarity of the concept to many developers and consumers, they will probably continue to hold a substantial proportion of the over 65 market. However, the proportionate share of continuing care facilities should rise dramatically, especially in areas where there is already some consumer awareness of the arrangement and its benefits.

(e) Unbundling of Service Packages

Service packages in retirement facilities traditionally have been provided on more or less of an all-or-nothing basis. A definite trend at this time is unbundling of services. A corollary tendency is toward the proliferation of services and service options. To some extent, the trends moderate each other, as facilities that offered it all tend to break up packages, and those adding services where there were previously none do so in small packaged options.

Continuing care facilities primarily have offered comprehensive service packages for a single monthly fee, with relatively few service options available on an à la carte basis, and little opportunity to receive credit for services available in the facility but not used by the resident. The recent tendency in these facilities is to provide more optional, and fewer mandatory, services. On the other hand, many facilities that tend toward the congregate housing model have had relatively few convenience services available, other than meals. In part, this latter fact is due to the low and moderate, federally financed roots of the congregate housing market. Now, these facilities are going uptown and upscale, and are offering more services, both à la carte and as a part of monthly fees. With ever-increasing competition, the range of service options between the all-included and the nothing-included extremes is rapidly being filled. At this point, rather than moving in one direction or the other, the industry appears to be filling in the middle ground.

Examples of the unbundling of services abound. With respect to health care, whereas traditional continuing care facilities have provided all needed health care, including hospitalizations, for the rest of a resident's life, some facilities are now limiting the scope and volume of health care services that

---

[115]Remarks of Dr. James Smith, Retirement Centers of America, Inc., at Sandy & Babcock seminar on "Proprietary Lifecare," San Francisco, July 19, 1985.

[116]*See* note 110, above. *But see,,* J. Howell, "Learning from Mistakes," National Association of Senior Living Industries 1987 Conference Proceedings, 29, indicating $5,000 to $7,000 per unit marketing costs for rentals.

[117]"What's Putting New Life Into 'Life Care' Communities," *Business Week*, March 3, 1986, 108.

will be available in return for an entrance fee, regular monthly fee, or other form of prepayment or predictable payment. Instead of full care, the facility may offer a limited number of skilled nursing days per year, or over the lifetime of the resident, without any additional charge. But if the resident requires additional nursing services, hospitalization, or other health care or personal services not included in the prepaid or periodically paid program, he or she will be charged for such additional care on a fee-for-service basis. Some alternatives to full health care guarantees have been categorized as follows:[118]

Percentage guarantee. The resident pays a percentage of the fee-for-service charges, with the retirement facility paying the balance.

Per day guarantee. The retirement community pays an established dollar amount per day and the resident pays the rest.

Cumulative day guarantee. The facility covers all charges up to a certain number of days per year and the resident is responsible for all extra days.

Cumulative dollar guarantee. The community pays for care up to a dollar limit per year, a lifetime limit, some percentage of the entrance fee, or a similar dollar amount.

See § 28.7 for examples of some of these types of provisions in resident agreements.

The trend toward more services and more service options should continue as retirement facility developers seek to fashion custom products that will help distinguish their projects from others and from existing facilities in their areas. As consumers become more educated to the various types of service programs available, and as competition increases and more choices are available, many will demand the ability to select from a menu of services and amenities, rather than being required to enroll in and pay for a complete service package that may contain elements they do not want or need. However, the pure à la carte approach can be costly, as anyone who has eaten at a French restaurant can attest. The elderly will want more services, but if economies of scale require mandatory participation, many will be willing to participate in limited mandatory programs.

A good example is meals. Three meals per day included as part of a monthly fee structure is becoming more and more rare. People want to have options to fix their own breakfast, or to go out to lunch or dinner with a friend or spouse without suffering an economic penalty. Therefore, facilities may offer one included meal per day, at the resident's choice, with additional meals available for an extra charge, or a choice between single and multiple meal plans. This is more of a Chinese menu approach, combining a set package with a pure à la carte option. It is representative of the probable model for many of the retirement facility programs to be developed in coming years.

[118]See, Winkelvoss and Powell, "Retirement Communities: Assessing the Liability of Alternative Health Care Guarantees," *The Journal of Long Term Care Administration*, Winter 1981, 9.

(f) New Payment Mechanisms

One change that will have the greatest impact on the business structure, marketing, and legal implications of any project is the development of new payment mechanisms for retirement facility occupancy and services. This trend has been generated largely by increased competition and the influx of real estate developers and other for profit entities in the retirement facility business. For example, real estate developers wishing to provide residents with some measure of security or predictability regarding the costs of future health care, but who are unwilling to bear the risk themselves, are turning to the insurance industry for products that will provide financial security at a fixed monthly rate, and on a noncancelable, lifetime basis. The insurance industry is responding, and custom-tailored insurance products designed to accommodate the needs of an individual retirement community are being created to bridge the gap between developers familiar primarily with real estate and the perceived eventual need of the consumer for health care and financial security (see § 27.2(c)(2)).

Another emerging concept is that of the refundable entrance fee for continuing care facilities. About 90 percent of continuing care facilities refund some portion of the entrance fee upon a resident's voluntary withdrawal from the community.[119] However, such refunds are generally limited to those who leave the facility within the first few years of residence, in which case the entrance fee is amortized to the facility owner at the rate of one to two percent per month of residence, and the balance refunded. Moreover, only about half of existing CCRCs refund any portion of the entrance fee upon the death of the resident.[120] Therefore, if a resident dies very shortly after admission, a substantial entrance fee could be lost in exchange for very little in terms of services actually received. (See § 21.6(c) for a discussion of the actuarial rationale for this system.)

Recently, however, some providers have experimented with the concept of a refundable entrance fee, whereby the entrance fee or some fixed percentage of it is fully refunded to the resident or the resident's estate upon the termination of occupancy of the retirement facility unit, without regard to the duration of residence or the reason for contract termination. This method of financing naturally requires a higher entrance fee upon admission to the facility, and the facility operator retains the income generated by the entrance fee for the period that the resident occupies the premises. A rule of thumb is that the refundable entrance fee is of necessity 25 to 50 percent higher than a nonrefundable entrance fee, in order to achieve economic equivalence. Nevertheless, many elderly people find the refundable entrance fee desirable because it does not result in a disinheritance of one's heirs, and provides an opportunity for the resident to recoup some of the initial payments in the event of a decision to terminate occupancy

---

[119]Raper, note 94, above, at 11.

[120]Winkelvoss and Powell, note 92, above, at 42.

after the first few years of residence. Variations upon the refundable entrance fee concept have included the sale of memberships, similar to country club memberships, as a means to give the resident an opportunity to
receive a return on investment through resale of the interest once occupancy is relinquished. In addition, some developers have offered residents
corporate stock, which can be redeemed at cost when the buyer leaves the
facility.[121]

It has been suggested that refundable entrance fee or membership types of
structures, in effect, act as private investment bonds, which can replace interim public bond financing.[122] Such a system puts the resident in a primary
position as creditor in the event of a failure, and may reduce bond counsel
costs.[123] But such fee structures may raise special securities registration issues (see § 24). In addition, refundable fees or arrangements where the developer promises to repurchase resident memberships, coop shares, or other
interests may be subject to reserve requirements to ensure that there is an
ability to make good on the promise (see § 21.5).

Some facilities applying unbundling of services thinking to their fee structures have offered residents the option of selecting a refundable or nonrefundable program. In one example, residents were able to choose between a
$67,125 fee, 94 percent of which is refundable upon death or withdrawal,
and a $44,750 fee, where 18 percent of it becomes nonrefundable per year of
residence, and all is lost upon death. The developer reports that most prospects are selecting the higher, refundable fee.[124] In another case, however,
where the entrance fee was the same for both the refundable and nonrefundable option, but where the refundable fee carried a higher monthly charge,
most residents chose the nonrefundable plan.[125]

Refundable fees are not without some controversy, however. One industry
spokesman warns that, "Whoever picks a refundable entrance fee is betting
he'll die early."[126] Nevertheless, a segment of the senior market will be willing to pay a premium to insure its investments against the possibility of death
or a change of heart before reaching actuarially calculated life expectancies.
While it may be more economical in the long run to choose a nonrefundable
fee structure, refundable fees, promises to repurchase resident stock or
memberships, and related plans will continue to grow in number.

---

[121] *See* note 117, above, referencing Life Care Communities Corp.'s Court at Palm-Aire, Pom-
pano Beach, Florida. *See also,* "A New Kind of Retirement Home," *Nation's Business,* Jan.
1986, 00.

[122] Caulfield, & Carlucci, note 78, above.

[123] *Id.*

[124] *Id.,* referencing Mediplex Group, Inc.'s Laurel Lake Retirement Community, Hudson, OH.

[125] Remarks of David Wildgen, of Charter House, Rochester, MN, at National Real Estate Development Center Conference, May 16–17, 1985.

[126] *See* note 117, above, quoting Lloyd W. Lewis, Kendal-Crosslands, Kennett Square, Pennsylvania.

Two

Project Planning and Implementation

The creation of any retirement facility requires the coordination of numerous tasks covering several disciplines, such as real estate development, finance, financial forecasting, law, health care services, management of operations, marketing, insurance, architecture, construction, and other fields. It is important to spend time early in the development process giving balanced consideration to all the major issues, and not to proceed too far with some parts of the project while letting others fall behind schedule.

Sometimes, developers can be too aggressive or impatient in their pursuit of certain aspects of the project with which they are most comfortable, such as the development of the physical plant. Prior to the commencement of marketing of any project, and certainly before commencing construction of any new structure, a developer must seriously consider, study, and resolve several additional issues that will determine the overall character of the project and that may make the difference between its success or failure. Important factors such as the size, characteristics, and preferences of the targeted market segment, the details of the service package, the tax and legal implications of business structures or resident payment mechanisms, or such regulatory matters as facility licensing must be addressed. If developers fail to pursue such topics concurrently with the routine real estate issues, they may find themselves in the embarrassing position of having to revise substantially their service package or business structure late in the development process, after having made public representations about the kind of project planned.

Successful development will depend in large part upon assembling the right group of advisors, establishing a comprehensive and well integrated schedule of tasks, and obtaining appropriate review of each successive phase of the development from concept to reality.[1]

§ 3   DEVELOPMENT TEAM FUNCTIONS

The components of any successful retirement facility development include a team of people from various disciplines who must work in concert to produce a balanced, cohesive product. Often, many of these team members are consultants hired by a developer or sponsoring organization to give advice or produce a study or design. Experienced retirement community developers and operators often employ some or all of the team members on a full time, in-house basis. In either event, regular communication among those performing the different functions described below is important, and in some instances can be critical to project success.

Although a few of the functions referred to in this Section may be performed by the same person or entity, each is a discrete role in which special expertise in retirement facility development and a concentration of staff resources should be brought to bear for maximum efficiency and effectiveness. The functions described usually do not involve a single task, but a series of analyses, recommendations, and tangible products that become increasingly detailed as project development proceeds.

§ 3.1   PROJECT COORDINATION

The role of project coordination is an obvious, but critical, one. Depending on the type of ownership and operation of the intended project, the coordinator may be an executive officer of a nonprofit sponsoring organization, a real estate developer, a hired "clerk of the works" type of consultant, or some other representative of the moving force or forces behind the project.

Whatever the facility format, it is important for the coordinator to adequately represent the interests of the owner and operator of the project, especially where these are multiple parties engaged in some form of joint venture. The coordinator should have experience in supervising the development of a real estate project and in working with consultants from a broad array of other disciplines, such as finance, law, architecture, construction, health care, and personal services management. Retirement facility operations experience is a plus. A coordinator must have the ability to develop a realistic timetable for the accomplishment of all the required tasks, to assign the necessary tasks to other team members and ensure follow-through, to keep all development activities, including financing, directed toward a clearly envisioned goal that is shared by all involved in the

---

[1]For a comprehensive review of retirement facility development issues, *see AAHA Development Manual: A Step-by-Step Guide for Trustees and Chief Executives Undertaking Development of Non-Profit Facilities for the Elderly,* American Association of Homes for the Aging, 1986.

process, and to be flexible enough to revise initial plans and overcome obstacles as the project evolves.

§ 3.2 MARKET FEASIBILITY STUDY

One of the most important steps in the development of almost every retirement facility is the creation of a market feasibility study.[2] Unless the developer is already acquainted with and has experience in the development of retirement facilities, an outside consulting firm with substantial experience and a good reputation in the retirement center industry should be retained to conduct a thorough study. The consultant performing the market study should not necessarily be the one performing the financial feasibility study.[3]

The need for a thorough market study increases as facilities become more specialized and complex. Although familiarity with different types of products may vary from one community to another, in general, continuing care facilities and other retirement centers that offer substantial service or health care packages may be more difficult to market and fill than simple rental housing. Therefore, the importance of a detailed market study, including consumer response to the specific project proposal, is heightened.[4]

The market study should identify the numbers of elderly persons within the various communities with sites that are candidates for development, as well as the surrounding primary and secondary market areas from which prospective residents might be drawn. Age subgroupings should be separately evaluated, as the circumstances, desires, and numbers of potential buyers may vary depending on age. The incomes of such age groups by locality should be included. If possible, some effort should be made to determine the general availability of illiquid assets of the elderly in each locale, for example, by reference to housing values in the particular area. The present residential, marital, religious, and other personal circumstances of elderly households should be referenced if possible. Groups that contain large numbers of elderly persons, such as social, religious, civic, and health care organizations, as well as other constituency groups, should be identified and described.

A good market study cannot be limited to demographics, however. A comprehensive report should include specific information about the types of services and amenities desired, and the forms of ownership or interest in real property preferred by the potential market. Questionnaires, telephone

---

[2]Studies may not be indicated, for example, where a group of prospective residents more than large enough to fill the facility is the driving force behind the project.

[3]Some commentators argue that the prospect of doing a financial feasibility study may bias a market analyst in favor of proceeding with development of a project. *See* McMullin, "Common Financial Problems Encountered by CCRCs," *Contemporary Long Term Care*, Feb. 1986, 50.

[4]*See* § 5.2, below, regarding how feasibility studies may make inaccurate assumptions that can jeopardize the project.

interviews, or face-to-face focus groups may be used to determine whether prospective residents are interested in facilities that provide medical care, dining, or other services; whether the respondents prefer to own, lease, or rent their units; what size units are preferred and what prices they can afford; whether they would be willing to pay an entrance fee or a fixed monthly insurance premium to cover the costs of unknown future health care liabilities; whether they would accept a high-rise structure as opposed to a low-rise multiunit or detached campus setting; and other preferences. The process of gathering this kind of information also serves as a valuable premarketing exercise that can identify many prospective residents.

The market study should also examine all the other facilities within the market area. Many developers find that the majority of their populations come from a relatively small area with a radius of approximately 25 miles of the site.[5] All other facilities within the region should be identified, whether or not they are the type that the developer intends to construct. The types of services offered at such facilities should be analyzed, as well as entrance fee rates or prices of units, monthly fees, sizes of the units, services available, occupancy levels, and length of waiting lists, if any. When possible, some effort should be made to determine what kind of success existing or planned facilities in the area have had in filling up their projects, and over what period of time. The study will identify a "penetration rate" which indicates the expected percentage of age- and income-qualified people in the area who can be expected to purchase a retirement facility product. Rates of 2 to 3 percent are commonly used, although in some areas where retirement facilities are more widespread, significantly higher rates have been achieved.

§ 3.3   FINANCIAL FEASIBILITY FORECASTING

The financial feasibility of any product is inextricably linked to the ability to market the product. In conjunction with the market analyst and management consultant,[6] the developer should develop an initial marketing plan that estimates, on a quarterly or even month-by-month basis, the expected numbers of sales of units in the project. It is generally accepted in the industry that rental projects are marketed faster than endowment or continuing care plans that require an entrance fee; therefore, a more precise analysis of the projected marketing strategy, together with a conservative time line for filling the project, is especially important in the latter cases. The financial feasibility study should include income and expense projections for the project during the development process and resident fill-up period. Many observers

---

[5] See, e.g., Laventhol & Horwath, The Senior Living Industry 1986, 33, 56, which reports that nearly 80 percent of the residents in both rental and entrance fee facilities come from within a 25 mile radius of the site.

[6] See § 3.6, below.

believe that it is during this phase of the project's life that the greatest risk of failure exists, particularly in the field of continuing care.[7]

The financial feasibility study should, of course, examine the projected income and normal expenses of operation once the facility has reached a stable level of occupancy, for example, 90 percent. Depending on facility type, a period of 5 to 20 years should be forecast.[8] Suggested sale prices, entrance fees, or rental rates for each type or size of unit should be determined, perhaps with the presentation of alternative pricing structures and their effect on the bottom line.[9] Projections should include a worst case scenario showing the financial impact of a lower than expected rent up. Of course, such an analysis requires a thorough understanding of the details of the proposed service package, necessary construction elements, staffing requirements, and other costly matters that may require architectural, legal, and marketing consultation.

For projects where the facility operator charges an entrance fee but retains ownership of the residential units or is otherwise dependent on income from resale of units,[10] income projections should include expected frequency of resales of the units. This projection should be based upon actuarial assumptions, plus experience concerning turnover in similar facilities. In a mature continuing care facility, unit releases may be expected to reach approximately eight percent per year.[11] However, it may take as long as 12 to 15 years for a new facility to reach maturity.[12] Apartment turnovers in rental facilities responding to one recent survey ranged from 8.6 to 14.7 percent per year, depending on facility age.[13] Of course, all these rules of thumb are based largely on traditional models, and assumptions may have to be modified for projects appealing to different age levels, or with different entry criteria or health maintenance programs.

A financial feasibility study should also take into account reserves required for debt service, future personal care or health care obligations, if any, building maintenance and replacement, working capital, and any reserves that may be required by state law. Of course, the numbers should take into account such other factors as inflation, construction contingen-

---

[7] See § 5.2, below.

[8] See AAHA Development Manual, note 1 above, at 31.

[9] For an example of different pricing methodologies, see §§ 6–8, below. See also Laventhol & Horwath, note 5, above, for a recent study of rental and entrance fee/monthly fee price ranges.

[10] E.g., in membership or real property sales formats where a portion of the sale price must be paid to the facility operator.

[11] See Winkelvoss & Powell, Continuing Care Retirement Communities: An Empirical, Financial, and Legal Analysis (Pension Research Council, Wharton School, University of Pennsylvania, Richard D. Irwin, 1984), 107.

[12] See McMullin, note 3, above.

[13] Laventhol & Horwath, note 5, above, at 26–27. Interestingly, the newer facilities experienced higher turnover, which may reflect increasing frailty of new admittees rather than resident lengths of stay.

cies, consultant fees, and all other projected or reasonably possible expenditures.

It is not necessary for the developer to have project financing in place in order to determine the initial financial feasibility of a project. It is, of course, advantageous to secure a financing commitment at the earliest possible stage and, if it is in place, the cost of servicing any debt should be factored into the feasibility study. Most likely, however, lenders will not be willing to look seriously at any project unless the developer can present a comprehensive development plan that includes a detailed market study, financial feasibility study, and general plan for the physical design and service package to be offered at the facility. Therefore, the typical financial feasibility study will be based upon various assumptions as to the cost of financing through identified or hypothetical sources.

A financial feasibility study can often be performed by an experienced facility developer and operator in consultation with the market analyst and any management consultant, especially in projects that do not offer an insurance type of product or that, for other reasons, require actuarial study. However, many consultants in the marketplace specialize in preparing financial feasibility reports, and they may have special expertise, particularly in fields such as continuing care, where state laws may require specific kinds of financial analyses and submission of those studies to the applicable state agency for review. It should be noted that financial feasibility and preparation of a market study are different disciplines, and the studies serve different purposes. While there may be some consultants who perform both functions well, the developer should be prepared to evaluate carefully the consultant's expertise and experience in each arena.

§ 3.4   LEGAL CONSULTATION

Two of the most frequently overlooked steps in the early stages of project development are a detailed review of the legal implications of various business plan and product development alternatives, and preparation of a proposed residence agreement. There are many legal issues with which the developer must become intimately familiar during the formative stages of the development plan. These include such issues as the tax implications, or implications upon tax exempt status, of various business and facility ownership structures, and the tax and legal advantages or disadvantages of sole ownership, joint ventures, lease transactions, or contractual relationships with other entities that may own or operate the facility.

In addition, the kinds of services offered at the proposed facility may determine whether, and to what extent, the facility, or portions thereof, must be licensed and operations regulated by state agencies. These legal consequences may have profound effects upon the structure and cost of the service package, its marketing, ability to obtain financing, tax exemption for financing, government loans or loan guarantees, construction standards, and even construction schedules. Of course, attorneys can also be of assistance in zoning and land use planning issues, obtaining financing, preparation and review of contracts, and other matters that are common in the development of any form of housing.

A most important aspect of early legal consultation is the development of a proposed residence agreement, which may be in the form of conditions, covenants, and restrictions upon the sale of real property, a lease or rental agreement, a continuing care contract, a membership agreement, a nursing facility admission contract, or another document that spells out the respective rights and obligations of the facility owner or operator and the resident.

Preparation of a residence agreement early in the planning stages of a project can serve several functions, especially in facilities that are service-intensive.

(1) It will force the developer to focus upon the details of the methodology by which the resident will be expected to pay for the residence, or use of the residence, and the services, possibly including health care, to be provided by the facility.

(2) It will help determine more precisely the services and amenities to be provided, the nuances of which can raise issues of business structure, pricing, right of title to, or possession of, the premises, licensing, securities registration, and other matters.

(3) The draft can serve as a tool for use in the latter stages of focus group discussions or other marketing activities.

(4) It can serve as the framework for the final document to be signed by residents and, if applicable, be submitted to state agencies for preliminary licensing review and approval.

(5) It may bring to light potential operational difficulties or needs that must be explored by management and marketing consultants. Often, for example, subtleties of contractual language can result in wide-ranging differences in the extent of state regulation, and it is in the preparation of the residence agreement that a balance is struck between the considerations of pleasing the consumer, operational practicality, financial feasibility, regulatory burden, and ease of marketing.

§ 3.5 EXPERIENCED ARCHITECTURAL AND CONSTRUCTION SERVICES

Architectural consultation is an obvious prerequisite to the development and marketing of any housing facility. With the elderly, more than many other groups, architectural services must deliver more than external "curb appeal." A sensitivity to the particular unit sizes, physical amenities, and interior design characteristics favored by retirement community residents is essential.[14] In addition, the development process may entail many unique rules and public approvals not present in other forms of housing.

[14] See discussion in § 2.2(a), above.

Nevertheless, developers sometimes employ those architectural consultants with whom they are most familiar, without regard to whether the architects have experience in designing retirement facilities of the type contemplated by the developer or indicated by the market study. Because retirement facilities are more than housing and may include dining, recreational, and even health facilities, the choice of architect, and even of construction contractor, is an important one.

For example, retirement facilities that contain areas used for the provision of health care or personal care may be subjected by state law to construction standards or fire safety requirements that are significantly more rigorous than those required of residential housing. Strengths and fire resistance ratings of building components, corridor and door widths, accessibility requirements, and mechanical specifications relating to heating, sanitation, or emergency power are among the many special considerations that may have to be addressed. Architects and contractors unfamiliar with these specialized construction standards might grossly underestimate the costs of construction, be required to do substantial research, or even substantially revise plans or completed building elements in order to comply with applicable laws.

§ 3.6   MANAGEMENT EXPERTISE

It can be helpful in the early stages of the project's development to obtain the services of a person who is familiar with the actual day-to-day operation of a retirement facility of the type under contemplation for construction. Such a person, who may ultimately become the administrator of the completed facility, can be extremely valuable in the formative stages of the project. An experienced manager may have first-hand knowledge of the senior marketplace and of the project's competition in the particular community. The manager will also have operations experience, which can be indispensable in developing the service package that will be offered to residents, verifying marketing and other assumptions, fleshing out the details of staffing needs and other projected operational expenditures for a financial feasibility study, and advising the developer about architectural details and amenities that experience shows are preferred by elderly people. Managers may also assist later in the development process in creating policies and procedures governing residence and operations of departments, such as dining, housekeeping, social and recreational activities, and health care.

§ 3.7   FINANCING

Financing is an essential ingredient of every development, but one that is often not as fully integrated into the process of product formulation as it should be. Often, the kinds of services offered at a facility, or the mechanisms used to obtain payment from residents for services or facilities, determines whether financing is available at all and, if so, from how many competitive sources.[15]

Some lenders, for example, have serious reservations about lending to facilities offering life care or assuming other long-term risks that may impair their ability to repay debt, while other lenders specialize in financing such facilities. The availability of financing in general should, therefore, be incorporated into the formulation of the initial project concept.

Assuming project financing is available, lenders have to be kept apprised of the progress of the development, and will want to take a careful look at the precise legal rights, if any, of the residents with respect to the improvements that are used as security for the debt. This is true particularly in unconventional or unfamiliar arrangements, such as life leases or memberships. In any case, lenders often have an interest in subordinating the contractual or other rights of residents to their own in the event of a default. Lenders' requirements must be taken into consideration when examining applicable license laws, preparing residence agreements, marketing, calculating reserves, and at other relevant steps in the process.

§ 3.8 MARKETING/ADMISSIONS

Unlike many other types of real estate developments, retirement facilities tend not to be built on speculation. Instead, retirement communities are often marketed, at least in part, before and during construction. In endowment projects, deposits from prospective residents may be used to assist in project financing. But even in rental projects, it has been found that substantial pre-construction sales activities take place.[16]

Although marketing may often be performed by the developer or other sponsor, or may be assigned to a facility management group, it is a function that can also require unique expertise. Marketing is a role that transcends the actual task of filling facility vacancies, and affects product and physical plant development, pricing considerations, development of residence agreements, creation and enforcement of admissions and waiting list policies, and other considerations that precede the closing of a sale.

Some consultants specialize in retirement facility marketing as distinguished from market feasibility studies, although there is some overlap between advanced feasibility study functions (e.g., focus groups), and the actual sales process. Of course, marketing is far more than advanced market feasibility study. Marketing consultants must become sensitive to the reputation, ideals, experience, and goals of the sponsor, developer, and operator, whether single or multiple entities. Likewise, they must recognize and respond to the needs and desires of prospective residents. Most importantly, marketing staff must communicate their concerns and ideas, and

---

[15] See, generally, Part VI, below.
[16] See Laventhol & Horwath, note 5, above, at 34.

their activities must be well coordinated with the other disciplines from early on in the development process. Finally, marketing consultants should have the requisite technical expertise to use communications media to the best advantage, and to follow up on a personal basis to obtain deposits or other commitments necessary to confirm sales.

§ 4 STEPS IN THE DEVELOPMENT PROCESS

No exact chronological process can be offered for the development of retirement communities generally. Many of the required tasks and inquiries are so interdependent that a casual attempt at sequencing the substantive groupings of tasks could lead one to conclude that everything should be done simultaneously. In reality, development progress over time really does not involve so much the movement from one kind of task or discipline to another, but is characterized instead by growth from a simple interplay of several disciplines to a more complex one. In other words, the members of the development team are all, to varying degrees, called on throughout the process to expand, rethink, and refine their work as the project evolves. This section attempts to outline, in a rough chronological format, milestones in a representative development process, and show how the talents of team members can be brought to bear on the various tasks. A sample critical path development timetable for a California life care project appears as Figure 4.1.

§ 4.1 BASIC CONCEPT STRUCTURING

(a) Team Selection

Selection of the following team members should occur at the beginning of the process:

Project coordinator

Architect for site review and conceptual drawings

Market feasibility consultant for basic demographic study of the area

Legal counsel for evaluation of business structure options, license requirements, tax consequences, zoning issues, drafting and review of documents, and so on

(b) Site Selection

Site selection should include such financial, marketing, operational, and legal considerations as:

Cost, seller financing

Location in relation to desirable community services such as transportation, shopping, health care, cultural and recreational activities

Location in relation to elderly population centers and other retirement facilities that may be competitive

Ability to retain an option on land pending initial project concept development

Topography, especially if a campus-style setting is desired

Zoning status and community atmosphere and attitudes toward multi-unit development or presence of a health facility

Certificate of need availability in the local health facility planning area

Location of potential joint venture partners, elderly constituency groups

(c)   Formulation of Basic Concept

All team members should share ideas concerning:

Basic architectural format, for example, high-rise, single family, campus

Basic service concept, for example, meals, housekeeping, laundry, social programs, transportation, health care, insurance product

Basic fee arrangements, for example, rental, entrance fee, purchase

Basic resident interest, for example, condo owner, monthly lessee, life lessee, coop owner, membership

Basic structure of owner and operator, for example, for profit, nonprofit, lease to operator, hire management company, joint venture, and so on

§ 4.2   CONCEPT TESTING AND REFINEMENT

(a)   More Team Members

Refinement of the basic concept may require input from additional sources:

A financial feasibility consultant to cost out preferred options

A marketing consultant to test and refine elements of the service package

A manager to point out operational difficulties and solutions

A financial consultant or broker to survey availability of funding

(b)   Financial Modeling

Different variations of the basic options being considered should be subjected to financial analysis and projection, taking into account:

Different pricing options, for example, all prepaid, prepaid plus à la carte, all fee-for-service, refundable versus nonrefundable fees

Balancing pricing levels, for example, size of entrance fee versus liberality of refund, lower costs of mandatory services versus higher priced optional programs

Figure 4.1 Sample Development Timetable: California Lifecare

STEP \ MONTHS	0	1	2	3	4	5	6	7	8	9	10	11
Consultant agreements, (feasibility study, legal, accounting, financial, architectural, construction, marketing)												
Preparation of overall business structure	-----	-----	-----	-----	-----							
Creation of new legal entity and preparation of joint venture agreements (if necessary)	-----	-----	-----	-----								
Obtaining tax exemption (if necessary)												
Application for plan approval and site data (nursing facility)			P	S	-----	-----	-----	-----	A			
Preliminary drawings and outline specifications (nursing facility)											P xxxxxxxxxx	S
Certificate of need (nursing facility)											P xxxx:	
State tax exempt financing approval (if necessary)										P xxxxxxxxxx		
Prelicensing application and questionnaire (personal care facility)								P $$$$$$$$$$$$$$$$$$$$$$$				
Basic legal documents (life care or residence agreement, deposit subscription agreement, escrow agreement)								P ++++++++	S	A		
Financial and occupancy projections												
License application (nursing facility)												
License application (personal care facility)										———		
Permit to sell deposit subscriptions												
Working drawings and final specifications (nursing facility)												
Environmental impact report												
Negative declaration								P **************	S	A		
Full review and certification								P *************************	S			
Land use permit												
Building permit												
Sale of deposit subscriptions												
Selection of bond counsel												
Bond marketing												
Closing on bond issue												
Construction of project												
Release of initial deposit subscription funds from escrow												
Occupancy permit												
License (nursing facility) (including preparation of written policies)												
License (personal care facility) (including preparation of written policies)												
Certificate of authority												
Signing of life care agreement												
Admission of residents												

12 13 14 15 16 17 18 19 20 21 22 23 24 25 26 27

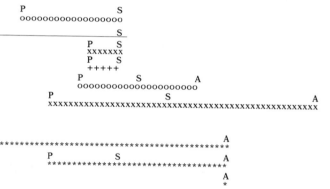

Legend

P = Preparation

S = Submission

A = Approval

xxx   = Skilled Nursing Facility
+++   = Personal Care Facility
oooo   = Life Care
****   = Local Land Use Planning
$$$$ = Financing
-----   = Preliminary Legal Work
———   = Activity or Event

```
            A
        xxx
              S         A
        xxxxxxxxxxxxxxx
              S         A
        xxxxxxxxxxxxxxx
          S         A
        $$$$$$$$$$


        P                 S
        ooooooooooooooooooo
                          S
                    P     S
                    xxxxxxx
                    P     S
                    +++++
                    P         S           A
                    oooooooooooooooooooooo
          P                   S                           A
        xxxxxxxxxxxxxxxxxxxxxxxxxxxxxxxxxxxxxxxxxxxxxxxxxxxxxxx


                                      A
----************************************************
            P             S           A
            ************************************
                                      A
                                      *
                            oooooooooooooooooooooooooooooooooooooooooooooooooo

              $$$$$$
                                    $$$$$$$$$$$$$$$$$$$$$$$$$$$$$$$$$
                                    $$$$$$
```

Figure 4.1 (*continued*)

STEP \ MONTHS	28	29	30	31	32	33	34	35	36	37
Consultant agreements, (feasibility study, legal, accounting, financial, architectural, construction, marketing)										
Preparation of overall business structure										
Creation of new legal entity and preparation of joint venture agreements (if necessary)										
Obtaining tax exemption (if necessary)										
Application for plan approval and site data (nursing facility)										
Preliminary drawings and outline specifications (nursing facility)										
Certificate of need (nursing facility)										
State tax exempt financing approval (if necessary)										
Prelicensing application and questionnaire (personal care facility)										
Basic legal documents (life care or residence agreement, deposit subscription agreement, escrow agreement)										
Financial and occupancy projections										
License application (nursing facility)										
License application (personal care facility)										
Permit to sell deposit subscriptions										
Working drawings and final specifications (nursing facility)										
Environmental impact report										
Negative declaration										
Full review and certification										
Land use permit										
Building permit										
Sale of deposit subscriptions										
Selection of bond counsel	ooooooooooooooooooooooooo →									
Bond marketing										
Closing on bond issue	$$$$$$$$$$$$$$$$$$$$$$$$$									
Construction of project										
Release of initial deposit subscription funds from escrow					A					
Occupancy permit					o					
License (nursing facility) (including preparation of written policies)									P	
License (personal care facility) (including preparation of written policies)									P xxxxxxxxxxxxxx +++++++++++	
Certificate of authority										
Signing of life care agreement										
Admission of residents										

38	39	40	41	42	43	44	45	46	47	48	49	50	51	52	53	54	55

Legend

P = Preparation

S = Submission

A = Approval

xxx	= Skilled Nursing Facility
+++	= Personal Care Facility
oooo	= Life Care
****	= Local Land Use Planning
$$$$	= Financing
-----	= Preliminary Legal Work
——	= Activity or Event

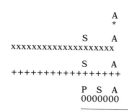

```
                        A
                        *
                  S     A
xxxxxxxxxxxxxxxxxxxx
                  S      A
++++++++++++++++++
                  P  S  A
                  0000000
```

Assessment of actuarial factors affecting future service liabilities and unit turnover

Rent up delays and effect on initial cash flows (monthly sales, income and expenditures projection)

Need for reserves for debt service, plant replacement, future health care obligations, other contingencies

State laws imposing financial disclosure or security requirements, such as liens, reserves, or bonding

Probable requirements of lenders

Review of the competition's practices and level of success

Costs of long-term care insurance or health plan enrollment, if applicable

Costs of special licensing requirements or elevated construction standards

Other usual costs, such as construction, interest, insurance, consultant fees, permits, staffing requirements, food and other supplies, and so on

(c) Premarketing

Prior to attempting to sell a fully defined product, it can be important to communicate with prospective residents and other interested parties.

Identify senior constituency groups

Survey preferences by questionnaire and selected interview regarding services and amenities, fee structures, unit sizes, and so on

Survey attitudes about the sponsor, project, resident's ability to pay, self-image as to physical and social needs, and so on

Establish relationships that will be useful in public approvals, and sales

Possibly approach local land use planning officials and neighborhood groups to test early reactions

Keep lists of all inquiries and prospects

Sell the sponsor and the basic concept

(d) Exploration of Financing

A financing commitment should be sought early on. Availability of construction financing and permanent financing depends on the type of project, and should include review of the following sources:

HUD loans or loan guarantees

State loan guarantees for health facility development

Tax exempt bond financing (often via municipal government)

Banks and other conventional lenders

Syndications

Pension funds

Resident funding via deposits toward entrance fees or sales of condominium interests, cooperative shares, or memberships

(e) Defining the Product

There will always be further adjustments, but by now a defined product should be identified for implementation, including:

Final determination of all owner/operator identities and relationships, including venture partners

Completion of proposed site plan, architectural design, unit sizes and mix

Drafting of a thorough proposed resident agreement with input from legal, marketing, management, and financial consultants, covering fees, services, resident transfer policies, and so on

Development of marketing materials with legal review for consistency with proposed agreement and sufficient breadth to accommodate moderate adjustments

Determination of how and by whom each basic service is to be provided, for example, in-house, by third party contract, on- or off-site, via a joint venture partner, and so on; include consideration of HMOs, insurance, and health facility transfer arrangements for health care services

Identification of all governmental approvals and legal steps necessary to implement the plan; check for licensing, zoning, securities offerings, subdivision approval, certificate of need, and so on

Identification of all remaining team members and responsibilities

Development of a realistic (i.e., conservative) timetable showing each task and its place in the overall development process

§ 4.3   INITIAL IMPLEMENTATION

Once the concept has been sufficiently refined, it is time to go public and begin implementation on several fronts. The priority and timing of these various steps may differ widely among projects, based on the duration of government review processes, identified problem areas, prerequisites demanded by lenders or by law, marketing strategies, and other considerations.

(a) Site Related Tasks

Commence the formal local land use planning approval process, zoning, environmental impact (can be time consuming)

Finalize working drawings and specifications

Put to bid for construction

Fund construction financing

Commence construction only after zoning, financing, sufficient presales or other market response, preliminary license approvals, contract reviews, and other essentials are in place

(b) Legal and Management Tasks

In general, these initial implementation steps should be performed by management and legal team members working together:

Complete all required organizational documents of sponsor, for example, new corporations or partnerships, joint venture agreements, leases, tax exemption applications, private letter rulings

During marketing phase, review questions about resident agreement and modify if necessary

Prepare or review contracts pertaining to construction, management, food service, housekeeping, finance, and so on

Prepare or review third party agreements concerning provision of health care, such as transfer agreements, health insurance policies, health maintenance organization agreements, contracts with medical director, home health agencies, and so on

Create and review policies and procedures of on-site health and personal care facilities

Create and review admissions and waiting list policies, with marketing input

Review issues concerning resident financial or medical qualifications, private pay agreements, resident trusts, powers of attorney, handicap discrimination issues

Prepare deposit agreements and other presales documentation

Review insurance needs of the facility, including general liability, directors' and officers', professional malpractice, employee bonding

(c) Marketing

Make draft of resident agreement and marketing materials available to prospects

Establish an admissions review team, with marketing and legal help, to establish age, health, and financial criteria for acceptance, and waiting list procedures

Begin intensive marketing, including taking of deposits on sales or entrance fee structures (check for licensing prerequisites)

§ 4.4   LATER DEVELOPMENT AND PROJECT OPENING

Project opening generally involves completion of the details of each ongoing element of the project, with a heightened emphasis on close coordination and timing.

Review and adjust budget and pricing assumptions in light of sales
   experience
Complete construction
Obtain certification for occupancy from local government
Obtain site inspections and certifications required for licensure of health
   or care facilities
Execute contracts with management company, and other vendors
Hire other necessary personnel
Collect final deposits from residents, and execute residence agreements,
   powers of attorney, and trust agreements, if any
Coordinate move-in of residents

§ 5   AVOIDING FINANCIAL PITFALLS

Although the vast majority of retirement facilities are run successfully, financial failures have received widespread attention in the press in recent
years.[17] Life care or continuing care communities, in particular, seem to
have attracted the most attention, although it is not clear that they have any
higher proportion of failures than other forms of retirement housing, such
as rental units, condominiums, or cooperatives.

Some commentators believe that the more spectacular failures of continuing care communities may not fairly represent the risks actually present in
the industry:

> Like the crash of a jumbo jet, the failure of a lifecare community attracts
> attention from the press and is brought glaringly into public scrutiny. Al-
> though statistics are not readily available to prove it, troubled facilities and
> failures in the lifecare industry may not occur with any greater frequency
> than in other segments of the real estate industry.[18]

One reason, of course, for the notoriety of life care community failures is
that residents or prospective residents typically make, as a condition of
admission, large lump sum payments to community developers or operators. Advance deposits or entrance fees used to help develop or operate
projects that eventually fail can often involve a substantial portion of the
elderly resident's life savings. Where life care entrance fees are protected
under state laws by escrow provisions or reserve requirements, residents
may not be at risk, but often bondholders become the victims of a default.

In contrast, developers and commercial lenders, rather than tenants and
bondholders, tend to bear the brunt of the financial risk that a rental project

---

[17]See, e.g., Rudnitsky & Konrad, "Trouble in The Elysian Fields," Forbes, Aug. 29, 1983, 58;
Topolnicki, "The Broken Promise of Life-Care Communities," Money, Apr. 1985, 150, and
other articles cited below.

[18]Curran & Brecht, "A Perspective on Risks for Lifecare Projects," Real Estate Finance Journal, Summer 1985, 64.

will fail. Moreover, resident expectations are reduced because of the limited term of the lease. While rental projects, as a more conventional form of real estate, tend, when they fail, to focus less attention upon the retirement home industry, as distinguished from housing in general, the usual presence of actuarial pricing considerations, future medical liabilities, higher intensities of services, and slower sales experiences of continuing care may help explain why it is a common element in many well publicized defaults. As non-continuing care facility programs become more complex, involving more extensive services and unusual payment mechanisms, and as public and governmental concern about transfers of persons in need of medical care becomes more acute, we may expect to see other types of retirement facilities bear a more representative share of attention to difficulties.

§ 5.1   EXAMPLES OF SERIOUS FINANCIAL DIFFICULTIES

The circumstances of several well known retirement facility bankruptcies have been discussed in the literature and press.

Probably the largest group of retirement homes to file for bankruptcy was the Pacific Homes corporation, which operated and now, after reorganization, continues to operate, several facilities located primarily in California.[19] Many of the homes' older life care contracts required payment only of an initial accommodation fee, or an assignment of the resident's assets, without monthly fees or other additional fees, in return for lifetime residence and services. Later contracts required payment of entrance fees plus a *fixed* monthly fee. Without the ability to adjust fees to keep up with inflation and meet rising operational costs, and due to use of capital funds for "capital expansion, speculative investment, and financing of operating losses,"[20] Pacific Homes soon needed to expand its facilities in order to sell new contracts and bring in new accommodation fees to cover obligations under prior contracts.[21] From 1969 to 1976, Pacific Homes' deficit grew from $17 million to $27 million. In 1977, it filed for bankruptcy.[22]

At least six lawsuits claiming damages in excess of $600 million resulted from the bankruptcy and related financial difficulties,[23] including suits

---

[19]For more detailed discscussions of the Pacific Homes cases, see "Continuing-Care Communities for the Elderly: Potential Pitfalls and Proposed Regulation," 128 U. Pa. L. Rev. 900 (1980); "Continuing Care Communities: A Promise Falling Short," 8 George Mason Univ. L. Rev. 47 (1985); *Matthews v. State of California*, 104 Cal. App. 3d 424, 163 Cal. Rptr. 741 (1980); *Barr v. United Methodist Church*, 90 Cal. App. 3d 259, 153 Cal. Rptr. 322 (1979), *cert. den.* 444 U.S. 973 (1979), *reh'g. den.* 444 U.S. 1049 (1980); *General Council, etc., of the United Methodist Church v. Superior Court*, 439 U.S. 1355 (1978); *In re Pacific Homes Corp.*, 1 Bankr. 574 (C.D. Cal. 1979); Senate Special Committee on Aging, Life Care Communities: Promises and Problems, S. Hrg. 98–276, 98th Cong., 1st Sess. (1983).

[20]*See* Comment, George Mason Univ. L. Rev., id.

[21]*Id., citing Bankruptcy Trustee's report, Oct. 15, 1979.*

[22]*Id.*

[23]United Methodist Communications News Release, Oct. 1979.

alleging that the United Methodist Church was an alter ego of Pacific Homes, Inc., and was liable for its contract obligations,[24] and that the state of California wrongfully failed to revoke Pacific Homes' life care license for failure to meet state-mandated reserve requirements.[25] Ultimately, Methodist Church groups contributed $21 million to settle the litigation, creditors have been repaid, and resident contracts have been renegotiated to permit operation on a fiscally sound basis.[26]

Another series of serious financial problems concerned homes operated by Reverend Jimmy Ballard and/or Reverend Kenneth Berg. In one case, Ballard was convicted in 1981 of securities fraud in connection with the sale of bonds for a proposed life care facility. Undisclosed to offerees was the fact that the bonds were to be encumbered by a debt from one of Ballard's previously failed life care projects.[27] In 1984, Berg was also convicted of securities fraud in connection with loans solicited from residents of the same troubled project.[28] In another massive, 1900 unit retirement community once operated by Berg, a lender paid $13 million to plaintiffs, $1 million to the facility, and $500,000 to plaintiff's lawyers, and forgave a $48.3 million mortgage on the facility to settle litigation concerning financial problems in the development of the project.[29] In all, Berg was involved with about 40 projects.[30]

The problems of securities fraud and overly restrictive pricing structures should be easily avoidable by a conscientious developer. However, most other cases of financial failure appear to involve individual facilities that cannot attract a sufficient number of residents to make the project financially feasible, but that are nevertheless financed and developed. Examples include a bond default involving an attempted conversion of Florida apartments into a continuing care project, allegedly with only 11 percent of the units presold;[31] a 300 unit Philadelphia area facility that had made only 16 sales when construction was completed in 1982;[32] and a 300 unit senior rental facility in California, for which only one apartment had been rented a year after the scheduled completion of construction.[33] While these individual failures do not always attract the kind of national media attention that

---

[24] See Barr v. United Methodist Church, note 19, above.

[25] Matthews v. State of California, note 19, above.

[26] Conversation with Mort Swales, president, Pacific Homes Foundation.

[27] See Topolnicki, note 17, above.

[28] Id.

[29] See John Knox Village (Lee's Summit, Missouri) news release, Dec. 11, 1985; In re Christian Services International, 102 F.T.C. 1338 (1983); Comment, George Mason Univ. L. Rev., note 19, above, at 53–55.

[30] Rudnitsky & Konrad, note 17, above.

[31] See Moore, "Major Southern Firms Swept Into Bond Default Litigation Net," Legal Times, Oct. 14, 1985.

[32] See Henriques & Holton, "Of Faith Misplaced: How Investors Lost Millions on Fiddler's Woods," Philadelphia Inquirer, (copy on file with author).

[33] See Pyle, "Bank Sues Over Maple Village Bonds," Fresno Bee, July 18, 1986, B-1.

is encountered by the bankruptcy of a chain of occupied facilities, or by the filing of criminal indictments, they probably constitute the pattern most representative of the real dangers to well meaning developers of retirement facilities.

§ 5.2   CAUSES OF FAILURES

Although no precise formula for success can be offered, commentators on the retirement facility industry have attempted to identify and address factors that account for the financial failures of some communities.[34]

In a preliminary survey conducted by the American Association of Homes for the Aging,[35] 70 facilities were identified as having experienced financial difficulty. Reasons that were identified were found to be subject to the following groupings:

Poor marketing/inadequate presales	23
Poor or inexperienced management	12
Poor financial planning	11
Fraud	3

Failure initially to fill up a new facility is surely one of the greatest causes of financial failure. It is important to study the market feasibility of a project before financing or construction,[36] but there is no substitute, especially in entrance fee styled projects, for actual presales of units with receipt and deposit into escrow of a substantial portion of the expected fee. Feasibility studies can make certain assumptions that turn out later not to be matched by actual consumer behavior. For example, studies may be overly optimistic about the percentage penetration of the age- and income-qualified marketplace that can be achieved.[37] Of course, percentages of market penetration may vary widely depending on such factors as consumer familiarity with the type of product, and the reputation of comparable facilities in the area. Studies may also make imprecise assumptions about the age group likely to be attracted to the facility,[38] about the ability to obtain licensure for health facilities,[39] or about other factors critical to sales and financial success. Feasibility studies are important, but should be

[34] See, generally, Wade & McMullin, "Lessons to Learn in Retirement Living," Contemporary Long Term Care, Oct. 1985, 21; McMullin, "Common Financial Problems Encountered by CCRCs," Contemporary Long Term Care, Feb. 1986, 50.

[35] Draft memorandum, dated May 15, 1986.

[36] See § 3.2, above.

[37] See, e.g., allegations reported in Philadelphia Inquirer, note 32, above.

[38] See, e.g., the allegation that a 79-to-82 age group, rather than the predicted 55-year-and-older segment, should have been targeted in one project. Fresno Bee, note 33, above.

[39] See allegations reported in Legal Times, note 31, above.

tested throughout the development process by identification of, and continuing contact with prospects plus, if possible, exaction of binding financial commitments from them.

Financial planning and management problems often tend to strike facilities years after the onset of operations, but their roots are frequently traceable to the initial development plan. Pricing structures should be flexible, to cover fluctuations in operating costs, allowing for adjustable periodic charges rather than only entrance fees, or periodic fees with dollar or percentage caps on increases.

However, the ability to adjust fees is not enough. If reserves for substantial health care costs, plant replacement, entrance fee refund obligations, or other liabilities have not been funded from the outset, a mature retirement community may find residents unable to absorb the increased costs via a sudden jump in monthly charges. Accordingly, it is important for initial financial feasibility studies to consider long-term obligations and establish a funding mechanism for them from entrance fees, monthly fees, or both.

In addition, where entrance fees are relied upon, financial feasibility studies should contain an actuarial component that conservatively predicts the rate of unit turnover. The unexpected longevity of residents in a facility relying on future entrance fee income from unit turnovers can spell financial disaster.[40] The often-quoted lament of the retirement facility administrator is: "I have two ladies who are 100 years old . . . and they're killing me!"

Other problems causing financial difficulties have included high mortgage interest rates, making it difficult for prospective retirement facility residents to sell their homes;[41] the loss of a nonprofit home's property tax exemption;[42] use of too great a portion of financing for purposes other than construction;[43] and the collection of deposits from prospective residents that are too small to assure that they will move in when the facility is ready for occupancy.

The Federal Trade Commission identified several problem areas in its investigation of fraud in one corporation's sale of life care contracts, but the Commission's points are worth noting by well intentioned developers of any retirement facility.[44] In summary, the problems were:

1. Use of entrance fees to cover construction costs, but not future increases in health care costs for the maturing population of the facility

[40] See, e.g., Swallow, "Agreement Near to Resolve Life-Care Homes' Bankruptcy," Washington Post, Oct. 13, 1984.

[41] See, e.g., "Shaky Lifecare Center Put Up for Sale," Modern Healthcare, Nov. 1980, 54.

[42] See, e.g., Smith, "Baptist Homes in Bankruptcy," Detroit News, March 19, 1977.

[43] See discussion in Rudnitsky & Konrad, note 19, above.

[44] See statement of Patricia P. Bailey, Hearing, Senate Special Committee on Aging, note 19, above, at 54–59.

2. Exploitation of the mortgage lender's reputation as an assurance to consumers of the project's financial soundness

3. Representations that monthly fee increases would be limited by a factor other than actual operating costs

4. Using reserves principally for lender's debt service requirements, while consumers believed future health liabilities were covered

5. Falsely implying a religious affiliation and a corresponding legal and moral obligation of some other organization for the facility debts

6. Failure to escrow resident presales deposits for refund in the event of project failure during development, resulting in dissipation of deposits for development costs

7. Use of entrance fees, monthly fees, or reserves from one project to fund expenses or cover losses at other, unrelated projects

While the problems encountered by failed or financially troubled retirement facilities can be avoided with careful planning, it is important, especially for new entrants in the marketplace, to study the failures as well as the successes of others, and to work with a development team with a proven record of long-term success.

§ 5.3   RECENT DEVELOPMENTS MAY REDUCE SOME RISKS

While certainly not a panacea, nor a substitute for careful market and financial feasibility work and the other planning steps discussed above, three recent trends may help to diminish the risk of failure in some retirement facility projects: (1) the growing availability of long-term care insurance, (2) more widespread state legislation, and (3) movement toward resident-equity structures.

Long-term care insurance has recently become more readily available, with more comprehensive coverages, than was historically the case.[45] By taking the actuarial forecasting responsibilities out of the hands of individual (and possibly inexperienced) facility developers, and by spreading the risk pool beyond the inhabitants of a single self-insured facility, the dangers of inaccurate predictions of future health care liabilities should be reduced. In addition, the economies of scale with which a commercial insurer deals can make long-term, noncancelable coverages available on a monthly premium basis, instead of using a lump sum entrance fee model that exposes more of the resident's assets to risk at the more vulnerable early stages of operation.

States have begun in recent years to adopt legislation dealing with continuing care, or other prepaid or long-term promises of care, at an accelerated rate.[46] While heavy regulation is no guarantee that financial failures

---

[45] *See* discussion in Part VIII, below.

[46] *See* § 21, below.

will not occur, [47] legal requirements such as financial disclosures and projections, escrows of resident deposits, minimum reserves, and presales
thresholds should reduce the incidence of financial difficulty.

Finally, the development of more resident equity models for retirement
facilities may have the effect of preserving more of the resident's investment
in the event of a failure. Theoretically, at least, structures using condominium, cooperative, membership, or even refundable entrance fee structures, if backed by a security interest, retain for the resident some legal interest in the assets of the facility or the provider. Of course, if the project is
financially unsound, the security of the resident's ownership interest may be
largely cosmetic in that construction lenders or other creditors will usually
have first priority in the event of foreclosure, and the project may often have
diminished value if it needs to be converted to some use other than the
planned retirement facility. Once initial lenders are paid off, however, resident equity can provide a degree of long-term financial security.

[47] For example, the Pacific Homes bankruptcy took place despite California's relatively strict
legislation.

Three

Program Business Structures

How the resident pays the facility operator for the shelter, food, medical care, and other services that may be made available at a retirement facility, plus the kind of real property or other interest acquired by the resident, has significant impact upon the business operations of the project and the tax liabilities of both facility operator and resident.

Historically, nonprofit operators have controlled the retirement facility industry, especially that segment of the business offering endowment or entrance fee programs, or continuing care for the resident. These facilities have for many years had special concerns relating to maintenance of their tax exempt status (see Part Four), but their structures have generally followed traditional patterns. The recent growth of for profit involvement in the industry is largely responsible for raising numerous new business, tax, and legal issues resulting in some creative structural solutions.

Several business and tax concerns have helped shape the emerging options. Relevant tax considerations may include the taxability of fees paid by residents to the facility owner or operator, the deductibility to the resident of all or some part of the fees, the ability of the resident to defer recognition of gain on the sale of a prior residence, and the characterization of payments as below market loans. Business considerations can range from the developer's profit opportunity, to operational control and ability to assemble desired services or amenities, to product attractiveness in the marketplace. The basic legal structure of the facility/resident relationship is of at least as much significance as architecture and operational expertise in determining how the project will sell and function. It should be one of the first decisions made in the development process, after careful consideration of the numerous alternatives that may be available.

Several of the issues discussed in this Part relate to more than one of the structures discussed below. However, they may be addressed in the context of only one structure.[1] This Part should be read as a whole, therefore, so that the interplay of the various issues and options is more fully appreciated.

§ 6   ENTRANCE FEE MODELS

§ 6.1   NONREFUNDABLE ENTRANCE FEES

(a)   Marketing and Business Issues

The traditional entrance fee format requires the resident to pay a substantial sum of money to the facility upon admission, in addition to monthly fees. One of the principal purposes of obtaining a relatively large entrance fee at the inception of the project is to help fund construction costs, or quickly retire construction debt, and possibly to set aside reserves for future medical care or other expenditures that may not be covered by routine monthly fees.

Usually, substantial entrance fees are collected in continuing care facilities in return for a long-term or lifetime promise of care and residence. Traditionally, most entrance fees paid to such facilities are not refundable either to the resident upon withdrawal from the facility, or to the estate upon death. A common exception is in the event of a resident's voluntary withdrawal from the community or termination for cause during the first five or six years of residence, in which case a pro rata portion of the fee, based on a declining amortization schedule of one to two percent per month, is refunded. However, when the resident dies, even during the first years or months after taking up residence, the life care contract is deemed to have been fully performed, and the resident's estate often receives no refund of the entrance fee or any portion of it. (See examples of contract provisions in § 28.11.)

Many concerns have been expressed about the fairness of nonrefundable entrance fees, and there has been some recent movement toward modified or other fee structures that permit some form of refund in the event of an early death or withdrawal. (See discussions in §§ 2.4(f) and 21.6(c).) The retention of the entrance fees of a resident who dies before reaching his or her life expectancy is economically justifiable in the self-insurance scenario of a typical life care facility, because the funds are needed to defray the costs of caring for those who will outlive the average life span. Nevertheless, in individual cases where many tens of thousands of dollars may have to be paid for a few days or months of residence and daily services actually received, many observers lose sight of the insurance dimensions of the transaction and find the payment unconscionable. (See § 21.6(c)).

The seeming unfairness inherent in some of the more extreme fact

---

[1]*E.g.*, at-risk rules, discussed in the rental section, apply to all real estate.

situations in part has led to more liberal partial refunds in the event of a death very early after taking up residence, and has also spawned the development of entrance fees that are refundable, in whole or in part, whenever the contract terminates, whether by voluntary cancelation, forcible discharge, or reason of death. However, the principal impetus behind the move away from nonrefundable fees has probably been the potentially drastic adverse tax consequences of nonrefundable fee systems upon the emerging for profit sector of the retirement industry.

(b)   Fees as Taxable Income

(1)   Treatment as Prepaid Rent or Service Fees

A for profit retirement facility that follows the traditional nonrefundable entrance fee format is likely to have the entrance fee treated by the Internal Revenue Service as prepaid rent or a prepaid service fee, which would be characterized as income in the year of receipt. Unless the developer sells the resident an interest in the real property, the money received from the resident cannot be offset by the developer's cost basis in the project and may be taxable in its entirety.

Assuming that a large majority of entrance fees will be received during the first year or two of operation, the financial impact of taxation on that income may significantly affect the developer's ability to pay down construction costs. Having to pass the additional costs to the consumer in the form of higher entrance fees or increased monthly fees would put the for profit facility operator at a competitive disadvantage with similarly situated nonprofit entities that do not have to pay tax on the entrance fees. In large, luxury projects, the amount of entrance fees that could be subjected to income taxation during facility fill-up can be as high as $50 million.

Under Treasury Regulation § 1.61-8, gross income includes rents received or accrued for the occupancy of real property, and specifically includes "advance rentals, which must be included in income for the year of receipt regardless of the period covered or the method of accounting employed by the taxpayer."[2]

In 1967, the Tax Court ruled in *Wide Acres Rest Home* that a stock transfer made by an elderly person to a rest home upon admission, in return for a promise of lifetime care, should be included as income in the year of receipt.[3] The home, an accrual basis taxpayer, argued that the payment did not constitute advance rentals under Regulation § 1.61-8 (presumably, they were characterized instead as service fees), and that the payment was not earned in the first year but should be received in income over the resident's lifetime. The court responded that the regulatory reference to advance rentals was only an

---

[2]Treas. Reg. § 1.61-8(b).
[3]*Wide Acres Rest Home*, 26 T.C.M. 391 (1967).

example of reportable prepaid income, and that the home's access to and use of the stock was unrestricted, compelling its treatment as income when received. Similarly, where there was neither a restriction on the use of advance payments received for services to be rendered in the future, nor any provision for refund, the payments were deemed taxable income when received.[4]

(2) Revenue Procedure 71-21

In general, prepayments for future services or prepayment of rent is treated as income in the year of receipt, even for accrual basis taxpayers.[5] Some exceptions are set forth in Revenue Procedure 71-21,[6] which permits accrual basis taxpayers providing services to defer income until the requisite service is performed, but only until the end of the following year. More interesting for retirement facilities is the provision in the Revenue Procedure that permits deferral of income, on the following basis, when received pursuant to an agreement requiring the taxpayer to perform contingent services:

(a) *On a statistical basis if adequate data are available to the taxpayer;* (b) on a straight-line ratable basis over the time period of the agreement if it is not unreasonable to anticipate at the end of the taxable year of receipt that a substantially ratable portion of the services will be performed in the next succeeding taxable year; or (c) by the use of any other basis that, in the opinion of the Commissioner, results in a clear reflection of income.[7] (Emphasis added.)

It can be argued that certain obligations of a continuing care facility are contingent upon the resident's need for health services, payment of monthly fees, and so on, and that actuarial statistics can be used to calculate the appropriate reflection of income. However, retirement facility prepayments, when required, are almost universally a condition of occupancy and could be characterized as prepaid rent, which is expressly excluded from the benefits of the Revenue Procedure.[8] For example, HUD payments are ineligible for deferral of recognition as income,[9] but payments for the occupancy of rooms where "significant services" are rendered to the occupant are not considered rent, and may be eligible for deferral under Revenue Procedure 71-21.[10]

One problem with the application of this entire analysis to lump sum retirement facility payments is that, although the actuarial statistics standard for deferral of income does not appear on its face to be limited in scope

---

[4]*Beaver v. Comm'r,* 55 T.C. 85 (1970).

[5]*See M.E. Schlude v. Comm'r,* 372 U.S. 128 (1963), 63-1 USTC ¶ 9284; and CCH, *Standard Federal Tax Reports* ¶ 2830.703.

[6]1971-2 C.B. 549.

[7]Rev. Proc. 71-21, § 3.06.

[8]*Id.* at § 3.08.

[9]*BJR Corp. v. Comm'r,* 67 T.C. 111 (1976).

[10]Note 7, above, at § 3.08.

or time, the intent of the Revenue Procedure in general is to permit accrual basis taxpayers to defer income for no more than one year.[11] However, one Revenue Ruling considered the application of Revenue Procedure 72-21 to a deferral of retirement facility entrance fees over the resident's life.

In Revenue Ruling 73-549,[12] the Internal Revenue Service considered whether an accrual basis retirement community offering lifetime contracts could defer recognition of lump sum entrance fees based on the resident's actuarially determined life expectancy. The financial arrangement was unusual in that two *separate* contracts were issued to residents. The first guaranteed lifetime use of an apartment and various common dining, recreational, medical, laundry, and other facilities in return for the entrance fee. A second contract was for provision of all the services in those facilities, in return for a monthly fee. Interestingly, the IRS, citing Revenue Procedure 71-21, found that recognition of the entrance fee income could not be deferred because the first contract had no service component and therefore the payment was rent. By implication, it can be argued, a lump sum payment under a single contract combining lodging and substantial services could be eligible for income deferral on an actuarial basis under Revenue Procedure 71-21.

Still, it does not appear that recognition of entrance fees as income can be spread out over the resident's life simply by characterizing the contract as one for services. In General Counsel Memorandum (GCM) 37019, Revenue Ruling 73-549 was briefly discussed in the context of a retirement facility transaction acknowledged to be a service contract that did not require payment of rent. The General Counsel did not find the distinction between prepaid rent and prepaid service fees to be of significance:

> In any event, whether the entrance fees are for rent or for rent and services, will make no difference in the determination of when the fee is taxable to the Corporation. In both cases such determination depends on when payment is received. See Rev. Rul. 60-85, 1960-1 C.B. 181, modified by Rev. Rul. 71-299, 1971-2 C.B. 218.

Thus, as in the *Wide Acres Rest Home* case, the analysis of whether entrance fees are earned as income should turn on whether the home's access to it is unrestricted when received, or whether there are restrictions upon its use based upon resident life expectancy or some other extended period.

(3) Security Deposits

It is generally recognized that where the parties intended that a payment is to be held as security for the future performance of the payor, there is

---

[11]*Id.*, at § 1.
[12]1973-2 C.B. 17.

sufficient restriction upon the payee's use of the payment that it need not be characterized as income when received.

Thus, security deposits received by a developer of residential rental property were not properly treated as income in the year of receipt.[13] Likewise, one year's advance rent received from a tenant on delivery of the lease was not income where the intent was that it would be held as security for the lessee's performance, interest was to be accrued, the balance was to be applied to last year's rent, and all was to be accounted for by the lessor to the lessee.[14]

On the other hand, where the landlord has insufficiently restricted access to the resident's deposit, or is not strictly bound to refund it, it is likely to be treated as prepaid rent. For example, deposits were treated as rent where they were refundable only in the event of destruction of the property[15] or were to be applied to the last month's rent but were commingled with the taxpayer's general funds,[16] or where the landlord had unrestricted use of the money pending occurrence of a limited refund contingency.[17] Detailed IRS guidelines have been established for reporting tenant security deposit trust account transactions.[18]

Entrance fees, if structured as security deposits, most likely could not be used to retire construction debt, or for ongoing operational expenses. On the other hand, if entrance fees are set at amounts designed to fund reserves for future contingencies such as for resident health care expenses, plant replacement or improvement, refund payments to residents or their estates, as an endowment for residents who run out of funds, or for other future obligations, it can be argued that they should not be received as income when initially paid to the facility. Of course, it would be important to have such entrance fees, or portions of fees, earmarked for the specific future uses and kept in segregated, restricted accounts.

(4) Trusts

One possible solution to the problem of receiving entrance fees as ordinary income over a short period of time is to establish a mechanism whereby the payments are distributed from the resident to the facility operator over a more extended time period. Although it is valuable to have all entrance fee monies available immediately to the developer for such purposes as retirement of the construction debt, another advantage of entrance fees is that the lump sum of money required to be paid is most

[13]Priv. Ltr. Rul. 7852009. Private letter rulings should not be relied on as precedent.

[14]*Clinton Hotel Realty Corp. v. Comm'r*, 128 F.2d 968 (5th Cir. 1942).

[15]*Hirsch Improvement Co. v. Comm'r*, 143 F.2d 912 (2d Cir., 1944), *cert. den.* 323 U.S. 750.

[16]*Shaucet*, TC Memo 1957-133.

[17]*Detroit Consolidated Theatres, Inc. v. Comm'r*, 133 F.2d 200 (6th Cir., 1942).

[18]Rev. Rul. 77-260, 1977-2 C.B. 466.

readily available at the time of admission, because the resident has most likely just sold his or her prior residence and liquidated a substantial amount of equity. It is desirable from the developer's point of view to tap that fund at the time of admission, before it is depleted. On the other hand, one may not want to tie up the funds in the manner of a security deposit arrangement, but receive distributions for retirement of debt and operational expenses.

One method for preserving entrance fee monies without realizing substantial taxable income in the first year is the establishment of a trust. Entrance fees can be paid into the trust by the resident in a lump sum at the time of admission and then be paid out to the facility in increments over a period of several years. As an alternative, the facility can borrow some or all of the trust corpus. The existence of a trustee can give added confidence, both to the resident and the facility owner, that funds will be available for payment to the retirement community, or for refund to the resident, when needed.

In general, funds placed in trust for services to be performed over several years are not income when transferred to the trust.[19] However, compensation paid into a trust for eventual distribution to a beneficiary may be deemed constructively received and taxable in the year of deposit where the right to payment is irrevocable and not subject to any contingency.[20]

The use of a trust as a device for avoiding taxation of retirement facility entrance fees was examined extensively in GCM 37019. There, an accrual method life care retirement facility required payment by residents of an entrance fee into an irrevocable trust, the income and principal of which was to accrue to the benefit of the corporate facility owner. A percentage of the trust corpus was to be paid to the corporation each month. The undistributed balance of the trust for each resident would be refundable to the resident or his estate only in the event of contract termination or death during the first 10 years. The trustee bank had general powers of management and control of the trust, but an advisory committee appointed by the corporation had authority to remove the trustee, as well as to give advice about investments and others matters. In addition, the trustee was to have no liability for mismanagement of the trust corpus.

The General Counsel's analysis first recited that income is taxable when received,[21] except that an accrual method taxpayer may elect to include income upon the earliest of (1) performance of the required service, (2) payment becoming due, or (3) payment being made.[22] Moreover, income is deemed constructively received where it is set aside for the taxpayer to

---

[19] *Harrison v. Comm'r*, 62 T.C. 524 (1974). *See also Meile v. Comm'r*, 72 T.C. 284 (1979).

[20] *E.T. Sproull v. Comm'r*, 16 T.C. 244 (1951), *aff'd.*, 194 F.2d 541 (6th Cir. 1952).

[21] I.R.C. § 451(a).

[22] Citing, Reg. § 1.451-1(a), and Rev. Rul. 74-607, 1974-2 C.B. 149, and *Schlude*, note 5 *supra*.

draw upon without substantial limitation or restriction.[23] The question, the General Counsel determined, is whether the payment into the trust is to be considered a payment, directly or constructively, to the corporation.

After discussing several cases, the Memorandum concludes that the corporation's dominion and control over the trust corpus, via the advisory committee's ability to terminate the trustee, plus the limitation upon the trustee's liability, eclipsed the fact that the corporation did not have actual possession or ownership of the entrance fee payments. For example, the corporation could in effect require the trustee, under penalty of removal, to invest funds in the exact manner the corporation would if it had actual title and possession of the trust corpus. Thus, the corporation was found to have constructively received the entrance fees when paid to the trust.

This conclusion does not mean that a trust for retirement facility entrance fees will always result in a finding that the payments are constructively received by the facility (see, for example, Letter Ruling 8326113, discussed in § 6.1(b)(5)). When setting up a trust for receipt of entrance fees, however, it is important to give the trustee the usual powers of dominion and control over the trust corpus, plus the concomitant responsibility for losses or mismanagement. If the trustee is to be subject to removal for cause, perhaps that decision could be made by a committee in which residents, or others not controlled by the retirement facility owner, participate. If the concerns of GCM 37019 are met, it appears that an entrance fee trust with periodic payments to the facility operator/beneficiary, conditioned upon continued performance of services and furnishing of lodging for the residents/grantors, can be effectively used to secure the resident's payments, without the facility immediately receiving taxable income on the entire amount set aside.

If the integrity of the trust is recognized, there are still some additional tax issues related to trust income. Trusts are themselves taxable entities, and income earned by the trust is subject to taxation. However, if income from the trust corpus is distributed to trust beneficiaries, the trust is treated as a conduit and the beneficiaries are taxed instead of the trust.[24] In the event the grantor of the trust has retained substantial powers over the trust, or a reversionary interest in the principal, the grantor, rather than the trust, could be treated as the owner and be taxed (presumably at a higher rate) on the trust income. Prior to the Tax Reform Act of 1986,[25] the major exception to this rule was for Clifford Trusts, in which a grantor with a reversionary interest could avoid taxation on trust income if the trust was irrevocable for at least 10 years. This longstanding rule has now been repealed, and a reversionary interest or other substantial control over the corpus will generally result in taxation of income to the grantor.[26]

[23]G.C.M. 37019, citing Treas. Reg. § 1.451-2(a).
[24]See I.R.C. §§ 643, 651, 661, CCH *Standard Federal Tax Reporter*, ¶ 3628.06.
[25]P.L. 99-514.
[26]I.R.C. §§ 673-675, CCH note 24 *supra*, at ¶ 3703.02, *et seq.*

Retirement facilities may wish to have trust income distributed to the operator, and this will normally lead to taxation of the income to the facility. However, if the entrance fee paid into the trust is refundable to the resident/grantor upon death or withdrawal from the facility, the income, even if distributed to the facility, is likely to be taxed to the resident when earned by the trust. In that scenario, there may be reason to pay the interest or other income to the resident. If the funds are borrowed from the trust, of course, income earned by the borrower thereafter is taxable to it.

(5)   Trust with Loan

In one private letter ruling,[27] the IRS examined in detail whether lump sum payments into a trust by "life tenant" retirement facility admittees would be treated as prepaid rents in circumstances where the trust later loaned the trust funds to the corporate facility owner. There, the elderly applicant was required to pay a lump sum initial rent amount into a grantor trust, plus monthly rent and a monthly service fee, in return for lifetime residence and services. However, the monthly rent obligation ceased after 15 years, and thereafter the resident could remain for life rent-free. Initial rent was not refundable after the first six months of residency, but was to be used, presumably, to prepay or offset the rental costs of those who stopped paying rent after 15 years. When the resident took occupancy, the trust was to loan a defined amount per resident to the facility.

The corporation agreed to repay the loan, with nine percent interest in equal monthly payments, over a period of 14 years, with a final balloon payment. The facility would further execute a negotiable promissory note to the trust, secured by a mortgage on the facility property, giving the trust a first lien, subordinate only to construction loans on the project. The loan proceeds paid to the facility were to be escrowed and used primarily for payment of construction debt, as well as for repayment of loans for residents who terminate early, and for administrative and other expenses. The trustee could make distributions of interest to residents, but most would have it applied automatically to monthly rent payments. Tenant interests in the trust could be sold, transferred, or assigned at the tenant's election. If a tenant elected to terminate the agreement, the corporation would not be relieved of its obligation to repay the loan from the trust.

The IRS noted that gross income includes advance rentals but, distinguishing Revenue Ruling 73-549,[28] found that the trust/loan arrangement amounted to a loan to the corporation, rather than prepaid rent. Importantly, the IRS noted that the corporation did not have unrestricted enjoyment of the funds, but was required to pay off its construction loan. In addition, however, the ruling emphasizes that unlike a rental situation, the resident will receive repayment of the principal plus interest. And if the

---

[27]Priv. Ltr. Rul. 8326113.
[28]See discussion in § 6.1(b)(2), above.

resident transfers the interest in the trust to a third party, the corporation's repayment of the loan will benefit the third party. The ruling concludes that, "A tenant will not, therefore, receive an apartment unit and other facilities for a deposit of a defined amount."

It is unclear whether transferability of the tenant's trust interest is a necessary, or even properly significant, factor in avoiding treatment as prepaid rent of amounts received by a retirement facility as a loan from a trust. If the right to payments from the trusts is sufficiently restricted, and loans are properly secured and subject to definite repayment schedules, the transaction should not result in taxation of entrance fees in the year of payment as prepaid rent or service fees.

An example of a trust fund entrance fee arrangement is one in which the resident is required to deposit one-half of the entrance fee in Trust *A* and the other half in Trust *B*. Trust *A* is distributed to the facility operator at the rate of 20 percent per year. Each year, the facility operator is paid 20 percent of Trust *A* (10 percent of the total entrance fee) as taxable income. The resident earns interest on the undistributed portion of the Trust *A* deposits. The half of the entrance fee deposited into Trust *B* is borrowed in its entirety by the facility operator immediately after deposit. In order not to burden the resident or trust with tax on imputed interest,[29] the developer pays interest annually at the federal borrowing rate upon the funds borrowed from Trust *B*. The borrowed proceeds of Trust *B* should not be treated as taxable income to the facility operator, and will be repaid to the resident upon withdrawal from the facility or death.

(c) Resident Tax Considerations

(1) Medical Deductions

From the resident's perspective, one of the advantages of a nonrefundable entrance fee is that, to the extent that a portion of the fee is a prepayment for future health care, the entrance fee may be deducted as a medical expense. After the Tax Reform Act of 1986, medical expenses incurred in any given year are now deductible only to the extent they exceed 7.5 percent (versus five percent) of the taxpayer's adjusted gross income.[30] At a time when it is becoming increasingly difficult to meet the test for deductibility of medical expenses in any given year, absent a catastrophic injury or long-term illness, the prepayment of medical expenses by means of an entrance fee creates a unique opportunity to incur a deductible expense that will exceed the threshold required by the Internal Revenue Code. Several IRS rulings expand upon the availability of the deduction.

---

[29]See discussion in § 6.2(b), below.
[30]I.R.C. § 213(a).

In Revenue Ruling 75-302,[31] a medical deduction was allowed, in the year paid by the resident, for that portion (about 30 percent) of a lump sum life care fee that the retirement facility could demonstrate from its prior experience was allocated to the provision of medical care, medicine, and hospitalization. A separate statement was issued to residents showing the medical expense. The IRS noted that the fee was refundable to the resident under certain circumstances (perhaps early withdrawal), and that in the event of a later refund, such amounts would have to be reported as income. It is unclear, however, whether a fee intended to be refundable whenever the contract terminates will ever qualify as a deductible expense when it is treated by the parties as a loan rather than a prepayment.

In a later ruling, the IRS approved a medical deduction for residents of a new life care facility with no prior experience as to its costs of medical services, where the facility used the financial information of a comparable retirement home to estimate its costs.[32] The IRS concluded that a portion of residents' fees was deductible because it was "made in order to secure medical services despite the fact that the medical services were not to be performed until a future time if at all."

In addition to physician and hospital care, nursing care and personal care may be considered a deductible medical expense.[33] However, portions of the entrance fee used for the construction of health care or personal care units in a retirement facility may not be deducted.[34]

In a recent private letter ruling, portions of nonrefundable resident fee payments to a retirement community offering nursing care when needed, could be deducted, where the calculation excluded construction debt service, and to the extent such payments were not compensated by insurance.[35] A 1986 ruling (No. 8630005) further clarified that medical expenses include staff costs, medications and supplies, pro rata shares of housekeeping, maintenance, utilities, administrative, and marketing costs, interest on indebtedness, real estate taxes, insurance, and depreciation of the nursing facility, and that these costs could be allocated among residents in order to place them on an equal footing with each other, taking into account variances in the cost of accommodations.

In addition to entrance fees, monthly fees may be deducted to the extent they can be shown to equal the retirement home's cost of providing medical care, medicines, or hospitalization.[36] The facility should keep records demonstrating what proportion of entrance and monthly fees is allocated to

---

[31]1975-2 C.B. 86.

[32]Rev. Rul. 76-481, 1976-2 C.B. 82. *See also* Priv. Ltr. Rul. 8221134.

[33]Reg. § 1.213-1(e)(1)(ii); Priv. Ltr. Rul. 8502009.

[34]Rev. Ruls. 76-481, 1976-2 C.B. 82, and 68-525, 1968-2 C.B. 112.

[35]Priv. Ltr. Rul. 8502009.

[36]Rev. Rul. 67-185, 1967-1 C.B. 70.

health services or health care reserves, and these records should be made available to residents for the preparation of their tax returns.

(2)   Section 1034 Carryover

One of the benefits of ownership of one's principal residence is the ability, under Internal Revenue Code § 1034, to defer the recognition as taxable income of some or all of the gain on the sale of the residence if, within two years before or after the sale, another qualifying residence is purchased.[37] A significant issue for retirement facilities is whether they qualify as residences that, when entered, permit the buyer to carry over or defer recognition of any gain on the sale of a prior residence. This can be an especially significant factor for facilities using entrance fees because they tend to rely upon the resident's sale of a prior residence as the funding source for initial fee payments. The amounts subject to tax can be significant for elderly persons whose mortgage-free homes may have undergone exponential rises in value over several decades of ownership. Moreover, the repeal of preferential tax treatment for capital gains under the 1986 Tax Act only exacerbates the problem.

Unfortunately, the Internal Revenue Service determined in Revenue Ruling 60-135[38] that a retirement facility furnishing a resident with living quarters and lifetime services such as meals, personal care, and medical care, did not qualify as a residence for purposes of exercising the Section 1034 carryover privilege. There, the resident paid a lump sum fee for living quarters, plus a deposit in a life care assurance fund that, together with monthly fees, covered the service component. No proprietary interest in the facility or any other asset was acquired by the resident as a result of the transaction.

Citing Revenue Ruling 55-37,[39] the Internal Revenue Service noted that Section 1034 does not apply to circumstances where the proceeds of the sale of the prior home are reinvested in a residence in which the taxpayer has no legal interest. Moreover, unlike cooperatives,[40] there is no specific provision granting the benefits of Section 1034 to such retirement facilities. The IRS found that "Such acquisition represents future support to the taxpayer rather than a purchase of an interest in the real property of a retirement home."[41]

It may be possible to distinguish this ruling in circumstances where the lump sum entrance fee payment is calculated to cover the costs of providing the housing, and only monthly fees are used to pay for services provided

---

[37]This rule is also discussed in §§ 7.1(d)(1), 7.2(b)(2) and 7.3(c)(2), below.

[38]1960-1 C.B. 298.

[39]1955-1 C.B. 347.

[40]See § 7.2(b)(2), below.

[41]Rev. Rul. 60-135; *id.*

at the facility. Still, absent some transferable resident interest, the IRS is likely to disallow income deferral.[42]

Another problem not discussed in the Revenue Ruling, but nevertheless apparent, is that application of Section 1034 to nonrefundable retirement facility entrance fees may result in the Treasury *never* being able to tax the gain from the sale of the prior residence. If proceeds of a sale are reinvested in a home owned by the taxpayer, the home remains an asset of the taxpayer, or of his estate, which will be subject to a final sale resulting in eventual recognition of taxable income. With the nonrefundable fee, however, there is no interest (real property or otherwise) left to sell, no resulting gain, and no opportunity for taxation.

All of the above points to some advantages for resident ownership of retirement facility units (including condominiums and cooperatives),[43] and possibly for some creative advocacy by owners of retirement facility memberships or, less likely, taxpayers with refundable entrance fees.

§ 6.2   REFUNDABLE ENTRANCE FEES

(a) Treatment as a Loan

The interest of for profit developers in continuing care facilities has resulted in special attention being paid to the concept of refundable entrance fees. A refundable entrance fee is one that is taken by the facility operator at the time of the resident's admission, and the entire fee, or some specified portion of it, is returned either to the resident whenever he or she leaves the facility or to the resident's estate in the event of his or her death.

Refundable entrance fees may well solve the income tax problem of proprietary facilities that receive entrance fees, in that the proceeds of the refundable entrance fee should be treated as a loan rather than as taxable income.

The Supreme Court, considering what constitutes income under Internal Revenue Code § 61, wrote that income is received "[w]hen a taxpayer acquires earnings . . . without the consensual recognition, express or implied, of an obligation to repay and without restriction as to their disposition."[44]

Although it seems elementary that a payment is not income to the payee if there is either an obligation to repay (a loan), or sufficient restriction on its use (e.g., a deposit), courts have carefully scrutinized the details of loans from lessees to lessors, and sometimes recharacterized the payments as prepaid rent.

[42] *See* discussion at § 7.3(c)(2), below.

[43] *See* § 7.1(d), below.

[44] *James v. United States*, 366 U.S. 213, 253 (1961).

In *Blue Flame Gas Co.*,[45] where a corporation leased its assets to its sole shareholder and received a loan from the lessee, the Tax Court found that the alleged loan constituted a payment of advance rent. The court noted that the loaned amount and the aggregate rent due under the lease were identical, the payment dates for each loan and lease installment payment were identical, and no payments actually exchanged hands, but were recorded by offsets recorded in the parties' books of account. Although there was a promissory note, the loan was noninterest bearing and unsecured, and it was an express condition of the lease transaction, prompting the court to call the transactions interdependent.

Likewise, where an accrual basis taxpayer received an advance payment from its lessee, the Tax Court determined, although the taxpayer contended that the payment was intended as a construction loan, that because the funds were not earmarked but commingled with general corporate funds, no promissory notes were executed, and no interest was charged, the payment constituted prepaid rent.[46]

In *United States v. W. B. Williams*,[47] where the lessee's loan had no specified repayment date, no promissory note was executed, and payments on the loan were to be made by the lessor out of yearly lease payments made by the lessee, the payment was treated as prepaid rent. In addition, the taxpayer made no attempt to seek a loan apart from the lease, and the amount loaned was directly related to annual rental payments. Although the lessor/borrower was obligated to pay interest on amounts due, the Fifth Circuit Court termed the charge "compensation for advance rent."

But, in *Illinois Power Co. v. Commissioner*,[48] the Seventh Circuit Court distinguished *U.S. v. Williams* and found that "[t]he underlying principle is that the taxpayer is allowed to exclude from his income money received under an unequivocal contractual, statutory, or regulatory duty to repay it."

Loans from residents to retirement facilities as a condition of admission certainly raise some of the issues addressed in the recharacterization cases discussed above. For example, the loan and resident agreement are generally interdependent, and the loans and lease payments are one and the same. Unlike a conventional loan, interest may not be paid and the date when payment is due may not be predictable.

However, the facts of the recharacterization cases also raised serious questions about whether there was an unequivocal intention and an enforceable obligation on the borrower's part to repay the amounts not taken into income. If retirement facility operators oblige themselves to repay loaned amounts upon the occurrence of some inescapable future event, such as death or contract termination, and secure that obligation, the

---

[45] 54 T.C. 584 (1970).
[46] *Harold Bell Co.*, T.C. Memo 1955-103, Dec. 20,1976.
[47] 395 F.2d 508 (5th Cir. 1968), 68-1 USTC ¶ 9394.
[48] 792 F.2d 683, 689 (7th Cir. 1986).

unequivocality of the repayment obligation should be the controlling factor.

The definiteness of the refund obligation was highlighted as the determinative factor in two Revenue Rulings involving refundable fees taken by swim clubs. In the first,[49] membership fees were treated as loans where they were to be refunded five years after the pool was constructed. In the second, however,[50] membership fees were treated as ordinary income where they were to be refunded only on a declining balance basis if the member moved out of the area within five years of joining. Distinguishing its earlier ruling where the club had a "continuing obligation to refund," the IRS found the declining refund arrangement to be "contingent" and club's repayment liability "not fixed."

Despite the dissimilarities between refundable entrance fees and conventional loans, the fees should not be considered income in a properly structured transaction where the repayment obligation is definite.[51]

(b) Imputed Interest

(1) Application of the Act

One of the most significant concerns regarding the refundable entrance fee structure stems from the Deficit Reduction Act of 1984.[52] The 1984 Act subjects below market loans to imputed taxable interest to the lender to the extent that the borrower pays no interest, or pays interest at a rate less than the short-term federal rate. This rate is determined from time to time by the Secretary of the Treasury, based upon average yields of outstanding obligations of the United States Government.[53]

If the imputed interest rules are applied to retirement facility fees, the Internal Revenue Service would pretend that the resident had received taxable interest income, at the federal borrowing rate, on the entire refundable portion of any entrance fee paid to the facility for each year that the loan exists. Because such lenders may be required to pay tax on income never actually received, the Act can pose serious problems for elderly residents, who are often on fixed incomes.

It should be noted at the outset that there is a significant question whether the imputed interest rules apply at all to retirement facility entrance fees. The Act specifically exempts loans made to "qualified continuing care facilities" prior to the effective date of the Act (October 11, 1985).[54] Although the

---

[49]Rev. Rul. 58-17, 1958-1 C.B. 11.

[50]Rev. Rul. 66-347, 1966-2 C.B. 196.

[51]*See also* the discussion of a loan from a trust in § 6.1(a)(5), above.

[52]P.L. 98-369, Section 172, 98 Stat. 494, amended by P.L. 99-121.

[53]I.R.C. § 1274(d).

[54]See P.L. 99-121, § 204(a)(2). Qualified continuing care facility is defined in I.R.C. § 7872(g). *See* § 6.2(b)(2), below, for discussion.

House-Senate Conference Committee Report[55] notes that the exemption for preexisting continuing care contracts is not intended to infer that the rules apply to such contracts entered into after that date, it remains to be seen if and how the rules will be applied.[56]

The Conference Agreement to the 1985 amendments to the Act clarifies that the Act also was not intended to apply to continuing care entrance fees where refunds are available only during initial occupancy periods for consumer protection purposes, or on a declining basis for the first several years of residence.

> In addition, the conferees understand that a payment to a continuing care facility pursuant to a continuing care contract frequently is wholly or partially refundable for a relatively brief period (e.g., six months) essentially for consumer protection purposes pursuant to State law or regulations. The conferees also understand that payments to a continuing care facility are often refundable on a declining pro rata basis over a somewhat longer period (often up to eight years). The conferees understand that such payments would ordinarily be treated as advance payment of fees and not as loans under present law.[57]

Having identified what is not covered by the Act, the analysis of whether and how other refundable retirement facility entrance fees would be covered by the rules becomes exceedingly complex.

As amended by the 1984 Act, the Code defines a below market loan according to whether it is a demand loan or a term loan. For demand loans, which are payable in full on demand of the lender, the loan is below market if the interest rate is less than the "applicable federal rate," which is the short-term rate under Section 1274(d).[58] All other loans are term loans, which are deemed below market if the amount loaned exceeds the present value of all payments due under the loan, using a discount value equal to the short-term federal rate.[59] Imputed interest for a demand loan is calculated annually for so long as the loan remains outstanding,[60] whereas the entire excess of the term loan over the present value of repayments due is subject to imputed interest in the year the loan is made.[61]

It is unknown whether refundable retirement facility entrance fees, if covered by the Act, would be categorized as demand loans or term loans. Although many of the newer forms of refundable fees generally are refundable

---

[55]Cong. Rec., June 22, 1984, H 6649.

[56]The IRS is expected to adopt implementing regulations in December 1987.

[57]*U.S. Code Cong. & Admin. News*, 99th Cong., 1st Sess., Vol. 2, pp. 451–452.

[58]I.R.C. §§ 7872(e)(1)(A), (f)(2)(B), (f)(5).

[59]I.R.C. §§ 7872(e)(1)(B), (f)(1), (f)(2)(A), (f)(6).

[60]I.R.C. § 7872(a)(1).

[61]I.R.C. § 7872(b).

in full,[62] and a refund may be triggered upon the option of the resident/ lender, the resident must give up the right to live and receive services at the facility in order to be repaid. Thus, more than a mere demand is required to obtain repayment, and refundable fees may well be characterized as term loans.

The law further divides below market loans into the following categories: (1) gift loans, (2) compensation related loans, (3) corporation-shareholder loans, (4) tax avoidance loans, and (5) other below market loans.[63]

The most likely category that retirement facility transactions would fall in is that of "other below market loans," which consists of loans not falling in the other categories, where the interest arrangements of the loan "have a significant effect on any Federal tax liability of the lender or borrower."[64] An example of a below market loan fitting the "other" category is given in the legislative history:

> The interest arrangement of a below-market loan has an effect on the tax liability of the borrower or the lender if, among other things, it results in the conversion of a non-deductible expense into the equivalent of a deductible expense. *For example, if a member of a club makes a non-interest bearing refundable deposit to the club in lieu of part or all of his or her membership fee, the member is paying the fee with money that has not been included in his income* (i.e., the investment income from the proceeds of the deposit), and has, in effect, converted the fee into the equivalent of a deductible expense.[65] (Emphasis added.)

The country club example is generally analogous to a retirement facility refundable entrance fee. However, several factors must be taken into account by the Treasury that may result in such entrance fees being determined not to constitute below market loans:

> The conferees anticipate that in determining whether an effect is significant, the Treasury will consider all the facts and circumstances including (1) whether items of income and deduction generated by the loan offset each other, (2) the amount of such items, (3) the cost to the taxpayer of complying with the provision and (4) any non-tax reasons for deciding to structure the transaction as a below-market loan rather than a loan with interest at a rate equal to or greater than the applicable Federal rate and a payment by the lender to the borrower.[66]

---

[62]For example, if a $100,000 fee is 90 percent refundable, the loan amount is only $90,000, and thus, the *loan* would be refundable in full.

[63]I.R.C. § 7872(c)(1).

[64]I.R.C. § 7872(c)(1)(E).

[65]*U.S. Code Cong. & Admin. News*, 98th Cong., 2d Sess., Vol. 3, pp. 1707–1708.

[66]*Id.*, at 1708.

Application of these criteria to retirement facility transactions may warrant a finding by the Treasury Department that they should not be considered below market loans. For example:

(1) To the extent entrance fees or the unrecovered interest thereon are for prepaid medical services (beyond the statutory threshold), there would be a tax deduction to offset some or all of the taxable interest income.

(2) The size of entrance fees on the average nationwide are relatively small (about $45,000 per lifetime).[67]

(3) The taxpayer's cost of compliance is especially large if the refundable fees are considered term loans, because the durations of such loans are unknown in advance and depend on the resident's life span or the date either party exercises contract termination rights, possibly resulting in the necessity of retroactive, amended tax returns.

(4) Most elderly residents are on fixed incomes, and may have difficulty paying tax on interest never received.

(5) Payments are usually made to charitable, tax exempt facilities operating at the lowest feasible cost.

(6) Life care residents are generally denied the opportunity to defer the recognition of gain on the proceeds of the sales of their prior residences, when used to pay entrance fees, while other similarly situated seniors who reinvest in a new residence owned in fee simple or in a cooperative may avoid taxation on those same proceeds for the rest of their lives.

(7) Public policy should, for fiscal[68] and humanitarian reasons, create incentives for private health self-insurance programs and senior living communities at least equal to incentives for the purchase of increasingly expensive homes with no services, by increasingly elderly people likely to need services in the near future.

Although there are arguments that the imputed interest rules should not apply to retirement facility fees, until clarifying regulations are issued, developers should seriously consider the potential impact of the rule for projects now in planning.

(2) $90,000 Exemption for Qualified Continuing Care Facilities

Amendments to the 1984 Act, passed in 1985, exempt from the imputed interest provisions of the Act the first $90,000 of entrance fees loaned to a "qualified continuing care facility for each year in which the lender or

---

[67]See § 2.3(d), above.

[68]*See, e.g.*, "Private Financing of Long Term Care: Current Methods and Resources," ICF Inc., Phase I, (1985), 6, submitted to U.S. Department of Health and Human Services, which suggests that the government could reduce federal health care expenditures by encouraging private financing of life care and other long-term care insurance programs.

lender's spouse has attained 65 years of age."[69] In determining the $90,000 threshold, the law requires aggregation of all outstanding loans from the lender and spouse to any qualified continuing care facility. The dollar amount of the exemption is to be adjusted annually after 1986, based on increases in the Consumer Price Index.

To qualify for exemption, the facility must permit the individual resident or spouse to use the facility for life. The resident(s) must first reside in an independent living unit with outside facilities available for provision of "meals and other personal care,"[70] but not be in need of "long-term nursing care." After entering the independent residential unit, the occupant must be provided, when needed, "long-term and skilled nursing care." The facility may not charge residents substantially more if they need "personal care services or long-term and skilled nursing care."

Finally, substantially all the facilities used to provide services required to be provided under the continuing care contract must be owned or operated by the borrower. Conventional nursing homes are not considered to be continuing care facilities.

The $90,000 exemption from the imputed interest rules is thus available primarily to traditionally styled life care communities that provide health and personal care services, when needed, as part of an actuarially determined, fixed or regular fee established at the time of admission (subject to adjustment). Long-term promises of priority access to facilities on the basis of the then-current fee-for-service, when the service is delivered in the future, do not qualify. In addition, residential facilities using other vendors of care services are ineligible, unless there is common ownership or operation.

The statute's references to "meals and other personal care" and "long-term and skilled nursing care" seem a bit out of step with jargon used in the trade and in state licensure laws. The principal question is whether qualified facilities must provide licensed personal care. It is not entirely clear from the statute whether licensed assisted living must be available to residents of independent living units, because the statute equates personal care with the generally unlicensed service of providing meals, and because residents in need of licensed personal care generally are not independent. When the resident can no longer remain independent, the law requires provision of long-term care, if needed, in addition to skilled nursing care. Long-term care is a generic term that usually includes skilled nursing care. It is thus unclear whether the law uses long-term care as a euphemism for licensed personal care,[71] whether it refers to other licensed long-term care,

---

[69] See P.L. 99-121, 99 Stat. 511-513 (1985), I.R.C. § 7872(g).

[70] I.R.C. § 7872(g)(3)(B)(i)(I). Note that meals are generally not considered personal care under state licensing laws. It is unclear, therefore, if licensed assisted living or personal care must be available while the resident is residing in the independent living unit.

[71] Many different terms are used by the various states to describe personal care. See § 20.3, below.

such as intermediate care, or whether the reference is simply to services that generally are unlicensed, such as meals, housekeeping, and laundry. Facilities with both licensed personal care and skilled nursing to supplement independent residences should be eligible for the $90,000 exemption. However, facilities with unlicensed services to supplement independent living, plus arrangements for skilled nursing care owned or operated by the same organization, arguably need not provide licensed personal care to qualify for exemption.

(3)   The $250,000 Entrance Fee Nonexemption

Hopes for a broader exemption from imputed interest rules were raised among nonprofit retirement facility operators in 1986 when the Treasury announced a proposed exemption for loans of up to $250,000 to nonprofit organizations.[72] Applied to refundable entrance fees, this would mean that if the borrower were a tax exempt organization, the first $250,000 loaned, interest free, as a refundable entrance fee would not be characterized as a below market loan.

Shortly after the initial announcement, however, the proposed rule was amended to state the original intention that only *gift* loans of up to $250,000 were to be exempted.[73]

This provision, as amended, clearly does not apply to those refundable entrance fees that are paid as a quid pro quo for admission to a retirement facility. Such fees are not likely to be characterized as gifts. (But see § 9.11 below, concerning deductible contributions to tax exempt retirement facilities.) Presumably, a truly charitably motivated interest-free loan of up to $250,000 to a nonprofit retirement facility would be eligible for exemption.

(4)   Coping with the Imputed Interest Rules

The possibility that imputed interest rules may be applied to refundable entrance fees has caused facility operators to have to address the problem before clarifying regulations are issued. Many facilities have structured transactions so that interest at the relatively favorable federal rate simply is paid to the resident. Others are paying no interest, and are leaving the matter between the resident taxpayer and the Internal Revenue Service.

An alternative may be for the facility not to pay interest, but to agree to pay any tax on imputed interest for which the resident may be obligated. This approach makes sense because the applicability of the rules is uncertain, and it is cheaper for the facility to pay the tax on imputed interest income rather than the interest itself, especially in light of the lower individual tax rates resulting from the Tax Reform Act of 1986.

[72]51 Fed. Reg. 25032, July 10, 1986.
[73]51 Fed. Reg. 28553, Aug. 8, 1986.

Although the taxation of refundable fees is technically between the taxpayer and the IRS, it may be prudent for facilities marketing refundable fee programs to advise prospective residents generally of the issue and to encourage them to seek private legal or tax accounting advice on the subject.

(c)   Securing the Refund

The nontax business issues, pro and con, relating to refundable entrance fees are discussed in several places in this book. Among the considerations and issues are the necessarily higher initial cost of refundable fees,[74] the financial benefits to the resident or the resident's estate in the event of an early death or withdrawal versus a long-term stay,[75] and the ability of the provider to make refunds when due.[76]

One way for a resident reasonably to be assured that the facility will have the substantial refund on hand when repayment is due is for the facility to set aside a reserve for that purpose. One state has adopted an interim refund reserve proposal,[77] but it remains to be seen in what circumstances a reserve should be mandated and how it is best calculated. Major corporate parents of a few retirement facilities, for example, may have sufficient assets to give reasonably reliable corporate guarantees that refund obligations of the subsidiary facility will be paid from the parent's funds whenever they become due. Some other facilities have secured the promise to make refund payments with mortgages or trust deeds upon the facility itself.[78] Of course, the problems with reliance on the building as security include the probable lien priority of construction lenders or others, the problems inherent in an individual resident undertaking a foreclosure and collection action against an operating retirement community, and the eventual deterioration of the building asset.

While these problems of the presence and reliability of security for the debt are inherent in any loan transaction, lenders usually are institutional enterprises with sufficient resources and expertise to evaluate thoroughly the individual borrower. Here, however, while elderly retirement facility applicants are often sophisticated and have professional advisors, as a group they are not well equipped to evaluate the financial strength of the retirement facility borrower. This fact will probably accelerate the proliferation of legislation dealing with reserve requirements, or strengthen the impetus in the private sector to establish strict, objective, and credible financial rating or accreditation systems for entrance fee styled retirement facilities. In the absence of reliable assurances that refunds will be paid, or

---

[74] *See* § 2.4(f), above.

[75] *See* §§ 2.4(f), above, and 21.6(c), below.

[76] See § 21.5 and discussion, below.

[77] See § 21.5, below.

[78] See trust/loan arrangement discussed in § 6.1(b)(5), below. Priv. Ltr. Rul. 8326113.

other contract obligations performed, or in the event of one or more dramatic facility failures, use of periodically funded long-term care insurance products as a substitute for entrance fee structures is likely to accelerate.[79]

§ 7 OWNERSHIP MODELS

§ 7.1 CONDOMINIUM OWNERSHIP

(a) In General

The central characteristic of condominiums is that their owners have fee simple interests in their residential units, and share with other owners an undivided interest in the land and other common areas of the project, such as hallways, entrance areas, and recreational facilities. Residents enjoy essentially all the practical and tax advantages of home ownership, and leave the burdens of maintenance and repair of the facilities to the homeowner's association.

On the other hand, the association's bylaws, together with deed restrictions or covenants, in addition to requiring payment of dues and adherence to procedural rules of operation, are likely to contain limitations upon the individual owner's ability to alter or improve the unit or to sell it to a buyer of the owner's choice. For retirement facilities, the issues of management control over operations and control over resales of individual units present the greatest challenges to long-term and harmonious functioning of the project in the manner originally intended.

Condominiums are generally financed by short-term construction loans, with unit owners each obtaining longer term financing on an individual basis. While some HUD mortgage insurance programs are available for condominiums, these are of limited usefulness.[80]

Condominiums also may be subject to federal and state securities registration laws or specific state statutes requiring filings and disclosures.[81]

(b) Business Issues

(1) Marketing

Home ownership is a cherished American opportunity of great attractiveness, especially to seniors, many of whom have become accustomed to being homeowners most of their lives. Most mature adults are familiar with the condominium ownership concept, and such a project probably does not

---

[79]See discussion in Part IX, below.
[80]*See,* Warren, Gorham & Lamont, *Housing & Development Reporter,* 25:0017–21.
[81]See discussion in § 24, below, and Rohan & Reskin, note 85, below, § 3.05.

require the degree of consumer education necessary for many entrance fee or membership formats.[82]

Providing the resident with ownership of the retirement facility unit creates several advantages for both developer and resident. From the developer's point of view, selling the unit permits the developer to receive a large amount of cash, similar to receipt of an entrance fee. However, unlike the nonrefundable entrance fee situation, the developer need not report the entire sales proceeds as income, but may offset the cost basis expended in development of the facility. Residents receive the tax benefits of homeownership, including the ability to carry over gain from the sale of a prior residence, and to exercise the one-time exclusion of $125,000 of gain upon sale of the condominium unit (see subsection § 7.1(d) below).

While condominiums may be familiar to consumers and their sale easier than some other models, retirement facilities with services create special problems of control, discussed below, that are not present in conventional developments, and that should be of considerable importance to the astute purchaser.

(2) Homeowner Management Concerns

Sale of the entire premises to condominium homeowners can result in a loss of control over the character and day-to-day operations of a retirement facility. If homeowners are able to resell their units without restriction or to exercise complete control over service management, the facility as envisioned by the developer could be compromised. Moreover, developers interested in operation of the facility could become powerless to maintain cohesiveness and clear direction.

Deed conditions, covenants, and restrictions may be effective in maintaining the character of a facility by controlling sales, for example, only to persons over a certain age who meet specific financial and health status standards set forth by the homeowners' association and reviewed by a committee of the association. Conflicts of interest may develop, however, when those who control the homeowners' association have to make decisions about such matters as the liability of the association to care for residents who have extraordinarily high medical expenses, or other problems that may have a financial or highly personal impact upon association members. The businesslike detachment of nonowner management with control over service facilities can help curtail the discord often evident in homeowner's associations. Its importance is only amplified in a facility with extensive personal and health services.

A few examples of resident-controlled condominiums operating with a continuing care format have arisen recently in the marketplace. Such a facility may have a health center that is commonly owned by the homeowners'

---

[82]See discussion in §§ 2.4(c) and (d), above.

association. The association then hires a management company to staff the facility and operate it. The homeowners' association has responsibility for developing facility policies and procedures, admission to the facility, and hiring and firing of management. As these facilities mature, it will be instructive to see how they cope with the potential problems of control in the face of differing resident needs. For those concerned with the long-term success of the project, it may be a mistake, however, simply to turn over unbridled control to the homeowner's association. Developers should seriously consider maintaining substantial control over operations and service areas, if state laws permit.

(3) Lost Resale Opportunity

From the facility developer's point of view, it may be more desirable to retain ownership of the residential units rather than to offer them for sale. Not only does retention of ownership alleviate concerns about control, discussed below, but the facility developer who elects to continue with operations of the community also maintains a continuing financial benefit from the project that goes beyond management fees. On the average, a mature continuing care facility, for example, can experience a complete turnover of population about once every 14 years. If there is some form of substantial entrance payment, the facility operator will in effect have the opportunity to "sell" a residential unit again once it is vacated. It is upon this resale of the unit, many years after the facility has been constructed and the costs of development substantially paid, that the developer/operator can expect to generate significant income over expenditures.

In some respects, the resident also benefits by this mechanism. The continued interest of the developer in keeping the project marketable should result in maintenance of high quality services and attractive facilities. In addition, to the extent that the developer may look forward to profit from the resale of units many years after construction, initial entrance fees or membership purchase prices can be reduced to encourage initial fill-up of the new project. These opportunities are lost when the facility is sold as condominiums or as some other form of fee simple ownership, unless substantial transfer fees, based on a percentage of appreciation value, can be worked into the transaction.[83]

(c) Developer Control Issues

(1) Management Contracts

Although the character of the condominium and its operations can be controlled to a limited degree by conditions, covenants, and restrictions contained in the deeds and by association bylaws and rules, homeowners'

[83]See discussion of membership structures, § 7.3, below.

associations often have a well deserved reputation for engendering discord and even lawsuits over relatively simple matters of maintenance of the premises. At least in theory, all homeowners' association governing members may have conflicts of interest between their personal welfare and that of the community at large. In a retirement facility, where services require more intensive day-to-day management oversight, and where decisions may have to be made about serious personal matters such as medical care benefits or the ability to remain in the residential unit with one's spouse, the homeowners' association may not be as well equipped to make important management decisions as an operator who maintains ownership of the facility.

In general, condominium developers establish the overall character of a property through its physical design and the creation of deed restrictions and homeowners' association bylaw provisions. Pending the sale of a majority of the units, the developer usually controls the homeowners' association and thus the facility management. Eventually, however, the association voting rights are turned over to the individual owners, and the extent to which the developer can retain control over or ensure perpetuation of the intended character of the community becomes an issue for all concerned.

Every state has some form of a condominium law[84] and, as interpreted by regulation or case law, these laws may place specific restrictions on the ability of a developer to maintain control over management of the facility after its transfer to the association.[85] For example, in California, homeowners' associations are prohibited, with limited exceptions, from entering into contracts for goods or services for a term longer than one year, unless a majority of the voting power of the association residing in members other than the developer approves the transaction.[86] Similarly, in Florida, where a developer had procured a management contract with the association while it was under the developer's control, once 75 percent of the units had been acquired from the developer, the association was able to cancel the contract, irrespective of whether it was a fair and reasonable contract, and without regard to whether the contract had been breached.[87] Interestingly, however, at least one Florida case has held that where the promoters, prior to selling units to individual purchasers, had the association enter into a 25-year management contract with them, the purchasers were deemed to have affirmed the existence of the long-term contract upon the sale of the units. Thus, the contract was deemed enforceable.[88]

[84]See, *Housing & Development Reporter*, note 80, above, 25:0151.

[85]*See, generally*, Rohan & Reskin, *Condominium Law & Practice*, (New York: Bender, 1987 [looseleaf, published annually]) ch. 10.

[86]10 Cal. Admin. Code § 2792.21(b)(1).

[87]*Tri-Properties, Inc. v. Moonspinner Condominium Ass'n., Inc.*, 447 So. 2d 965 (Fla. Dist. Ct. App. 1984).

[88]*Point East Management Corp v. Point East One Condominium Corp.*, 282 So. 2d 628, 284 So. 2d 233 (Fla. 1973), *cert. den.* 415 U.S. 921 (1974) *See also Plaza del Prado Condominium Assoc. v. Del Prado Management Co.*, 298 So. 2d 544 (Fla. 1974).

Other attempts to limit developer management contracts have been based on general concepts of fairness and policies against self-dealing. For the most part, such attacks have been unavailing.[89] Thus, individual state statutes must be reviewed to determine the extent of restrictions on management contracts with developer/promoters.

The federal Condominium and Cooperative Abuse Relief Act of 1980[90] also restricts operation, maintenance, or management contracts of more than three years, and unconscionable leases, benefiting developers or their affiliates, entered into in *conversion* of projects from rentals to condominium or cooperative units, and where the developer at the time had control of the owners' association. Although the Act creates judicial relief for alleged violations, actions respecting unconscionable feases had to be brought prior to October 9, 1984, so the law has little impact at this time.

(2)   Common Use Areas and Amenities

An alternate or additional method of retaining control over the service and amenities aspect of a retirement facility condominium project is for the developer to own common areas such as dining, recreational, and health care facilities, in which such services are provided, and/or to include deed covenants requiring payment for such amenities or common services.

In a recent Illinois case,[91] for example, a covenant was upheld that required condominium owners to pay annual dues to an adjacent sports facility owned by the developer. The court rejected arguments that the deed restriction was unconscionable, a restraint on alienation, and did not run with the land, and upheld the sports club's lien against the condominium unit owner for unpaid dues because the covenant was part of the original deed, and known to the purchaser, and the club was part of the same complex of buildings.[92]

However, where a developer executed a lease of recreational space to himself on behalf of the homeowners' association before it was officially formed, and without subsequently obtaining the association's ratification, the association was not bound to honor it.[93]

In addition, statutes requiring that recreational leases or management contracts must be fair and reasonable, if entered into before unit owners control the association, can preclude long-term leases to the promoter.[94]

[89]See, Annot. "Self-Dealing By Condominium Developers," 73 A.L.R. 3d 613, § 3.

[90]P.L. 96-399, § 601; 15 U.S.C. §§ 3601-3616.

[91]*Stream Sports Club, Ltd. v. Richmond*, 99 Ill. 2d 182, 457 N.E.2d 1226 (1983).

[92]*See also, Point East Management Corp. v. Point East One Condominium Corp.*, note 88, above.

[93]*Berman v. Gurwicz*, 189 N.J. Super. 89, 458 A.2d 1311 (1981), *aff'd.* 189 N.J. Super. 49, 458 A.2d 1289 (1983), *cert. den.* 94 N.J. 549, 468 A.2d 197 (1983).

[94]*See, e.g., Point East One Condominium Corp v. Point East Developers, Inc.*, 348 So. 2d 32 (1977) (99 year lease); Fla. Stat. Ann. § 711.66(5)(e).

For facilities interested in providing mandatory long-term care insurance, there is some precedent for mandatory insurance assessments against condominium owners.[95] However, where the mandatory services, amenities, or facilities are not a usual and integral part of a condominium project, there is a danger that the transaction may be viewed as an arrangement involving the tying of two products for sale in violation of federal antitrust or state unfair competition laws.[96] Generally, unlawful tying arrangements occur when a seller with market control over one product conditions its sale upon the purchase of another product. Therefore, while leases of common areas, or assessments for property insurance or maintenance, might more readily be considered part of a single condominium product, assessments for dining or medical facilities and services may be considered a separate product unlawfully tied to the condominium purchase. Potential plaintiffs may include the residents themselves, as well as competitors in the tied product business, such as health care providers.

Condominium unit owners have successfully initiated legal actions against developers on antitrust theories in an effort to overturn long-term management contracts or leases.[97] However, where approval of a long-term lease with the developer for garage space, in effect before the condominium association was formed, was made a condition of initial purchase of the units, at least one court viewed the transaction as the sale of a single product and merely a limitation on the estate purchased.[98]

Although no clear pattern emerges from the cases, and specific state laws may yield different results, some potential condominium retirement facility arrangements appear less vulnerable to challenge than others. Of course, making payment for facilities and services optional is the most legally secure alternative. If developers retain ownership of adjacent or on-site properties where dining, recreational, or medical facilities are available, but their use is not mandatory, the mere convenience of their location could be sufficient to make them economically successful. If mandatory resident support of the facilities is desired, it seems safer to include such requirements in deed restrictions, rather than resorting to leases or other contracts between the developer and homeowners' association. Mandatory services and amenities should be integrated as much as possible into the project to create a unified product resistant to tying arrangement claims. This can mean more than merely physical integration. For example, if the financial arrangements are such that a fixed, overall fee covers dining,

---

[95] *Sun-Air Estates Unit 1 v. Manzari,* 137 Ariz. 130, 669 P.2d 108 (1983) (blanket policy on condominium unit).

[96] See discussion of antitrust arguments against mandatory meals in HUD-subsidized projects in § 22.5(d), below.

[97] *See, e.g., Mission Hills Condominium Assoc. v. Corley,* 570 F. Supp. 453 (N.D. Ill. 1983); *Miller v. Granados,* 529 F.2d 393 (5th Cir. 1976); *Imperial Point Colonnades Condominiums, Inc. v. Mangurian,* 549 F.2d 1029 (5th Cir. 1977).

[98] *Johnson v. Nationwide Industries, Inc.,* 450 F. Supp. 948 (N.D. Ill. 1978).

availability of different levels of health care facilities, housekeeping, recreational programs, and other services, the transaction is more likely to be treated as a single, comprehensive program rather than as a series of separately priced, but tied, products. In addition, blanket state licensure of the entire program (e.g., as a life care facility) can give weight to the single product concept.

(3) Resale Restrictions

A fundamental requirement for any retirement facility condominium is the ability to restrict occupancy to elderly people. Where health care or other substantial services are included, it may also be necessary to establish financial and health criteria for occupancy. Unlike entrance fee, rental, or even cooperative formats, the individual unit ownership characteristic of condominiums raises special questions about the developer's ability to place limits on the owner's freedom to use or sell his or her own property.

Federal and state laws may prohibit age discrimination in the sale or rental of housing. However, with some restrictions, exceptions generally have been recognized for senior citizen housing projects, due to the perceived special needs of the elderly to live together among their own age group.[99] This theme can have enhanced validity where a health insurance program is offered, or where licensed health facilities catering to elderly needs are offered as part of the overall program.

Courts have upheld deed restrictions that provided for a residential association's right of first refusal to ensure "a community of congenial residents."[100] On the other hand, arbitrary refusal to consent to a transfer without provision for compensation of the unit owner has been determined to be an unreasonable restraint on alienation.[101] Rights of first refusal exercisable by condominium associations have raised issues concerning violation of the rule against perpetuities.[102] And a statute was upheld that created a rebuttable presumption of unconscionability for any covenant or bylaw provision that gave the association a right of first refusal.[103]

Covenants that limit residence to members of, or those sympathetic to, a particular religious or philosophical sect have been found to be

---

[99]See, e.g., O'Conner v. Village Green Owner's Ass'n., 33 Cal. 3d 790, 191 Cal. Rptr. 320 (1983), and discussion in § 23.1, below.

[100]Chianese v. Culley, 397 F. Supp. 1344, 1346 (S.D. Fla. 1975).

[101]Aquarian Foundation, Inc. v. Sholom House, Inc., 448 So. 2d 1166 (Fla. App. 1984).

[102]See Cambridge Co. v. East Slope Investment Corp., 672 P.2d 211 (Colo. App. 1983), rvsd, 700 P.2d 537 (Colo. 1985), in which the Colorado Supreme Court upheld such a right of first refusal even though it technically violated the rule against perpetuities. Some states have by statute exempted condominium rights of first refusal from application of the rule against perpetuities. See Rohan & Reskin, note 85, above, § 10.03(2).

[103]Berkley Condominium Assoc. v. Berkley Condominium Residence, Inc., 185 N.J. Super. 313, 448 A.2d 510 (1982).

unenforceable.[104] Discrimination in the sale of homes on the basis of race, color, religion, sex, or national origin is also prohibited by federal law.[105]

In general, retirement facilities should be able to enforce deed covenants that restrict resales to persons meeting age, health, and financial criteria that are reasonably related to some required or fundamental component of the service program offered at the community. If the developer or homeowners' association seeks to place restrictions on resales without objective standards based on program features, a right of first refusal may present a legitimate vehicle to accomplish that end.[106] However, state laws and court opinions must be reviewed to identify any particular limitations that may be applicable.

(d)   Tax Issues

(1)   Resident Ownership Tax Advantages

Because a condominium structure allows the resident to obtain a real property interest in the retirement facility unit, he or she may enjoy several tax advantages that attach to the ownership of real property used as a principal residence. To the extent any gain is received from the sale of a principal residence occupied prior to entering the retirement facility, recognition of the profit as taxable income can be deferred to the extent that it is reinvested within two years in another principal residence in which the taxpayer has an ownership interest.[107]

The Internal Revenue Code also permits persons over the age of 55 to exercise a one-time lifetime exclusion from income of $125,000 of capital gain from the sale of a principal residence.[108] If, as is often the case, an elderly person has sold his or her residence prior to entering the retirement facility, and the retirement facility unit is leased rather than owned, the taxpayer may be forced to exercise the $125,000 exclusion in the year of admission to the retirement facility. However, in a condominium, the taxpayer will have the option of exercising the lifetime exclusion at a later date, upon sale of the retirement facility unit.

Finally, residents may deduct real estate taxes and mortgage interest.[109] Membership fees and dues are not likely to be deductible.[110]

---

[104]See, e.g., Taormina Theosophical Community, Inc. v. Silver, 140 Cal. App. 3d 964, 190 Cal. Rptr. 38 (1983), State v. Celmer, 80 N.J. 405, 404 A.2d 1 (1979); "The Rule of Law in Residential Associations," 99 Harvard L. Rev., 472 (1985).

[105]See 42 U.S.C. §§ 3601–3631.

[106]See, generally, Annot., "Validity, Construction, and Application of Statutes, or of Condominium Association's Bylaws or Regulations, Restricting Sale, Transfer, or Lease of Condominium Units," 17 A.L.R. 4th 1247.

[107]I.R.C. § 1034.

[108]I.R.C. § 121. Lesser ownership interests, such as life estates, are also eligible. Rev. Rul. 84-43, 1984-1 C.B. 27.

[109]I.R.C. §§ 163, 164; Rev. Rul. 64-31, 1964-1 C.B. 300.

[110]I.R.C. § 262.

(2) Homeowners' Association Exemption

Section 528 of the Internal Revenue Code creates an exemption from taxation for homeowners' associations, including a "condominium management association."[111] The association qualifies if: (1) it is organized and operated to provide for the acquisition, construction, management, maintenance, and care of association property; (2) at least 60 percent of its gross income consists of dues, fees, or assessments from owners of residential units; (3) at least 90 percent of its expenditures are for the acquisition, construction, management, maintenance, and care of association property; (4) no part of the net earnings inure to the benefit of any private individual; and (5) the association files an election form with the Internal Revenue Service for each taxable year.[112] Income from sources other than membership dues, fees, and assessments is taxable at the rate of 30 percent.[113]

§ 7.2 COOPERATIVES

(a) Cooperative/Condominium Differences

Cooperatives have been used as a form of multiunit ownership, including retirement facility developments, for many years. In most respects, cooperatives are similar to condominiums: (1) residents have the right to occupy specific units and to use common areas, (2) a governing body administers general services, such as maintenance and repairs, and the residents share these expenses, (3) residents' interests are transferable, and (4) tax deductions related to real estate ownership are available to individual occupants. Like condominiums, cooperatives may be subject to federal and state securities registration requirements or specific state disclosure requirements.[114]

However, unlike a condominium, where each resident can be the fee simple owner of the individual residential unit and an undivided portion of common areas, cooperatives generally are corporations that own the entire project and sell transferable memberships or shares to tenant-stockholders, entitling them to occupy a residential unit and use the common areas. Several practical differences between cooperative and condominium development and operations result from this basic difference in structure.

Because the residents' ownership interest is in a corporation, rather than in real estate, cooperatives tend to have more control flexibility than many condominiums. The cooperative's board of directors can more easily control who is admitted to residence in the building, and is not subject to the rules prohibiting unreasonable restraints on alienation (conditions upon

---

[111]See I.R.C. § 528(c)(2); Treas. Reg. § 1.528-4(c).

[112]I.R.C. § 528(c)(1)(A)–(E).

[113]I.R.C. §§ 528(b), (d).

[114]See discussion at § 24, below.

transfer) of real property interests such as condo ownership.[115] Because coop residents generally have a leasehold interest in their units, association rights of first refusal over the transfer of coop shares are not likely to be subject to the rule against perpetuities.[116]

In addition, blanket mortgage financing is more readily available to cooperatives, which have a single owner, than to condominiums, which have numerous owners, each of whom may be required to obtain separate financing.[117] This advantage can be of special importance when contemplating conversion of an existing rental apartment facility or other structure into a resident ownership structure, because existing mortgages, assuming they have favorable low interest rates, may be assumed by the cooperative.[118] On the other hand, in the event of a default in payments by an individual resident, the cooperative must absorb any financial loss, whereas condominium owners would bear individual responsibility.[119]

(b)   Tax Treatment of Cooperatives

(1)   Tax and Interest Deduction Passthrough

A tenant-stockholder of a cooperative housing corporation may deduct real estate taxes and interest on indebtedness incurred in the acquisition, construction, alteration, rehabilitation, or maintenance of the land or building, to the extent of the tenant's proportionate share of the cooperative's expense.[120]

Prior to the adoption of the Tax Reform Act of 1986, shareholders' pro rata deductions could be based only on the percentage of the total stock they owned, irrespective of unit size. Now, any basis reasonably reflecting the corporation's cost for the stockholder's unit may be used.[121]

Section 216(b) of the Internal Revenue Code defines a "cooperative housing corporation" as a corporation (1) having only one class of stock outstanding, (2) each of the stockholders of which is entitled, solely by reason of ownership of stock in the corporation, to occupy for dwelling purposes a house, or an apartment in a building owned or leased by such corporation, (3) no stockholder of which is entitled to receive any distribution that is not out of earnings and profits of the corporation, except on a

---

[115]*See, e.g.*, Kazlow & Schrager, "Cooperative, Condominium Ownership Compared," *The National Law Journal*, June 16, 1980, 19, and discussion, § 7.1(c)(3), above.

[116]*See* Rohan & Reskin, note 85, above, at § 10.03(2).

[117]Kazlow & Schrager, note 115, above.

[118]*Id.*, discussing New York law requiring existing blanket mortgages to be paid off in a condominium conversion.

[119]*See, generally, Housing & Development Reporter*, note 80, above, 25:0011.

[120]I.R.C. § 216(a).

[121]I.R.C. § 216(b)(3)(B).

complete or partial liquidation of the corporation, and (4) 80 percent or more of the gross income of which, for the taxable year in which the taxes and interest for which the deduction is sought are paid or incurred, is derived from tenant-stockholders.

However, in Revenue Ruling 62-177,[122] the cooperative *leased* a parcel of land in an existing apartment building for a period of 70 years. Although the estimated useful life of the building and improvements was substantially shorter than the term of the lease, the Internal Revenue Service held that because the lessor was benefiting from the building and improvements through rental payments, the cooperative lessee was not entitled to sole enjoyment of the entire worth of the building and improvements, and was not entitled to deduct real estate taxes. Accordingly, its residents also were not entitled to deduct taxes.

Revenue Ruling 62-178[123] dealt with similar facts, except that the cooperative lessee was directly liable on the loan procured to finance the construction of the building, and the lessor received no rental income from the building. The lessee, in that ruling, enjoyed the entire worth of the building, and the obligation to pay tax was that of the lessee and not the landlord. Consequently, the tenant stockholders were entitled to the deduction. On the other hand, taxes levied on recreational facilities owned and operated by an organization other than the cooperative could not be deducted by coop members.[124]

(2) Section 1034 Carryover

Another possible resident tax advantage of cooperative membership is the ability under Internal Revenue Code Section 1034 to defer recognition of gain when entering a coop after having sold a principal residence. The regulations indicate that "[p]roperty used by the taxpayer as his principal residence may include a houseboat, a house trailer, or stock held by a tenant-stockholder in a cooperative housing corporation."[125] Several Revenue Rulings have upheld the application of Section 1034 to the ownership of stock in cooperative housing.[126] In Revenue Ruling 60-76,[127] for example, the IRS noted that where the coop owner was obligated, under the terms of the lease, to pay his or her proportionate share of principal and interest payments on the lease, and where his or her stock interest was pledged as security on the note, the transaction was identical to a purchase of real property subject to an indebtedness, and the cost of the new residence for

---

[122] 1962-2 C.B. 89.

[123] 1962-2 C.B. 91.

[124] Rev. Rul. 69-76, 1969-1 C.B. 56.

[125] Treas. Reg. § 1.1034-1(c)(3)(i).

[126] *See, e.g.*, Rev. Ruls. 85-132, 1985-2 C.B. 182; 64-31, 1964-1 C.B. 300; 60-76, 1960-1 C.B. 296.

[127] 1960-1 C.B. 296.

purposes of the application of Section 1034 would include debt-financed portions of the purchase price.

(3) $125,000 Exclusion

The one-time exclusion of $125,000 of gain from the sale of a principal residence for persons over age 55[128] also applies to cooperative shares because the definition of principal residence is the same as that used in Section 1034.[129]

§ 7.3 MEMBERSHIPS

(a) Business Considerations

A few retirement facilities have been developed with a membership format similar to that employed by health clubs or country clubs. Rather than sell an interest in the real property of the retirement community, as condominium developers do, an intangible personal property membership is sold to the resident. The facility operator or developer retains ownership of the apartment unit or other real property. Unlike a cooperative, however, there is no share in a business interest. Instead, membership confers the right or license to use facilities and receive services.

Whenever the resident determines that he or she wishes to leave the facility, or in the event of death, the membership may be sold to a new resident who meets the age, financial, health status, and other prerequisites of admission to the facility. The selling member may reap a profit or suffer a loss upon the sale of the membership. The facility developer may be entitled to some share of any appreciation in the value of the membership upon its resale. This gives both developer and resident an economic incentive to ensure that there will be appreciation in the value of the membership, which should promote quality management of the facility, maintenance of the facilities, and cooperation in establishing a desirable place to live.

One of the advantages of the membership format is that, like the refundable entrance fee concept, it gives the resident an opportunity to recover some or all of his or her original investment in the retirement community. There is even an opportunity to make a profit. Of course, the down side of this equation is that the resident stands to lose money if the facility is a failure, or if for other reasons the value of the membership declines. The opportunity for profit and the risk of loss inherent in a membership structure may raise particular questions about whether the transaction constitutes a security under federal or state laws.[130]

[128]I.R.C. § 121.

[129]See Reg. § 1.121-3(a).

[130]See discussion at § 24, below.

(b) Taxation of Sales Proceeds

Several cases have considered whether membership fees should be considered income to the organization receiving them or a capital contribution.

In *Washington Athletic Club v. United States*,[131] a membership athletic club charged substantial initial fees plus monthly fees to members in return for a membership that could be terminated only by voluntary resignation, vote of the board of governors, or nonpayment of dues. No refund was available at termination of membership except in the event of dissolution of the club. Memberships could be transferred under limited circumstances upon payment of a transfer fee to the club. The club established a capital improvement fund and characterized membership fees deposited into it as capital contributions exempt from taxation. The court rejected the club's position, finding that the motivation of members was not to make a capital contribution, but to pay a fee that was a condition of entitlement to use the club's facilities.[132] The court found that, due to the absence of significant refund rights, there could be no significant, long-term investment motive.[133] Moreover, it distinguished cooperative cases where shareholders' payments are considered capital contributions because they amortize the cooperative's mortgage payments and increase the shareholders' equity.[134]

Although retirement facility memberships that can be resold by retirement facility residents for a profit have some of the characteristics of a capital investment, it is doubtful that such memberships will be treated as a capital contribution rather than as income.[135] The resident's primary purpose for retirement facility membership will most likely be for the privilege of receiving services and using the facilities of the retirement community, rather than for investment reasons. While the same may be said of stock cooperative housing associations, coop shareholders have an equity interest in the real property owner, voting rights and management control, and special opportunities to take pro rata deductions for real estate taxes and mortgage interest, which is distinguishable from the license type of interest typically extended to a club member.

Treatment of membership fees as income poses a problem for the proprietary facility operator in the form of a substantial tax obligation for fees received during the initial sell out of the project. Assuming that the membership sale does not involve the sale of an interest in the real property of

---

[131]614 F.2d 670 (9th Cir. 1980).

[132]*Id.*, at 675.

[133]*Id.*

[134]*Id.*, at 676, citing *Lake Forest, Inc.* 36 T.C. 510 (1961), *rvsd, other grounds*, 305 F.2d 814 (4th Cir. 1962), and *Eckstein v. U.S.*, 452 F.2d 1036, 1048 (Ct. Cl. 1971). In *Eckstein*, it was noted that cooperatives are viewed as pass-through organizations by the IRS, allowing shareholders to deduct mortgage interest expense and property taxes.

[135]*See, e.g., Affiliated Government Employees' Dist. Co. v. Commissioner*, 322 F.2d 872 (9th Cir. 1963), *cert. den.* 376 U.S. 950; *Oakland Hills Country Club*, 74 T.C. 35 (1980).

the retirement facility, the developer/owner will not be able to offset its cost basis in the property against membership fee income, which may therefore be taxable in full. As a result, membership structures so far generally have been used by nonprofit entities or in for profit/nonprofit joint ventures (see § 12.3).

(c)   Resident Tax Considerations

(1)   Imputed Interest

While the membership format contains some of the advantages of the refundable entrance fee from a consumer viewpoint, it should not be subject to the imputed interest concerns that face a retirement facility operator offering refundable fees. Because the transaction can be characterized as a sale, it should be distinguishable from loan transactions, even though the resident may have an opportunity to recoup all of the money originally expended as a condition of admission to the retirement facility. A key to preserving the characterization of the transaction as a sale, rather than a loan, is to ensure that the facility developer or operator has no obligation to repurchase the unit from the resident who wishes to sell a membership. If the facility owner or operator assumes such an obligation, its position appears indistinguishable from that of a borrower obligated to repay a loan on the happening of a condition, such as the lender's death or withdrawal from the facility.

(2)   Section 1034 Carryover

The membership format, as a transaction involving intangible personal property, is not as likely to hold for the resident the tax benefits inherent in the purchase of a real property interest in the retirement facility, such as the Section 1034 carryover of gain on sale of a principal residence.

However, memberships that can be resold by the retirement facility resident or his estate straddle the middle ground between conventional nonrefundable entrance fee arrangements, which have been found ineligible for Section 1034 benefits,[136] and real property ownership interests eligible for carrying over of gain.[137]

A nonrefundable entrance fee payment, which in the view of the Internal Revenue Service ensured the resident's future support rather than the purchase of an interest in the retirement facility property, has no residual value at the end of the contract term. Thus, there is nothing to resell, and no sales proceeds subject to taxation. On the other hand, a transferable membership can be structured as an interest that has significant residual value or even

---

[136] See § 6.1(c)(2).
[137] See §§ 7.1(d)(1) and 7.2(b)(2).

increased value even after all services are rendered to the resident. Upon its resale, there are likely to be proceeds subject to taxation, just as in the sale of a house, condo, or coop.

In a series of revenue rulings, however, the Internal Revenue Service has suggested that in order to take advantage of Section 1034, the taxpayer must have a legal interest in the property sold or acquired for such property to be considered an eligible residence. Thus, for example, a new home to which a taxpayer's daughter had title was not a "residence" to the taxpayer.[138] The IRS, referring to the predecessor of Section 1034 (Section 112), noted that the purpose of the section:

> Is to defer recognition of all or a part of the gain realized on the sale of the "old residence" to a future taxable event. This is accomplished under Section [1034 (c)] by deducting from the basis of the "new residence" the non-recognized gain realized from the sale of the "old residence," and using this adjusted basis in computing taxable gain, if any, upon the subsequent sale or exchange of the "new residence."

In that ruling, the taxpayer had reinvested the proceeds of the sale from the old home in a home in which she had no legal interest, but to which her daughter held title. Thus, in a subsequent sale, her daughter, rather than she, would be taxed on any gain realized from the sale of the new residence. Therefore, if Section 1034 were applicable, the mother would never pay tax.

While interpretive rulings have largely assumed that the taxpayer must own a fee simple interest in the real property to qualify for the carryover, the Code refers merely to sales of property used by the taxpayer as his principal residence.[139] It is clear from the rulings that the taxpayer, and no other, must have the salable interest in the residence, but whether that must be a fee interest in unclear. Stock cooperatives are the only kind of nonfee interest specifically mentioned as eligible for Section 1034 treatment, but other forms may be possible under the general statutory language. Because transferable memberships can function, for tax purposes, in almost the identical manner as a cooperative, they arguably may be entitled to Section 1034 benefits.

§ 8   RENTALS

§ 8.1   BUSINESS ISSUES

Rental retirement facilities have the advantages primarily of (1) being easy to understand and market in comparison to entrance fee structures, (2)

---

[138]Rev. Rul. 55-37, 1955-1 C.B. 347.

[139]I.R.C. § 1034(a). Note also that life estates receive certain favored tax treatment usually reserved for owners. See note 108, above.

requiring relatively small commitments of consumer capital, (3) being relatively easy for the consumer to leave, (4) having fewer problems of owner flexibility and control concerning program content or transferability of units, (5) generally not being subject to life care laws or securities registration, and (6) having HUD financing or loan insurance programs more readily available to them.

Among the disadvantages are (1) the absence of a long-term commitment by either party, which could result in the unavailability of shelter and health care or other services when most needed by the elderly resident, and greater fluctuations in occupancy levels for the owner, (2) inability of the developer to tap the home equity of seniors leaving single-family residences, and (3) the unavailability of resident tax benefits, such as tax and interest deductions, carryover of gain on the sale of a principal residence, and deductions for prepaid medical expenses.

Since the adoption of the Tax Reform Act of 1986, the once-favorable tax treatment given to residential rental housing investment is now absent. Nevertheless, rental retirement housing is still considered by some to have excellent investment potential.[140]

§ 8.2   TAX REFORM ACT OF 1986 CHANGES

(a)   Passive Loss Rules

Residential rental housing was one of the enterprises most dramatically affected by the Tax Reform Act of 1986.[141] Under the Act, losses of individuals and certain closely held corporations from "passive activities," which consist of any business in which the taxpayer "does not materially participate," may be deducted only to the extent income is received from other passive activities.[142] Thus, except for one circumstance described below, such losses cannot be offset against income from wages, investment portfolios, or active businesses, but must be carried into future years until they can be offset against passive income. Passive activities expressly include "any rental activity,"[143] which is further defined as activities "where payments are principally for the use of tangible property."[144]

There is also a limited exemption from the passive loss rules that applies only to persons who actively participate in rental real estate activities. If such persons have an adjusted gross income of $100,000 or less, they may offset nonpassive income with up to $25,000 of tax deductions or credits

---

[140]*See, e.g.*, Smith, "Syndication Topics: Rental Retirement Housing," 16 *Real Estate Rev.* 4 (Winter 1987),10.

[141]H.R. 3838, P.L. 99-514.

[142]*See, generally*, I.R.C. § 469.

[143]I.R.C. § 469(c)(2).

[144]I.R.C. § 469(j)(8).

from such active real estate interests.[145] However, the $25,000 exemption is reduced by 50 percent of every dollar of the taxpayer's adjusted gross income over $100,000, so that a person earning $150,000 or more receives no exemption.[146] If the tax credit for which exemption is sought is for certain low income housing projects,[147] the phaseout does not commence until the taxpayer's income exceeds $200,000.

These tedious rules raise some fundamental issues when applied to the retirement housing field. If rental retirement facilities have a sufficiently high proportion of services, for example, can they avoid the passive income rules altogether on the ground that payments are not "principally for tangible property," but for the services? Or does service component income need to be separated from rental income? The Senate Report notes that certain short-term rental activities with heavy user turnover and a significant service component (e.g., a hotel) should not be covered by the passive loss rules.[148] The Report also mentions, as another factor indicating an activity that should not be treated as a rental activity, circumstances where "the expenses of day-to-day operations are not insignificant in relation to rents produced by the property, or in relation to the amount of depreciation and the cost of carrying the rental property."[149]

Rental retirement facilities should not meet the short-term occupancy criterion that might exempt hotels, but they may qualify for an alternative exemption where daily operations expenses (e.g., staffing costs, food and medical supplies) are significant when compared to depreciation, debt service, taxes, insurance, and other costs related to pure real property ownership. Regulations have yet to be issued clarifying these matters, but it is anticipated that many rental retirement facilities should be able to avoid characterization as rental activities automatically subject to passive loss rules.

Nevertheless, even if not characterized as rental property (automatically considered passive), investors still must materially participate in the retirement facility activity in order to avoid general application of the passive loss rules.[150] This means that the taxpayer's involvement must be regular, continuous, and substantial.[151] Limited partnership interests are not to be considered material participation, except as the forthcoming regulations may specifically allow.

---

[145]I.R.C. § 469(i).

[146]I.R.C. § 469(i)(3)(A).

[147]*See* discussion below.

[148]*See, A Complete Guide to the Tax Reform Act of 1986*, (Englewood Cliffs; Prentice-Hall 1986), at 4075.

[149]*Id.*

[150]I.R.C. § 469(c)(1).

[151]I.R.C. § 469(h)(1).

(b) At-Risk Rules

At-risk rules limit the amount an individual or closely held corporation can deduct for a particular activity in any tax year, to the amount the taxpayer is at risk for the activity.[152] Prior to the 1986 Tax Reform Act, real property was exempt from the at-risk rules,[153] permitting real estate limited partners to take deductions in amounts greater than the total of their investment at risk in the enterprise.

The 1986 Act eliminates the real estate exemption, but adds a new rule that should neutralize the impact of the new law for most conventionally financed facilities.[154]

Under the current Code, the taxpayer's share of qualified nonrecourse financing for a project is considered at risk. Eligible financing is that borrowed with respect to holding real property, and that is made by a qualified person such as a bank or savings and loan, or is made or insured by a governmental entity, for which no person is individually liable, and that is not convertible.[155]

For retirement facilities with conventional nonrecourse loans, inclusion of the loaned amount as an amount at risk permits the investor to take a pro rata share deduction up to the project value, even though it was built or purchased with borrowed funds. However, if the property is seller financed, or financed directly via residential deposits and entrance fees, it is unlikely that the nonrecourse financing exception applies.[156]

(c) Conclusion

The at-risk and passive loss rules certainly establish some serious impediments to those seeking to use limited partnership syndications as tax shelters for investor's employment income or portfolio interest or dividends. However, if investors have other passive investment income against which to offset losses, or if the project does not generate significant losses but is entered into for economic value, or if investors participate in project operations, the new rules should cause little concern. Moreover, corporate investors are unaffected. Retirement facilities should be well suited to attracting investors seeking value rather than tax shelter.

---

[152]I.R.C. § 465(a)(1).

[153]Former I.R.C. § 465(c)(3)(D).

[154]See Holtz & Brecht, "Tax Reform Will Hit Retirement Housing," *Retirement Housing Rep.* 1, No. 1, (Sept. 1986), 12–15.

[155]I.R.C. § 465(b)(6).

[156]*See, generally,* Holtz & Brecht, note 154, above.

§ 8.3 LOW INCOME HOUSING TAX CREDIT

The 1986 Act adds Section 42 to the Internal Revenue Code to create a substantial tax credit for certain low income rental housing projects.

The credit for conventionally financed facilities placed in service in 1987 is in the amount of up to nine percent per year of the owner's qualified basis in the property for a period of 10 years, for new construction or for rehabilitation where the costs equal at least $2000 per unit.[157] The credit is designed to have a present value of 70 percent of the basis.[158]

For federally subsidized facilities financed with tax exempt bonds or below market federal loans, and for nonrehabilitated existing buildings in service more than 10 years, the credit is four percent per year, with an intended 30 percent present value.[159]

After 1987, the Treasury will set credit rates designed to reflect the 70 percent or 30 percent present values.[160] There is no credit for property placed in service after 1989.[161]

To qualify, a facility must require that 20 percent of its total units be occupied by persons with income of 50 percent or less of the area median income, or that 40 percent of the units be occupied by persons with 60 percent or less of median income.[162] In addition, units counted to qualify for the credit must be rent-restricted so that the gross rent charged each tenant is no more than 30 percent of the applicable 50 or 60 percent of median income limitation.[163] The 30 percent limit does not apply to Section 8 rental assistance payments.[164]

Qualified projects must commit to adhering to the eligibility criteria for a period of 15 years, or else the credits will be recaptured.[165]

Credits available to taxpayers in each state are limited to an aggregate sum equaling $1.25 per state resident, except for certain tax exempt bond financed projects. Taxpayers generally must apply to the designated state agency for credit approval, and states must reserve at least 10 percent of their credits for projects in which nonprofit organizations materially participate.[166]

Rental retirement facilities with services probably can qualify for the credit if compliance is financially feasible. Although nursing homes, hospitals,

---

[157]I.R.C. § 42(b)(1)(A), (e)(3), (f)(1).

[158]I.R.C. § 42(b)(2).

[159]I.R.C. § 42(b)(1)(B), (i)(2).

[160]I.R.C. § 42(b)(2)(B).

[161]I.R.C. § 42(n).

[162]I.R.C. § 42(g)(1).

[163]I.R.C. § 42(g)(2).

[164]*Id.*

[165]I.R.C. § 42(i)–(j).

[166]I.R.C. § 42(h)(5).

hotels, and trailer parks do not qualify, related facilities can be covered where their purpose is subordinate to the provision of residential rental units.[167] However, each unit must have full facilities for "living, sleeping, eating, cooking, and sanitation."[168]

Meeting the tenant income and rent restriction criteria can be difficult without use of the Section 8 rent subsidy. Except for existing projects with subsidies in place, this is a relatively scarce benefit.[169] However, fees for services such as meals, recreational programs, or health care probably can be charged to tenants without regard to the 30 percent limit on rents, assuming that separate service fees are not considered rent.[170]

---

[167] See Senate Report, reported at CCH, *Standard Federal Tax Reports*, at 11,286.

[168] *Id.*

[169] See discussion at § 22.3(b), below.

[170] See discussion of this issue at § 22.5(d), below.

Four

Tax Exempt Operation

§ 9 FEDERAL TAX EXEMPTION

Tax exempt organizations have been responsible over the years for the bulk of development in the retirement housing field, especially in the more heavily service-oriented end of the spectrum (see § 2.3). These facilities are largely owned by or affiliated with religious and fraternal organizations that qualify for exemption as public charities under Section 501(c)(3) of the Internal Revenue Code. Often, such organizations engage in a wide variety of activities that are charitable in nature and recognized as tax exempt activities, such as furnishing health care in hospitals or nursing facilities. Generally speaking, however, the mere fact that such a tax exempt organization may own and operate housing for the elderly does not make the ownership and operation of that housing a tax exempt activity, and income may be subject to taxation.

Historically, merely providing market rate elderly housing, without care and services, has not been considered a tax exempt activity, even if the owner or operator is already a tax exempt charitable organization. While there may be a tax exemption available when such housing is offered on a charitable basis or at below-market rates (see discussion in § 9.3), operation of market rate housing for the elderly, in and of itself, does not justify a tax exemption. Even such housing composed of low- and moderate-income units is not necessarily eligible for tax exemption.

However, if a retirement facility follows certain specific guidelines set forth by the Internal Revenue Service, even a luxury facility designed for the wealthy elderly may qualify for exemption from income tax under Section 501(c)(3) of the Code.

§ 9.1   BASIC TESTS FOR TAX EXEMPTION

While Section 501(c) of the Internal Revenue Code sets forth numerous specific exemptions for various types of organizations, Section 501(c)(3), dealing generally with charitable organizations, is most relevant for those contemplating development of a retirement facility. That section provides a basis for exemption for:

> Corporations, and any community chest, fund, or foundation, *organized and operated exclusively* for religious, *charitable,* scientific, testing for public safety, literary, or educational purposes, or to foster national or international amateur sports competition (but only if no part of its activities involve the provision of athletic facilities or equipment), or for the prevention of cruelty to children or animals, *no part of the net earnings of which inures to the benefit of any private shareholder or individual,* no substantial part of the activities of which is carrying on propaganda, or otherwise attempting, to influence legislation (except as otherwise provided in subsection (h)), and which does not participate in, or intervene in (including the publishing or distributing of statements), any political campaign on behalf of any candidate for public office. (Emphasis added).

(a)   Organizational

To qualify as an exempt charitable organization under Section 501(c)(3), a corporation must be both organized and operated exclusively for a charitable purpose. The regulations explain that, to meet the organizational test, the corporate articles must (1) limit the purposes of the organization to one or more exempt, charitable purposes, and (2) not empower it to engage, except to an insubstantial extent, in activities that do not further an exempt purpose.[1] The term *charitable* is used in its generally accepted legal sense, and may include:

> [r]elief of the poor and distressed* or of the underprivileged; *advancement of religion;* advancement of education or science; erection or maintenance of public buildings, monuments, or works; *lessening of the burdens of Government;* and *promotion of social welfare* by organizations designed to accomplish any of the above purposes, or (i) *to lessen neighborhood tensions;* (ii) *to eliminate prejudice and discrimination;* (iii) to defend human and civil rights secured by law; or (iv) *to combat community deterioration* and juvenile delinquency. [Reg. § 1.501(c)(3)–1(d)(2); (emphasis added.)]

Retirement facilities may fit under one or more of the examples of charity, as is discussed more fully in the following sections.

In addition, the organization must be structured so that it is not expressly empowered to participate in any political campaign for a candidate,

---

[1]Reg. § 1.501(c)(3)-1(b)(1).

or devote more than an insubstantial part of its activities to attempting to influence legislation.[2] A third major criterion of the organizational test is that the organization's assets must be dedicated to an exempt purpose, so that on dissolution, for example, they would go to another 501(c)(3) exempt organization or the government.[3]

(b) Operational

The operational test requires the exempt organization to engage primarily in activities that will accomplish the exempt purposes, provided that no more than an insubstantial portion of the activities can be other than in further-ance of the exempt purpose.[4] This apparently confusing test seems even less intelligible in light of the statute's requirement that operations be exclusively for charitable purposes. However, it is important to note that the Code looks to the exclusivity of the charitable *purpose*, and not to whether the organiza-tion's *activities* are exclusively charitable.[5] Therefore, under the statutory language, it is possible for an organization with a purely charitable purpose to engage in activities that, standing alone, are not charitable endeavors, but that are performed by the exempt organization solely to further its charitable purpose. The regulations further expand this distinction by requiring only a primary devotion to charitable *activities*, yet an all-but-insubstantial part of the total activities must be in furtherance of charitable *purposes*. This dis-tinction may be of significance in analysis of retirement projects containing mixed uses, such as low and moderate income units (see § 9.4).

The second principal aspect of the operational analysis is called the pri-vate inurement test, which requires that no part of the *net* earnings of the organization benefit private shareholders or individuals.[6] This requirement can have particular significance for retirement facility joint ventures or con-tract relationships involving taxable and nonprofit entities (see §§ 12.1(b), 12.1(d)).

§ 9.2 HOME FOR THE AGING TAX EXEMPTION

(a) Revenue Ruling 72-124

In 1972, the Internal Revenue Service issued a landmark revenue ruling for the retirement housing industry. Revenue Ruling 72-124[7] considered the

---

[2]Reg. § 1.501(c)(3)-1(b)(3).

[3]Reg. § 1.501(c)(3)-1(b)(4).

[4]Reg. § 1.501(c)(3)-1(c)(1).

[5]*See* Hopkins, B. *The Law of Tax Exempt Organizations*, 4th ed. (Wiley, 1983), 201–208, for a good discussion of this distinction.

[6]Reg. § 1.501(c)(3)-1(c)(2).

[7]1972-1 C.B. 145.

application for exemption of a church-sponsored home providing housing and medical care for persons over 65. Rather than serving poor persons, the home admitted only those who were able to pay the entrance fees and monthly fees charged by the facility. However, net earnings were used to provide services, and a limited amount was set aside as reserves for expansion or unforeseen expenses. Most importantly, the home had a policy of maintaining in residence any person who subsequently became unable to pay the monthly charges.

The IRS distinguished prior rulings that had based exemptions on below-cost charitable services[8] and concluded that the elderly experienced forms of nonfinancial distress that could be alleviated by means other than providing free or below-cost services. Citing to the Older Americans Act of 1965,[9] the ruling declared that the need for housing, physical and mental health care, civic, cultural, and recreational activities, and for an overall environment conducive to dignity and independence, were also causes of elderly distress. The ruling concluded that a home for the aging qualifies for charitable tax exempt status if operated in a manner designed to satisfy three primary needs of retired persons: the need for housing, health care, and financial security.

(1) Housing Element

Under Revenue Ruling 72-124, residential facilities must be provided that are specially designed for the elderly and that meet some combination of their physical, emotional, recreational, social, religious, and similar needs. Revenue Ruling 79-18[10] later interpreted this standard to have been met where apartment units were constructed with fire-resistant materials and equipped with such amenities as indoor and outdoor recreation areas, skid-resistant floors, ramps, grab bars, wide doorways, 24-hour emergency call systems, and similar features. Presumably, a structure designed for general public use could not qualify under this test without some remodeling or special accommodation for particular elderly needs.

The housing element of a retirement facility is clearly provided when the owner or operator of a continuing care facility makes a residence available to the elderly person on a rental or life lease basis, as was the case in the home for the aged being considered in Revenue Ruling 72-124. However, it is unclear from a reading of that ruling whether a facility in which residents purchase their units in fee simple meets the housing element of the IRS's three-prong test. The concern is that by turning ownership of the housing over to a resident, the facility developer and operator are arguably no longer providing the housing when that resident at some later date resells

[8] See § 9.3, below.
[9] 42 U.S.C. § 3001.
[10] 1979-1 C.B. 194.

the unit to another person. Moreover, a recent IRS General Counsel's Memorandum has concluded that the financial security requirement of Revenue Ruling 72-124 was not met by a facility selling condominium units in a life care facility (see § 9.2(b)(3)).

Another situation that may pose a problem in meeting the housing test arises where the resident more clearly provides his or her own housing. For example, if a developer establishes a mobile home park for the elderly, with health care and other services available on the premises, but the residents supply their own mobile home units on land leased from the developer, it is doubtful that the arrangement would meet the provision of housing requirement of Revenue Ruling 72-124. Similarly, if a management company goes into an existing senior housing development, where residents already own their own homes, and begins to offer health care and service programs to those residents, there is a substantial question as to whether the arrangement will meet the housing test.

In most circumstances, however, the housing element is probably the easiest of the three tests set forth in Revenue Ruling 72-124.

(2)   Health Care Element

The second prong of Revenue Ruling 72-124 requires that a retirement facility must directly provide "some form of health care, or in the alternative, maintain some continuing arrangement with other organizations, facilities, or health personnel, designed to maintain the physical, and if necessary, mental well-being of its residents."

Many retirement facilities directly provide skilled nursing or other health care to residents in facilities owned and operated by the organization supplying housing. However, it is sufficient for the facility to help its residents access health care in the community by means of establishing ongoing transfer agreements, or other preferred relationships, with hospitals or other related health care facilities already existing in the community. It also appears that an arrangement with a health maintenance organization or other form of prepaid plan for health care should qualify.

In Revenue Ruling 79-18, a senior housing facility's provision of 24-hour nonmedical emergency aid and referral, plus transportation for medical examinations and treatment, were enough to satisfy the test. Some facilities specifically exclude provision of mental health care from coverage under their health plans, but this runs afoul of the literal language of Revenue Ruling 72-124. (See contract examples in § 28.5.)

An unanswered question in the interpretation of Revenue Ruling 72-124 concerns application of the health care test to long-term care insurance or other forms of health insurance.[11] If, for example, a facility operator obtains a group insurance policy with special provisions, coverages, and

---

[11] *See* § 27.2, below, for a discussion of long-term care insurance.

premiums geared to the particular needs of the individual retirement facility's population, and arranges for premium payments as a part of the regular monthly fee, that developer is truly assisting the resident population in obtaining access to health care in a way that a mere health facility transfer agreement could not accomplish. Although an insurance policy is not an arrangement with a direct provider of health services, the insurer often has arrangements with preferred providers of health services. Thus, the establishment of a group health insurance policy should qualify as a "continuous arrangement . . . designed to maintain the physical and . . . mental well-being of the residents." While the specific facts of Revenue Ruling 72-124 and its progeny have not dealt with the question of long-term care insurance or the provision of similar benefits, the IRS should consider such services to satisfy the health care element of the home for the aging exemption, in that they can serve the specific health care needs of the elderly at least as well as other methods already approved by the IRS.

(3) Financial Security Element

To qualify for the home for the aging tax exemption, a facility must provide for the financial security needs of its elderly residents. The financial security test may be met by (1) having a policy that permits residents to remain at the facility, even though they may run out of funds, and (2) operating the facility at the lowest feasible cost.

(A) No-Eviction Policy

The first aspect of the financial security test of Revenue Ruling 72-124 requires that facilities have a policy that permits residents who run out of funds or otherwise become unable to pay their charges to remain at the facility.[12] The policy may be accomplished by drawing upon reserve funds, contributions, federal or state assistance payments, or other sources. Revenue Ruling 79-18 amplifies slightly upon this rule by approving a plan that would retain residents unable to pay, but only to the extent the facility was able to do so. A facility need not place itself in financial jeopardy in order to adhere to its no-eviction policy.[13] The no-eviction policy may be informal, and need not be set forth in the resident contract.[14] Of course, those who are able but refuse to pay or to abide by reasonable rules governing residence should be subject to eviction without jeopardizing the exempt status.

One exception to the no-eviction policy standard of Revenue Ruling 72-124 is for "an organization that is *required* by reason of Federal or state

[12]*See also* Priv. Ltr. Rul. 8022085. Note that private letter rulings are not to be relied on as precedent.

[13]*See* Priv. Ltr. Rul. 8405083.

[14]Rev. Rul. 72-124, above.

conditions imposed with respect to the terms of its financing agreements to devote its facilities to housing *only aged persons of low or moderate income* not exceeding specified levels *and* to recover operating costs from such residents." (Emphasis added.)

The ruling then cites section 236 of the National Housing Act[15] as an example of a financing program with such requirements. Unfortunately, Section 236 financing is unavailable today, and other federal housing programs for the elderly currently in vogue, such as 221(d) and 232, do not limit admissions solely to low and moderate income elderly persons. The exception is probably still applicable to Section 202/Section 8 elderly housing projects, for which limited federal funds are still available (see discussion in §§ 22.1–22.4).

(B) Operation at Lowest Feasible Cost

Revenue Ruling 72-124 requires that the facility operate at the lowest feasible cost. However, this criterion does not require that the facility operator generate no excess income over expenditures. In fact, facilities are permitted to set aside reserve funds for the payment of indebtedness, for subsidization of residents unable to pay, for future contingencies and expenditures, and for expansion or improvement of the services or facility.[16]

One situation that may create problems in meeting the lowest feasible cost test can occur when a charitable organization in another business, such as the operation of a hospital, establishes a retirement community as an expected profit center for the hospital. For example, a nonprofit hospital looking to expand its revenue base may desire to set up a nonprofit subsidiary to operate a retirement facility on land adjacent to the hospital. Normally, a nonprofit subsidiary could donate any net income to the nonprofit parent without jeopardizing the subsidiary's exempt status. However, if a retirement facility corporation, exempted from taxation pursuant to Revenue Ruling 72-124, were simply to make an unrestricted gift of surplus funds to a parent hospital corporation, such an action would arguably run afoul of the operation at lowest feasible cost criterion. However, the retirement facility could use surplus funds to improve services to its residents and perhaps to expand even the hospital's health services or facilities that are devoted to the residents of the retirement facility.

Revenue Ruling 72-124 provides further that if there is doubt that the facility operates at the lowest feasible cost, the fact that it makes some units available at less than its usual charges for persons of more limited means constitutes additional evidence of meeting the test. The amount of entrance fees or monthly fees charged to residents is not per se determinative of whether the

---

[15] 12 U.S.C. § 1715z-1.

[16] *See* Rev. Ruls. 72-124, 79-18. However, *see Onderdonk v. Presbyterian Homes of New Jersey,* 85 N.J. 171, 425 A.2d 1057 (1981), which held that a life care provider could not base residents' fee increases on expenses incurred in the defendants' other operations.

lowest feasible cost test is met. (See Revenue Ruling 64-231,[17] which provides that, for purposes of determining if a retirement facility's fees are below cost, entrance fees are to be amortized over the expected lives of each resident.)

(b)   Practical Methods of Coping with Revenue Ruling 72-124

Revenue Ruling 72-124, and particularly its no-eviction policy, seems so restrictive that one may think that only traditional charities, with a substantial base of endowments or contributions, can as a practical matter qualify for the exemption and embark on development of a facility. On the contrary, many such facilities are self-starting, self-sustaining, and may eventually generate enough revenue to fund development of additional projects.

(1)   Building Luxury Projects

Many nonprofit facilities that qualify for the home for the aging exemption can be and are structured as luxury retirement facilities. Nothing in Revenue Ruling 72-124 requires that nonprofit tax exempt facilities be made available to the elderly residents at below-market rates, or that lower or middle income residents be targeted to occupy the facility. Provided that such facilities meet the housing, health care, and financial security needs of the elderly residents they serve, tax exempt retirement facilities may cater to middle and upper income clientele and provide the finest of services and accommodations. Facilities can even make some services available to the general public without treatment of the income as unrelated business taxable income.[18]

(2)   Financial and Health Screening

For retirement facilities that are tax exempt and yet operate on a market rate basis, a significant concern is whether residents will run out of funds, thus obligating the facility to provide for their food, shelter, and medical care for life without compensation. A further concern is that a person may come into the facility who is suffering, or is likely to suffer, a protracted, serious illness shortly after admission to the facility that will substantially deplete reserves.

To help reduce the risk of such large financial drains upon the facility's operations, most providers require residents to undergo a thorough financial and health status screening prior to their acceptance as residents. Financial screenings usually require a listing of all assets as well as a statement of retirement income. Usually, a review of tax returns will be warranted. In

[17] 1964-2 C.B. 139.
[18] Priv. Ltr. Rul. 8030105.

addition to a health questionnaire completed by the resident, most facilities require a physical examination and report from the applicant's physician. While these measures do not eliminate the risk of resident insolvency or illness, they help screen out the worst-case applicants. Most resident agreements provide that any misstatement in the financial or health questionnaire is ground for automatic termination of the contract and dismissal. (See § 28.11 for forms of such contract provisions.)

(3)   Maintaining Control over the Premises

Generally, the facilities meeting the no-eviction test of Revenue Ruling 72-124 are continuing care or life care facilities, which are designed to care for all residents for life, and utilize entrance fees to help fund reserves for those who become unable to pay fees. However, monthly rental facilities may also be structured to meet the criterion if rents are set high enough to create a reserve, or if reserves are available from contributions or are set aside from borrowed funds. In both cases, the facility does not relinquish title to, or control over, the property to be occupied by the resident.

However, the IRS found in at least one case that retirement facility units offered to residents on a fee simple ownership basis could not qualify for exemption under Revenue Ruling 72-124. In a 1985 General Counsel Memorandum,[19] the requirements of Revenue Ruling 72-124 were analyzed in connection with a life care facility where residents purchased residential units as condominiums, but were also required to purchase a full program of lifetime medical care, meals, housekeeping, recreational and social programs, and related life care services for an initial payment plus a monthly fee. Membership in the program was limited to those who met the nonprofit operator's admissions criteria, and the organization retained a right of first refusal respecting any proposed resale of a unit. The organization had a policy of maintaining in residence those who became financially unable to pay ongoing charges. Sales of some of the units were financed via loans from third party lenders, secured by mortgages on the units.

The IRS General Counsel observed that where the housing was sold to residents, the endowment and monthly fees paid to the nonprofit operator for lifetime services could not guarantee the resident a continued right to housing. If the resident were to default on a loan secured by the condominium, the nonprofit operator would be powerless to prevent foreclosure and keep the resident in the community. Therefore the General Counsel concluded that the no-eviction facet of the financial security test articulated in Revenue Ruling 72-124 could not be met.

A further issue raised by the IRS was that a fee simple sale would conflict with a community accessibility requirement, on the ground that, once the organization sold a unit, it lost control over the pricing of the unit upon

---

[19]GCM 38478, Aug. 6, 1985.

resale by the resident. The General Counsel's concern, however, was not that the resale price might rise, but that the organization would lose control over access to the community. The reference to a community accessibility requirement appears to be a reference to dictum in Revenue Ruling 79-18 that the project there in question set rental charges at a level "within the financial reach of a significant segment of the community's elderly persons." No such requirement is discernible in Revenue Ruling 72-124, however, and a community accessibility requirement does not definitively appear to be a prerequisite to exemption.

General Counsel Memorandum 38478 does not seem to pose insurmountable difficulties for a facility seeking to sell units to residents and still qualify for the home for the aged exemption. The concerns raised in the GCM could be met by leaving in the hands of the nonprofit organization control over facility access, and over any encumbrances upon the resident's title. Thus, for example, deed restrictions could require only cash sales, or permit financing only by the organization or a controlled entity. In addition, all buyers of units would have to be prequalified for residence by the organization.

Finally, membership structures, or stock cooperatives,[20] which give the operating organization more control over resales, would probably not violate the provisions of GCM 38478, provided there is no independent, third party financing.

(4)   Prohibitions against Private Pay Agreements

Many facilities across the country, including nursing facilities, have sought to obtain the agreement of an elderly person's family to guarantee payment of the charges incurred in caring for the relative residing in the facility. While it is often the case that elderly persons being considered for admission may be closer to financial dependency than their sons or daughters, and the children are quite willing to execute such a guarantee, such circumstances must be handled with extreme caution.

The Social Security Act fraud and abuse provisions prohibit any facility that provides services under the Medicaid program from requiring, as a condition of a Medicaid-eligible patient's admission or continued stay in the facility, any payment for covered services that is supplemental to that paid by the Medicaid program. Violation of this requirement is a federal felony that carries with it substantial criminal sanctions of fines and imprisonment.

Section 1909(d) of the Social Security Act[21] provides:

(d) Whoever knowingly and willfully—

---

[20]See §§ 7.2 and 7.3, above.
[21]42 U.S.C. § 1396h(d).

(1) charges, for any services provided to a patient under a state plan approved under this subchapter, money or other consideration at a rate in excess of the rates established by the state, or

(2) charges, solicits, accepts, or receives, in addition to any amount otherwise required to be paid under a state plan approved under this subchapter, any gift, money, donation, or other consideration (other than a charitable, religious or philanthropic contribution from an organization or from a person unrelated to the patient) (A) as a precondition of admitting a patient to a hospital, skilled nursing facility, or intermediate care facility, or (B) as a requirement for the patient's continued stay in such a facility, when the cost of the services provided therein to the patient is paid for (in whole or in part) under the state plan, shall be guilty of a felony and upon conviction thereof shall be fined not more than $25,000 or imprisoned for not more than five years, or both.

An obvious violation would occur when a facility approaches the relative of a patient who is receiving assistance for skilled nursing services under the Medicaid program and requires that the relative pay the difference between the Medicaid rate and the facility's usual charges for care, under threat that the facility will otherwise discharge the patient. The Social Security Act obligates the facility to accept the Medicaid payment as payment in full for the nursing services.

While this obvious kind of abuse can be easily avoided by a facility operator, a more subtle problem can arise under the statute. For example, if a person seeking admission into a retirement facility is not yet eligible for the Medicaid program, but it appears that in the next several years the person's assets might be depleted substantially, the facility operator might approach a son or daughter and obtain that person's agreement to pay the resident's charges for the duration of her stay at the facility (a private pay agreement). At the time such an agreement is entered into, it probably does not violate at least the letter of the Social Security Act, because the resident is not yet eligible for the Medicaid program. However, when the elderly resident does run out of funds several years later, and seeks a determination of eligibility under the Medicaid program, it is possible that the relative's agreement will not be considered an asset of the resident, and the resident will be eligible to enroll in the Medicaid program. At that point, if the facility seeks to enforce the private pay agreement as a condition of the resident's continued stay at the facility, that conduct could very well constitute a felony violation of the fraud and abuse statute.

There is a question as to whether the facility could lawfully seek to enforce the agreement against the resident's relative, without threatening eviction of the Medicaid enrollee residing at the facility. Technically, such a practice may be permitted by the literal language of the fraud and abuse statute, but providers in this circumstance should exercise extreme caution and consult legal counsel.

Several other opinions have held that nursing facilities cannot require that patients seeking admission, or their relatives, enter into private pay agreements as a condition of admission, even though the applicant is not yet eligible for Medicaid benefits and without regard to whether discharge was threatened. In *Glengariff Corporation v. Snook*,[22] a nursing home that required the son of an applicant for admission to sign a contract agreeing to pay the full private room rate for a specified period of years was found to have violated Congressional intent underlying the fraud and abuse amendments to the Social Security Act. In that case, the patient was able to apply for and be determined eligible for Medicaid even though the son had previously signed the private pay agreement. The court determined that as soon as the patient became eligible for Medicaid, the private pay agreement became unenforceable under the terms of the fraud and abuse amendments.

In Maryland, the state Department of Health and Mental Hygiene determined that, under the federal fraud and abuse provisions, nursing homes could not require private pay agreements as a condition of admission of *any* person.[23] It further found that such an agreement would conflict with the patient's bill of rights, which is applicable to all patients in Medicaid certified nursing homes, regardless of private or public pay status.[24] Finally, the Maryland decision concluded that the continued use of private pay agreements would amount to a deceptive and misleading practice under federal law in that the patient was likely to be unaware that the clause is unenforceable.

In Wisconsin, the Attorney General issued an opinion that likewise found that private pay agreements obtained prior to the patient becoming eligible for Medicaid violated federal law and applicable state laws, both civil and criminal.[25]

In an opinion dated May 28, 1986, the Rhode Island Attorney General determined that a nursing home may not require Medicaid eligible individuals or their families to sign private pay agreements or to show ability to pay the private rate for a period of time prior to any conversion to Medicaid. The opinion found that any state laws that appeared to authorize such private pay agreements were void pursuant to the supremacy clause of the U.S. Constitution, and further found that the practice violates federal criminal law and state laws prohibiting fraud.[26]

It is clear that private pay agreements with relatives become unenforceable when the patient becomes Medicaid eligible. While some states have

---

[22] 93 A.D.2d 900, 122 Misc. 2d 784 (N.Y.S. Ct. 1984).

[23] *Matter of Summit Nursing Home* (1984), C.C.H., *Medicare and Medicaid Guide*, ¶ 33,977.

[24] 42 C.F.R. § 405.1121(k).

[25] OAG 4-86, March 7, 1986; C.C.H. *Medicare and Medicaid Guide*, ¶ 35,317. *See also*, Ohio Attorney General Opinion No. 85-063, Sept. 24, 1985 (C.C.H. *Medicare and Medicaid Guide*, ¶ 34,988).

[26] C.C.H., note 23 above, ¶ 35,441.

made general pronouncements against all agreements with relatives, it is not clear that agreements with relatives are unlawful when the patient is not Medicaid eligible.

A strategy for facilities seeking to ensure that a resident will be able to pay the full charges for the duration of his or her stay at the facility is to attempt to ensure that the elderly resident will never become eligible for the Medicaid program. A way to do this, assuming there is a relative with sufficient finances to tap, is to have the relative give money to the applicant for residence, place it in trust, or purchase an annuity, so that the elderly applicant will have legal or beneficial title to the funds. At least one state prohibits requiring a financially responsible cosigner or payment of a security deposit as a condition of admission of a Medicaid-eligible patient, but the statute does not apply, on its face, to such practices before the patient becomes eligible.[27]

Each state's Medicaid eligibility criteria and nursing home licensure standards differ, and a provider should consult counsel to determine what lawful methods will help prevent the elderly applicant for facility admission from running out of funds and becoming dependent upon the Medicaid program.

(5) Endowment Funds

Many nonprofit facilities establish endowment funds geared primarily to solicitation of contributions from facility residents. Most residents of retirement facilities feel that they are part of a community of friends and neighbors with whom they share a strong attachment. A facility with such an atmosphere is a natural object of bequests in residents' wills. Such endowment funds may be used to care for those who may run out of funds, or to improve or expand facilities and services in the retirement community. Although one must be careful to avoid the problems of the fraud and abuse statute discussed above, relatives of residents may also be good prospects for contributions to an endowment fund. (See § 9.11 regarding the tax deductibility of contributions.)

(6) Charity Services

Many facilities comply with Revenue Ruling 72-124 by providing free or below-cost services to a substantial number of residents within the facility. Facilities that serve the middle and upper income population, however, tend to require that all residents pay market rate fees, except in the rare case when a resident runs out of funds. These facilities have found it prudent, however, to engage in certain charity services that may be directed to the outside community. An example is "Meals on Wheels" served to the

---

[27] *See* 1986 California Statutes Ch. 1073, adding Welf. & Inst. C. §§ 14110.8 and 14110.9.

elderly urban poor from the facility's kitchens. Such services provided in connection with a market-rate luxury facility may also be helpful in preserving tax exemption benefits under state laws.

(7) Transfer to Related Facilities

As noted above, the facility's required policy of keeping residents who run out of funds need not be absolute, but must be enforced only to the extent of the financial ability of the sponsor.

One interesting application of this exception is discussed in IRS Private Letter Ruling 8117221. There, the organization planned to maintain in their apartment units residents who could not continue to afford monthly fees, but only for so long as contingency funds and public contributions permitted. When funds ran out, the facility planned to transfer residents who could not pay to the organization's adjacent nursing facility, and in no event would they be turned out of that location. The IRS found that the plan constituted a sufficient commitment to keep in residence those who become unable to pay, and qualified for exemption.

By transferring a destitute resident to a controlled nursing facility, the exempt organization at least can take advantage of Medicaid reimbursement, which is not available for living in an apartment setting.[28] Of course, the placement should be medically appropriate and not motivated solely by financial considerations, as was implied in the facts of Letter Ruling 8117221.

§ 9.3   HOMES OPERATED AT LESS THAN COST

When Revenue Ruling 72-124 was issued, it departed from precedential rulings that confined the privilege of tax exempt status to retirement facilities providing services at substantially below their actual cost. These earlier rulings continue to represent an alternative route to exemption.

Revenue Ruling 61-72[29] considered whether a retirement facility that did *not* provide free care, and that did *not* reduce the charges of those who became unable to pay, could qualify for exemption. The organization offered care and assistance, as well as food and shelter, to its residents, and sought to serve elderly persons without the financial means to adequately care for themselves without hardship. It screened applicants to determine that they would be able to pay the charges, but charges were set at a level that resulted in operational expenses 35 percent higher than resident revenues. The deficit was made up with gifts and contributions.

Relying upon rulings relating to hospital services, the Internal Revenue Service determined that free services were not necessary, and found the organization to be making a gift to a charitable class where (1) it is dedicated to, and does furnish care and housing to the aged who would otherwise be

---

[28]See § 26.1(c), below, for a general discussion of Medicaid coverage.
[29]1961-1 C.B. 188.

unable to provide it for themselves without hardship; (2) it renders such services to all or a reasonable proportion of the residents below cost, to the extent it is financially able; and (3) the services are of a type that minister to the needs and relief of distress of the aged.[30]

Three years later, in Revenue Ruling 64-231,[31] the IRS considered an argument that retirement home entrance or membership fees should not be considered in determining whether fees are set below cost. The rationale advanced by the home was that the entrance fee constitutes a capital contribution, as distinguished from the costs of care. The IRS noted, however, that the payments were prerequisites to obtaining services at the facility, gave no ownership interest to residents, and were partially refundable in the event of contract cancelation. Therefore, they could not be considered a capital contribution, but must be included in the determination of whether services were being rendered at a level below actual cost. In calculating the relationship of fees to costs, entrance fees are to be amortized over the actuarial life expectancies of each of the residents, using annuity tables appearing in federal regulations.

These rulings leave open the question of whether the capital contribution distinction can have validity under appropriate circumstances. For example, it seems possible that an arrangement involving the fee simple sale of a housing unit, plus the provision of below-cost services, could qualify for exemption under Revenue Rulings 61-72 and 64-231. This is of particular interest because of the difficulty the IRS has with the concept of a fee simple sale qualifying for exemption under the more modern home for the aging criteria of Revenue Ruling 72-124 (see § 9.2(b)(3)).

§ 9.4 LOW AND MODERATE INCOME HOUSING

While the provision of low and moderate income housing for the elderly is commonly thought of as a tax exempt charitable activity, the availability of a broad exemption for such projects is unclear, and relevant IRS pronouncements do not disclose a single, unifying path to tax exemption. Low income housing is not automatically charitable. Where a low income project gave admission preferences to employees of a particular proprietary organization, exemption was denied on the basis that a private, rather than public, interest was served.[32] It should be noted that low and moderate income housing units are not necessarily, nor commonly, offered at below-cost rates, nor are residents who run out of funds and fail to pay rent usually permitted to stay. This class of facility is therefore analyzed with the assumption that it does not meet the criteria set forth in Revenue Rulings 72-124 (see § 9.2), or 61-72 (see § 9.3).

---

[30]*See also* Priv. Ltr. Rul. 7916068.
[31]1964-2 C.B. 139.
[32]Rev. Rul. 72-147, 1972-1 C.B. 147.

(a) Revenue Ruling 70-585

Revenue Ruling 70-585[33] sets the tone for consideration of tax exempt status of low and moderate income housing projects. In it, the Internal Revenue Service reviews the Treasury Regulation[34] that defines *charitable* to include relief of the poor and distressed or of the underprivileged, and the promotion of social welfare by organizations designed to lessen neighborhood tensions, to eliminate prejudice and discrimination, or to combat community deterioration. The Ruling then sets forth four illustrative scenarios and examines the charitability of each circumstance.

In the first example, new and renovated homes are sold to *low* income families who qualify for loans under a federal housing program. The organization also provides financial aid to those unable to assemble the down payment. The organization seeking exemption is funded through federal loans and public contributions.

The second hypothetical involves the sale of new units to *low and moderate* income persons with preference given to racial and ethnic minority groups previously located in ghetto areas.

Situation three concerns an organization planning to rehabilitate a deteriorated area and rent apartment units at cost to *low and moderate* income families, with preference given to those already living in the area.

The last circumstance involves the rental of housing, at cost, to *moderate* income families, in a community where there is a shortage of affordable housing. Federal and state funds, and public contributions, finance the project.

According to the Ruling, the first three situations result in a tax exemption because, respectively, they (1) relieve the burdens of the low income poor, (2) help eliminate prejudice and discrimination and lessen neighborhood tensions, and (3) combat community deterioration. It is not clear from the Ruling whether moderate income facilities meeting the social welfare test of the Regulation must, for example, rent at cost, or duplicate other factors set forth in the examples.

The fourth project is not eligible for exemption because, even by serving moderate income persons in need, it does not cater to the poor or serve the specific kinds of community social welfare purposes articulated in the Regulation.

What is clear from Revenue Ruling 70-585 is that (1) the fact that the organization qualifies for federal or state funding for housing programs does not make the activity tax exempt; (2) what constitutes service to the low income (poor and distressed) population is to be determined on an individual case basis; (3) moderate income housing is charitable if combined with low income housing *and* if a social welfare purpose, such as

---

[33] 1970-2 C.B. 585.
[34] Reg. § 1.501(c)(3)-1(d)(2).

elimination of neighborhood tension, prejudice, or community deterioration, is met; and (4) not for profit provision of affordable moderate income housing that is needed and may be otherwise unavailable through private sector initiative is not a charitable activity.

Thus, a demonstration program designed to aid low income families living in deteriorating neighborhoods, by studying the feasibility of housing rehabilitation, was deemed to serve a charitable purpose.[35] Similarly, provision of interest free loans to low income homeowners for the purpose of rehabilitation of a deteriorated neighborhood is charitable.[36] (But see Revenue Ruling 77-3,[37] which held that an organization leasing housing to a city *at cost* for temporary free occupancy by displaced victims of fire was not charitable.)

(b) Hybrid Projects

Revenue Ruling 70-585 presents a real problem for the hybrid low and moderate income elderly housing projects typically encountered in the marketplace. Often, facilities with HUD insurance programs such as Section 202 (see § 22.3(a)), or those seeking to qualify for the low income housing tax credit (see § 8.3), reserve only 20 to 40 percent of their units for low income occupancy. The remainder may be rented at market rates for moderate income or even higher income use. Unless such projects are part of a community redevelopment plan, or can demonstrate aggressive minority group outreach, Revenue Ruling 70-585 on its face appears to be an obstacle to tax exemption.

(1) Elderly Distress

An argument can be made that the moderate income elderly, while not poor, are "distressed," and in that way fit the language of the Regulation defining charitable activities. Revenue Ruling 70-585 dealt with moderate income housing in general, not projects for the elderly. Indeed, that the nonpoor elderly may be "distressed" is a principle on which the home for the aged basis for tax exemption rests.[38] Unfortunately, the applicable Revenue Rulings set out the precise kinds of distress to which the elderly are susceptible and the specific steps that must be taken to relieve that distress, such as the arrangement for health care, operation at lowest feasible cost, and retention in residence of those who run out of funds.[39] The requirement

---

[35] Rev. Rul. 68-17, 1968-1 C.B. 247. *See also* Priv. Ltr. Rul. 8101009, and GCM 33671.

[36] Rev. Rul. 76-408, 1976-2 C.B. 408.

[37] 1977-1 C.B. 140.

[38] See Rev. Ruls. 72-124 and 79-18; § 9.2(a), above.

[39] *See* GCM 38478 (8/6/85), which confirms that the housing, health care, and financial security tests must be met to relieve elderly distress.

of Revenue Ruling 72-124 that a facility retain in residence those unable to pay does not apply to facilities required to serve only low and moderate income elderly pursuant to federal financing restrictions, but this exception is of limited use.[40] The elderly-as-distressed argument is therefore of little comfort for low and moderate projects that do not independently meet the criteria of Revenue Ruling 72-124.

(2)   Low Income Presence; Low Income Purpose

It is still possible under Revenue Ruling 70-585 that the presence of a low income component in a project could warrant an exemption for the project even though it also contains moderate income units, but it is difficult to find authority for this proposition. Letter Rulings granting exemption to combined low and moderate income housing projects do not appear to rely on the presence of the low income housing component as a basis for exemption. In Letter Ruling 7823072, for example, where the project was designed for 25 percent low income, 55 percent moderate income elderly or handicapped, and 20 percent moderate income families, the IRS found a charitable purpose, but focused almost exclusively on the fact that it was a redevelopment authority project designed to "combat community deterioration."[41] The existence of a substantial low income component, or of a senior/handicapped set aside for the majority of units, did not ostensibly enter into the government's analysis. However, less than half of the units in that example were for low income use.

It is theoretically possible that a project making less than all of its units available for low income residents can qualify for tax exemption on the basis of relief of the poor, without independently meeting one of the social welfare tests, the home for the aged exemption, or some other separate basis for exemption. The fact that Section 501(c)(3) requires the organization seeking exemption to pursue a charitable purpose "exclusively" does not necessarily mean that all its activities be charitable. As discussed in Section 9.1(b), above, it is possible to engage in a hybrid, exempt and nonexempt activity that is exclusively charitable in its ultimate purpose. The regulations [42] require merely that the organization's *primary activity* be charitable, provided that all but an insubstantial portion of the total activities serves the charitable purpose. Therefore, a housing project with more than 50 percent low income units arguably could qualify for exemption if it is demonstrated that the exclusive purpose of providing the other, non-low income units is charitable, for example, that they are economically necessary to support the development and ongoing provision of the low income units. It is possible, but

---

[40] *See* § 9.2(a)(3).

[41] *See also* Priv. Ltr. Rul. 8101009, which similarly uses the community deterioration rationale for exempting a 20 percent low income housing project.

[42] Reg. § 1.501(c)(3)-1(c)(1).

more difficult, to apply this reasoning to projects with a majority of moderate or other noncharitable units, where their sole purpose is to make possible the provision of a lesser proportion of low income facilities.

§ 9.5   HEALTH FACILITIES

Although there is no specific reference to it in the Internal Revenue Code or Treasury Regulations, the promotion of health has come to be recognized as a charitable purpose under Section 501(c)(3). Most of the legal authority for this exemption has evolved in the context of hospitals.

As was the case with retirement facilities, early Internal Revenue Service rulings required that exempt hospitals furnish free or below-cost care.[43] This position changed in 1969, when it was recognized that promotion of health, even for private pay or insured patients, was inherently charitable, provided care was available to the community at large, for example, via an emergency room open to all.[44] Of course, exempt health care facilities must serve a public purpose and cannot benefit private interests.[45]

Even hospitals without emergency rooms have been found to be exempt where they had a community board of directors, an open medical staff policy, patients paying their bills with the aid of government programs such as Medicare and Medicaid, and the application of surplus funds to improvement of facilities, care, education, and research.[46]

In 1972, the Internal Revenue Service ruled that a home health organization providing professional nursing and therapeutic services primarily to elderly persons in their homes, pursuant to a physician-prescribed course of treatment, promotes health and is eligible for exemption.[47] Skilled nursing facilities also appear to be routinely granted exemptions.[48]

Prepaid health plans generally have been treated as Section 501(c)(4) social welfare organizations, rather than as charitable organizations, because of the preferential treatment given to members (a private inurement problem) and because the prepayment is viewed as a form of insurance, which is a noncharitable activity.[49] The Tax Court has ruled that a health maintenance organization can be exempt from tax under circumstances where it provided care facilities directly, carried on research, made services available to those unable to pay, and where the class of members was large enough to constitute a community.[50] There, the Tax Court found that

[43]Rev. Rul. 56-185, 1956-1 C.B. 202.
[44]Rev. Rul. 69-545, 1969-2 C.B. 117.
[45]See, *Sonora Community Hospital v. Comm'r*, 397 F.2d 814 (9th Cir. 1968).
[46]Rev. Rul. 83-157, 1983-2 C.B. 94.
[47]Rev. Rul. 72-209, 1972-1 C.B. 148. *See also* Priv. Ltr. Ruls. 8427078, 8510068, and 8534089.
[48]*See, e.g.*, Priv. Ltr. Ruls. 8616095, 7948104.
[49]*See* Hopkins, note 5 above, at 94.
[50]*Sound Health Association v. Comm'r*, 71 T.C. 158 (1978).

while the *activity* or providing insurance was commercial and nonexempt, the organization's purpose of promoting health was charitable.[51]

However, the Tax Reform Act of 1986 has made it clear that entities otherwise qualifying under Sections 501(c)(3) and 501(c)(4) will be denied tax exemption if any substantial part of their activities consists of providing "commercial insurance."[52] Although the prohibited activity does not include "incidental health insurance provided by a health maintenance organization of a kind customarily provided by such organizations,"[53] the congressional committee reports [54] make clear that only those HMOs providing services to their own members, with their own employees, in their own facilities (the Kaiser model), will remain eligible for exemption. Those engaged primarily in insurance for health services rendered by others (Blue Cross model) will be taxable.[55]

Promotion of health is a concept that may be of limited usefulness in obtaining an exemption for a retirement facility. Many facilities, while arguably designed to promote the general health of their residents, offer primarily independent housing and are not licensed in their entirety, if at all, as health facilities. This class of facility is probably preemptively covered by the criteria of Revenue Ruling 72-124 and related rulings (see §§ 9.2 and 9.3).

It may be possible, however, to obtain an exemption on the basis of health promotion for facilities that are primarily dependent-care oriented, such as assisted living facilities. While these technically are not health facilities under most state license laws, they are at least primarily directed toward the provision of care, rather than housing. In Letter Ruling 8506116, the Internal Revenue Service found a "long-term care facility for the elderly" to be eligible for exemption. Although it reviewed the criteria for a home for the aging exemption under Revenue Ruling 72-124 (housing, health care, and financial security), the IRS also noted that the organization would operate exclusively for the "charitable purpose of promotion of health."

Whether or not the housing aspect of a retirement facility can be subsumed under the banner of an overall charitable purpose of health promotion, the concept presents opportunities for facility developers. Where housing facilities are to be combined with health services, it may be possible to establish a separate organization for the health care provider and obtain an exemption for it on its own merit. Thus, the residents of nonexempt, independent senior housing, offered at market rates, could be

---

[51]*Id.*, at 189.

[52]I.R.C. § 501(m).

[53]I.R.C. § 501(m)(3)(B).

[54]Reported at CCH, *Standard Federal Tax Reporter*, 1987, at 37,022–37,023.

[55]*Id.*

served by an exempt home health agency, health maintenance organization, or nearby nursing facility.

The exempt health promotion purpose of a given facility may also be used to justify otherwise nonexempt activities, such as the provision of housing. For example, Revenue Ruling 81-28[56] found that the provision of free, temporary, modest housing for relatives of patients in neighboring hospitals and nursing facilities served a charitable promotion of health purpose in that visitation of patients had therapeutic value. Similarly, condominium units provided on a temporary basis to patients of a medical clinic who had to travel considerable distances to receive treatment were not unrelated to the organization's exempt health purposes.[57] While neither of the referenced rulings permits permanent housing as an adjunct to a health promotion purpose, a plausible argument can be made that retirement housing can, for example, serve the health promotion purposes of an adjacent sponsoring hospital.[58]

§ 9.6   CHURCH GROUPS

Religious organizations, as well as charitable ones, are eligible for tax exemption under Section 501(c)(3). Churches are included among the groups to which a contribution may qualify for a charitable deduction.[59] It is clear, however, that the concept of a church is not limited to the house of worship itself, but may also include such entities as schools owned by church groups.[60]

An integrated auxiliary of a church is defined in regulation as a tax exempt organization that (1) is affiliated with a church (i.e., is controlled by the church or shares common religious bonds and convictions with it), and (2) whose principal activity is "exclusively religious."[61]

The test of exclusive religiosity is not met if the organization has an independent basis for exemption. Thus, a charitable home for the aged, even though it limits admissions to members of the church, is not a religious organization where it is entitled to a separate home for the aging exemption.[62] However, examples given of integrated church auxiliaries include men's or women's organizations and mission societies.[63]

---

[56] 1981-1 C.B. 328.

[57] Priv. Ltr. Rul. 8427105.

[58] *See, e.g.,* the discussion of construction of medical office buildings as exempt activities of hospitals (§ 12.1(b)(2)).

[59] Reg. § 170(b)(1)(A)(i).

[60] *See, St. Martin Evangelical Lutheran Church v. South Dakota,* 451 U.S. 772, 101 S. Ct. 2142 (1981).

[61] Reg. § 1.6033-2(g)(5).

[62] Reg. §§ 1.6033-2(g)(5)(ii), (iv) (Ex. 4).

[63] Reg. § 1.6033-2(g)(5)(iv).

While it is conceivable that a retirement facility can be considered exempt as part of a church, the strict test set forth in the regulations would probably disqualify all but the most unusual cases. For example, a mountain lodge operated for religious retreats was found not to be engaged in an exclusively religious activity where religious activities were optional and not regularly scheduled, and usual recreational activities were available.[64] On the other hand, a church that spent over 20 percent of its disbursements on a medical plan for church members was found by the courts to be serving a sufficiently religious purpose.[65] Thus, a noncharitable retirement home with regularly scheduled religious services probably could also provide medical and other secular services, and qualify for exemption on a religious basis, provided that the religious purposes and activities are sufficiently pervasive to dominate the home's character. Rent free housing for retired missionaries in financial need has been found exempt, but probably on the basis of its charitable, rather than religious, nature.[66]

It should be noted here that retirement facilities affiliated with major church groups may qualify for inclusion under a group exemption by means of a listing in the church's national directory of related organizations.[67] Application is made to the church group for listing, and not to the Internal Revenue Service. Upon listing, the organization is automatically deemed exempt pursuant to the church's blanket ruling. While this may be a convenience for the applicant organization, it is not carte blanche to engage in otherwise nonexempt activities in the name of a church, and it is incumbent upon the organization to demonstrate to the listing church the basis for qualification as an exempt organization.

§ 9.7 EXEMPT SERVICES

Several activities benefiting the elderly, but not involving the furnishing of housing or health care facilities, have been deemed charitable. (Health services such as home health and prepaid health plans have already been discussed in § 9.5.)

Nonhealth services may also qualify for exemption. For example, in Revenue Ruling 76-244,[68] a Meals on Wheels service designed to provide meals at cost to elderly persons in their homes was found to be tax exempt and charitable. Although it charged a fee, the organization used volunteers for deliveries, and would reduce the charge or continue free service to those who could not afford the usual charge. Interestingly, the Ruling did not

---

[64]*Schoger Foundation*, 76 T.C. 380 (1981).

[65]*Bethel Conservative Mennonite Church v. Comm'r*, 746 F.2d 388 (7th Cir. 1984), *overruling* 80 T.C. 352.

[66]Priv. Ltr. Rul. 7718008.

[67]See Rev. Proc. 80-27, 1980-1 C.B. 677.

[68]1976-1 C.B. 155.

focus entirely upon the financial relief afforded to those unable to pay, but took an expansive approach and considered in general the nonfinancial distress of the elderly. Although similar to the analysis of Revenue Ruling 72-124 (see § 9.2), this Ruling infers that one can relieve the nonfinancial distress of the elderly without providing housing and health care, as Revenue Ruling 72-124 dictates.

A senior center that provides referral and counseling services regarding health, housing, finances, education, and employment and that maintains a senior recreation center is exempt, where there is no membership requirement as a prerequisite to use of the facilities and services.[69]

Exemption was also granted to a publicly supported rural rest home that, for a nominal charge, admitted elderly poor from nearby metropolitan areas for two-week stays, including food and recreational programs.[70]

In Revenue Ruling 77-246[71] it was held that the provision of transportation services to the elderly and handicapped is an exempt activity. The Ruling referred to the elderly as a "charitable class."

However, there are definite limits on what services the IRS will consider to be charitable in nature. In Revenue Ruling 70-535,[72] it was held, rather summarily, that a nonprofit's mere management, for a fee, of low and moderate income housing owned by tax exempt nonprofit organizations does not amount to promotion of the common good and general community welfare sufficient to qualify the organization for exemption as a Section 501(c)(4) social welfare organization. The IRS found that its primary activity was the carrying on of a business with the general public in a manner similar to for profit organizations.

Similarly, in *Senior Citizens Stores, Inc. v. United States*,[73] an organization engaged in retail sales on a nonprofit basis, which used proceeds of sales to provide training, jobs, and recreational activities to seniors, was found to be ineligible for exemption because a substantial portion of its activities was not in furtherance of an exempt purpose.

While no definitive pattern emerges from the authorities, it is clear that some activities that do not meet elderly housing needs can qualify for tax exemption. However, they should have recognized charitable characteristics, like health promotion, or include free or below-cost services, as did the Meals on Wheels program of Revenue Ruling 76-244, and not be too similar to businesses normally operated for profit.

In the context of a retirement facility, it may therefore be possible to reduce program costs by structuring or working with nonprofit service organizations that cater to residents of a nonexempt housing facility. (For a

[69]Rev. Rul. 75-198, 1975-1 C.B. 157.
[70]Rev. Rul. 75-385, 1975-2 C.B. 205.
[71]1977-2 C.B. 190.
[72]1970-2 C.B. 117.
[73]602 F.2d 711 (5th Cir. 1979).

full discussion of for profit and nonprofit ventures and relationships, see Part V.)

§ 9.8 HOMEOWNERS' ASSOCIATIONS

Recently, service oriented retirement facilities have been structured as condominiums or subdivision units in which the homeowners' association acts as the provider of services to the owners. Internal Revenue Code Section 528 makes certain income of a qualifying homeowners' association exempt from taxation.

Exempt function income includes amounts received as dues or assessments from owners of the condominium units or other real property.[74] However, to be exempt, at least 90 percent of the annual expenditures of the organization must be for the "acquisition, construction, management, maintenance, and care of association property."[75] Examples of such expenditures are given in regulation, including upkeep and repair of streets, signage, recreation areas, and hallways, hiring security and management personnel, legal and accounting fees, property insurance, and property taxes.[76] It therefore appears that homeowners' associations that spend more than 10 percent of their expenditures for nonproperty related services to residents, such as meals, housekeeping, and health care, will be subject to taxation of income received as dues or assessments.

Nevertheless, it appears possible to use a tax exempt homeowners' association to provide property oriented services, in combination with a nonprofit organization that provides other exempt services, such as health care or low cost meals or recreational programs, via individual contracts with resident owners (see §§ 9.5 and 9.7).

§ 9.9 AVOIDANCE OF PRIVATE FOUNDATION STATUS

Tax exempt retirement facilities should be structured to avoid classification as private foundations because contributions to private foundations generally are tax deductible to the donor to a lesser degree than contributions to public charities. Private foundations are also subject to an excise tax on investment income, must file more complex reports than other exempt organizations,[77] and are subject to a battery of taxes for certain proscribed activities.

The tests for avoidance of private foundation classification are set forth in Internal Revenue Code Section 509(a). Three relevant types of public charities are defined in the Code:

---

[74]I.R.C. § 528(d)(3).
[75]I.R.C. § 528(c)(1)(C).
[76]Reg. § 1.528-6(c).
[77]See, generally, I.R.C. §§ 170 and 4940 et seq.

(1) A religious, charitable, or otherwise exempt organization normally receiving a substantial part of its support (other than income from an activity constituting the basis of its exemption) from a government source, or from contributions from the general public.[78]

(2) An organization (a) normally receiving more than one-third of its annual support from a combination of gifts, grants, contributions, or membership fees, *and* gross receipts from admissions, sales, performance of services, or furnishing of facilities, in an activity that is not an unrelated trade or business, but not including receipts from any one person or entity to the extent they exceed $5000 or one percent of the organization's annual support; and (b) normally receiving one-third or less of its annual support from gross investment income (e.g., interest, dividends, rents) and the excess of unrelated business taxable income over the tax on such income.[79]

(3) An organization operated exclusively for the benefit of, or to function for, and that is controlled, operated, or supervised by one or more Type 1 or Type 2 organizations.[80]

The first, publicly supported organization category is not a likely vehicle for most retirement facilities. The test may be met by showing that at least one-third of the organization's total support is from public contributions or government sources,[81] or that at least 10 percent is from such sources, there is an ongoing solicitation program, and other facts and circumstances exist.[82] Although membership fees are included in the computation of public support,[83] exempt function income is not.[84] In *The Home for Aged Men v. United States*,[85] a federal district court found that entrance fees required to be paid to a life care type of retirement facility as a prerequisite to admission are funds derived from running the business of caring for the aged and are therefore exempt function income, rather than membership fees. Therefore, such fees were not counted as public support and the organization was characterized a private foundation. Most retirement facilities that rely primarily on resident fees for their income will likely face a similar fate under this analysis.[86]

The second type of public charity can rely upon gross receipts from admissions, sales, performance of services, or furnishing of facilities, as well as contributions, in meeting its one-third test. Therefore, entrance fees, monthly fees, sale prices of condominiums or memberships, and related

[78] I.R.C. §§ 509(a)(1), 170(b)(1)(A)(vi).

[79] I.R.C. § 509(a)(2).

[80] I.R.C. § 509(a)(3).

[81] Reg. § 1.170A-9(e)(2).

[82] Reg. § 1.170A-9(e)(3).

[83] Reg. § 1.170A-9(e)(7)(iii).

[84] Reg. 1.170A-9(e)(7)(a).

[85] CCH, 80-2 U.S.T.C. ¶ 9711 (N.D. Va. 1980).

[86] *See also, Williams Home, Inc. v. U.S.*, 540 F. Supp. 310 (W.D. Va., 1982).

receipts from furnishing or operating an exempt facility will count toward qualification. Medicare and Medicaid income in connection with the exempt activity should also count as gross receipts that are credited toward meeting the one-third test.[87] However, income from any single source does not qualify to the extent it is in excess of the greater of $5000 or one percent of the organization's total support. As a practical matter, this dictates construction of larger facilities, for example, of 100 units or more, so that no resident contributes more than one percent of total income.

The third category is that of a support organization. The niche can be of use where an existing Type 1 or Type 2 organization, such as a hospital, spins off a controlled organization to operate the retirement facility. The supporting organization need not independently meet the public support criteria of the other two categories if it (1) is operated, controlled, or supervised by the supported organization (parent-subsidiary model), (2) shares common supervision or control with the qualifying public charity (brother-sister model), or (3) is operated in connection with the public charity in that it takes over a function of the charity, or pays 85 percent or more of its income to the organization, which must be sufficient to assure a significant voice in the charity's investments, and the charity is responsive to the supporting organization.[88]

For an example of a retirement facility employing all three types of public charity status, see Letter Ruling 8506116, where a long-term care facility for the elderly (X) transferred all its fund-raising activities to one related organization (Y) and all its investment income producing activities to another (Z). The government found that X was a Type 2 entity, which could qualify on the basis of its exempt operations income, Y a Type 1 entity supported by the public, and Z a Type 3 support organization.

§ 9.10   UNRELATED BUSINESS TAXABLE INCOME

(a)   Unrelated Trades or Businesses

An exempt organization can be subject to payment of tax on income from a trade or business that is not substantially related to the exercise of its charitable or other exempt purpose.[89] The regulations explain that the unrelated trade or business must be regularly carried on[90] and generally involves the generation of income from the sale of goods or performance of services.[91] In addition, if unrelated activities become too substantial a portion of the

---

[87]*See* Rev. Rul. 83-153, 1983-2 C.B. 48.
[88]*See* Reg. § 1.509(a)-4.
[89]I.R.C. §§ 511-514.
[90]Reg. § 1.513-1(a).
[91]Reg. § 1.513-1(b).

organization's overall activities, the tax exempt status of the entity can be jeopardized (see § 9.1(b)).

In Revenue Ruling 81-61,[92] the IRS considered whether the operation, at market rate fees, of beauty and barber shops for older people by a nonresidential senior citizens center was an exemption related activity. The activity was deemed to be related to the exempt purpose, which included ministration to elderly persons' social, recreational, physical, and health needs, because it was conveniently located for those who might have impaired ability to travel, and met the psychological and health needs of area elderly by supplying their grooming needs.

However, in a companion ruling,[93] the government held that a senior citizen center's sale of heavy duty appliances to seniors was not related to any exempt purpose because, unlike hairstyling, appliance purchases need not be conducted in person and are a sporadic, rather than ongoing, need. Thus, the organization did not relieve any significant form of elderly distress by selling appliances.

To avoid tax on income, therefore, activities should directly serve the object of the exempt purpose—the residents—rather than simply line the coffers of the organization, even if that income is ultimately dedicated solely to the benefit of the aged.[94] However, elderly residents need not be the exclusive users. In the nonprofit hospital context, for example, gift shops, cafeterias, and parking lots, while not patronized exclusively by patients, were deemed exemption related activities.[95] The theory was that facilities fostering patient visitation by relatives and friends contributed to the patients' well being, and that staff use of such facilities enabled the institution to accomplish its exempt purposes more efficiently. Similar logic can be applied to retirement facility restaurants, recreation centers, transportation, or other amenities open to visitors or even the public on a limited basis.

Similarly, a long series of IRS pronouncements has established that hospitals' construction of adjacent medical office buildings does not result in unrelated business income because these buildings serve the organization's exempt purposes by encouraging physicians to locate nearby and refer patients.[96]

It is conceivable to stretch the relatedness point so that, for example, a nonprofit hospital could argue that its adjacent retirement facility, which otherwise would not qualify for exemption, serves the *hospital's* exempt purpose on the ground that it establishes a potential new patient base,

[92] 1981-1 C.B. 355.

[93] Rev. Rul. 81-62, 1981-1 C.B. 355.

[94] *See, e.g.,* Rev. Rul. 55-449, 1955-2 C.B. 599, which found that a church group's sale of housing to raise revenue was an unrelated activity.

[95] *See* Rev. Rul. 69-267, 69-268, 69-269, 1969-1 C.B. 160.

[96] *See, e.g.,* Priv. Ltr. Ruls. 8134021, 8201072, 8301003, 8312129.

attracts physicians, and promotes cost efficient sharing of services. Unfortunately, there is little, if any, direct authority for such a proposition. In Letter Ruling 7733070, a residential retirement center to be built and operated by a hospital near its medical complex was found not to generate unrelated business income, but the Internal Revenue Service recited criteria and qualifying facts, including continuing service for those who became unable to pay, sufficient to gain a home for the aged exemption under Revenue Ruling 72-124 or 79-18 (see § 9.2(a)). Although one encounters occasional unpublished decisions where exemption has been granted for retirement facilities without strict compliance with precedent, or as an apparent bootstrapping from an existing exempt activity, it appears that retirement centers generally have been so comprehensively discussed in IRS rulings as to warrant independent analysis of their exempt purposes.

(b) Rental Income

Rental income from real property generally is excluded from the definition of unrelated business taxable income.[97] Therefore, a retirement facility, or land on which a retirement facility is to be built, may be leased by a nonprofit property owner to another person or entity who operates the facility for profit or for some other purpose unrelated to the owner's exemption, without taxation of rental income or jeopardy of the lessor's exempt status.

However, rental income will be subject to inclusion as unrelated business income when the amount of the rent is based on income or profits derived from the leased property, unless it is a fixed percentage of receipts or sales,[98] or includes substantial personal property.[99] Therefore, a nonprofit's rental income from property used in an unrelated business can be a fixed rate, or a percentage of gross revenues, but not a share of profits or net revenues.

The rental income exemption does not apply at all to income received from debt financed property.

(c) Debt Financed Property

Income from debt financed property is subject to taxation as unrelated business income.[100] Debt financed property is that which is held to produce income, and for which there was an acquisition indebtedness outstanding at any time during the taxable year.[101] The principal exception is for property, substantially all of the use of which is related to the organization's charitable or other exempt purpose.[102] The purpose of taxing debt financed property

---

[97] I.R.C. § 512(b)(3)(A)(i).
[98] I.R.C. § 512(b)(3)(B)(ii).
[99] Reg. § 1.512(b)-1(c)(2)(iii)(a).
[100] I.R.C. §§ 512(b)(4), 514(a)(1).
[101] I.R.C. § 514(b)(1).
[102] I.R.C. § 512(b)(1)(A)(i).

income is primarily to prevent use of a nonprofit as a straw man buyer/lessor to fund a bootstrap property sale from future operating income, generated by a lessee related to the seller,[103] where the nonprofit's use of the property is unrelated to its exempt purpose.

Most retirement facility rulings dealing with debt financed property have concerned property to be used as the site for the facility itself. Therefore, if the retirement facility is eligible for exemption, operating income derived from it is related to the exempt purpose, and not subject to taxation, even though the acquisition may have been debt financed.[104]

§ 9.11 DEDUCTION OF PAYMENTS TO EXEMPT FACILITIES

Contributions to charitable organizations are generally deductible to the donor for purposes of calculation of income subject to taxation.[105] Early on, however, the IRS held that no part of a founder's fee paid by a taxpayer to a nonprofit home in return for life care in the home was deductible.[106]

However, in 1962, the federal Eighth Circuit Court of Appeals, in *Wardwell v. Commissioner*, determined that a "room endowment" paid to a tax exempt home for the aged, on the day before the taxpayer moved into the facility, was deductible.[107] The home solicited endowments of $5000 per room and generally permitted the donor to occupy the room or designate its occupant. The Internal Revenue Service had argued successfully before the Tax Court that the payment was made with the motive and expectancy of securing occupancy in the home, was a quid pro quo arrangement, and not the result of a detached charitable intention. The Eighth Circuit reversed, finding that the taxpayer's motive on the date the *payment* was made was not relevant, but that her intention on the date the gift was made was relevant. Although the payment in this case had been made prior to moving in, it had been pledged, in writing, after the taxpayer's application for residence had been approved by the home. The court concluded that a legally binding pledge was made regardless of any expectation about her admission.

The *Wardwell* ruling was criticized by the IRS in its Revenue Ruling 72-506,[108] where it denied the deduction for a "sustainer's gift" payment solicited by a retirement facility from all applicants who were "financially able,"

---

[103]For example, *A* sells income producing property to *B* (a nonprofit) for a small down payment. *B* leases to *C*, which is related to *A*, for a rent based on a share of operating profits. *B* pays off the debt to *A* out of rents from *C*. *C* gets a rent deduction. *A* generates more after-tax income (capital gains) than if it had continued to operate the property and take ordinary income. *B* eventually acquires the property for virtually no investment. *See* Hopkins, note 5, above, at 682ff, and *Comm'r v. Brown*, 380 U.S. 563 (1965).

[104]*See, e.g.,* Priv. Ltr. Ruls. 8025132, 8117221.

[105]I.R.C. § 170.

[106]Rev. Ruls. 54-430, 1954-2 C.B. 101; 58-303, 1958-1 C.B. 61.

[107]301 F.2d 632 (8th Cir. 1962).

[108]1972-2 C.B. 506.

varied according to the size of each unit. The Service found the "gift" to have been made with an "expectation of benefits." It also disagreed with *Wardwell* insofar as the case could be interpreted to preclude denial of the deduction unless the donor had a legal right to admission in return for the payment.

The reasoning of the IRS was followed in *Sedam v. United States*,[109] in which the Seventh Circuit found that where payments were made with the intent to induce admission to a facility, there was no gift, even though there was no legal obligation to make the payment. However, in *Dowell v. United States*,[110] the Tenth Circuit found a charitable gift where the sponsorship gift was solicited during the process of application for a residence, but after acceptance to the facility had been granted.[111]

Nonprofit retirement facilities should not hesitate to solicit contributions from applicants for admission, or from their relatives, except under the circumstances described in Section § 9.2(b)(4), above, concerning Medicaid fraud and abuse. However, facilities should not represent to applicants for admission that payments made to the home are deductible, especially when solicited or paid prior to acceptance at the facility, as the IRS has consistently taken a negative view of such payments. Of course, solicitation of existing residents does not present the kinds of problems addressed above. If a facility is concerned that applicants will be dissuaded from making truly voluntary contributions because of the uncertainty of their deductibility, it may wish to devise a carefully crafted solicitation program along the lines of the *Wardwell* and *Dowell* criteria, taking no pledges or payments prior to acceptance for admission, and making no guarantees of any quid pro quo. One might even seek a blanket Internal Revenue Service letter ruling, although the IRS may feel compelled to analyze the individual facts of each contribution to determine the taxpayer's donative intent. (For a review of the deductibility of a portion of entrance fees or monthly fees as a medical expense see § 6.1(c)(1).)

§ 10   STATE TAX EXEMPTION

§ 10.1   IN GENERAL

Approximately 16 states have enacted statutes specifically addressing the availability of a tax exemption for homes for the aging.[112] About 20 states

---

[109]518 F.2d 242 (7th Cir. 1975).

[110]533 F.2d 1233 (10th Cir. 1977). However, *see Klappenbach v. Comm'r*, 52 T.C.M. 437 (1986), in which the Tax Court distinguishes *Dowell* and rules against the taxpayer.

[111]*See also* 34 A.L.R. Fed. 840 for a general survey of cases.

[112]M. Sweterlitsch, State Tax Exemptions: Homes for the Aging (Sept. 1986) (unpublished survey on file with Community Health and Nursing Services, Columbus, OH, and the author).

have laws dealing with state tax exemptions for nonprofit-owned, low in-come, or federally subsidized housing projects.[113] Often, where facilities have a mixture of low income and market rate units, a pro rata exemption is available. In addition, virtually every state has a general law exempting from state taxes those activities deemed to be charitable in nature.[114]

One must look principally to case law in the various states to determine how these general and specific statutory pronouncements have been inter-preted in the contexts of different retirement facility types.[115] If an exemp-tion is available, it can result in avoidance not only of state income taxes but, more importantly, of local ad valorem real property taxes.

In general, a retirement facility's exemption from federal income tax is no guarantee of state tax exemption. To the contrary, most states have developed much stricter standards for retirement projects than the IRS. Thus, for example, while the federal government exempts self-supporting, often luxury, elderly projects that follow the standards of Revenue Ruling 72-124 (provision of housing, health, and financial security), an apparent majority of states that have considered the question deny tax exemptions where the facility charges residents rents sufficient to meet expenses.

§ 10.2 APPROACHES IN VARIOUS STATES

A brief survey of selected contemporary case law and statutes from many of the states that have considered tax exemptions for homes for the aging follows.

(a) Arizona

Arizona statute provides for a property tax exemption for residential apart-ment house facilities that are designed to serve the handicapped or elderly, and where the operating expenses are substantially subsidized by either federal, state, or local governments, or by nonprofit organizations.[116] Con-sequently, senior citizen apartments that were owned and operated by a hospital to provide low rent housing and medical care for aged persons, and that were not designed to make a profit, constituted a charitable institution for the purposes of a property tax exemption.[117]

---

[113]*Id.*

[114]*See, e.g.* citations to Idaho, Illinois, Iowa, Minnesota, Missouri, and Nebraska Statutes, below.

[115]A detailed review of case law regarding state tax exemption for homes for the aged and for nursing homes appears at 37 A.L.R. 3d 565 (1971) and 45 A.L.R. 3d 610 (1972).

[116]Ariz. Rev. Stat. Ann. § 42-271(13) (1986).

[117]*Memorial Hospital v. Sparks*, 453 P.2d 989 (1969).

(b) California

California Revenue and Taxation Code Section 214(f) provides an exemption for elderly housing owned and operated by an entity exempt from federal income tax pursuant to Section 501(c)(3) and that was:

1. Financed by the federal government through one of several specified HUD programs, or
2. Offers care or special services designed to meet the particular needs of the elderly.

The second provision was added by amendment in 1984 to provide specifically that non-HUD facilities that offer services specially tailored to meet the needs of the elderly be exempted from real property tax.[118]

Prior to that amendment, there were a number of cases in the courts interpreting the earlier version of the statute. The courts had determined that the mere provision of housing to the elderly at market rates would not qualify for the tax exemption, even though the facility owner was a nonprofit corporation.[119] The courts had also made clear that, in situations involving nonprofit continuing care facilities, the provision of personal care to the elderly would make even a market rate upper income facility eligible for property tax exemption.[120] The very liberal amendment to Revenue and Taxation Code Section 214(f) now makes it possible for facilities that do not necessarily provide care, but that have some specialized service program for their elderly residents, to qualify for the exemption. It remains to be seen in California what kinds of specialized services will be required in order to meet the test of the amended statute.

(c) Colorado

Colorado statute provides an exemption for homes for the aged over 62 years whose income is up to 150 percent of the limits for low income public housing,[121] as well as for charity-run health care facilities.[122] Accordingly, a nursing home for elderly persons where all residents need nursing care, and those unable to pay are given a reduced rate or not charged, is exempt from tax.[123]

---

[118] Stats. 1984, c. 1102, at 22, § 1.

[119] *Martin Luther Homes v. County of Los Angeles*, 12 Cal. App. 3d 205, 90 Cal. Rptr. 524 (1970).

[120] *John Tennant Memorial Homes v. City of Pacific Grove*, 27 Cal. App. 3d 372, 382-85, 103 Cal. Rptr. 215 (1972).

[121] Colo. Rev. Stat. § 39-3-101(II)(A) (1982).

[122] *Id.* at § 39-3-101(I)(B).

[123] *Stanbro v. Baptist Home Assoc.*, 475 P.2d 23 (1970).

(d) Florida

Florida statute exempts nonprofit elderly and HUD facilities where residents meet certain income limits, and nursing homes.[124] A facility that is the equivalent of a high-priced condominium providing luxury living does not qualify for tax exempt status as fulfilling a charitable purpose, even though its use is limited to older persons and it is operated by a licensed nonprofit organization.[125]

(e) Hawaii

The Hawaii statute provides an exemption for nursing homes and federally subsidized housing for seniors.[126] However, a church-run retirement facility that accepted only reasonably healthy persons and that required all residents to pay established charges was also entitled to exemption, since the primary purpose of such charges was to further the residence's objectives of providing housing and services for elderly persons, and not to produce income.[127]

(f) Idaho

An Idaho retirement facility with residential units and an intermediate care facility was found not to be a charitable institution eligible for exemption from Idaho real property tax, because the $25,000 entrance fee and monthly fees charged to residents were sufficient to cover current operating expenses and to retire the home's debt.[128]

(g) Illinois

Illinois has established particularly strict standards of charitability. The organization must show, among other things, that funds are derived mainly from private and public charity, and that charity is dispensed to all who need it and apply.[129] In one case, an exemption was denied where applicants for residence were required to pay a substantial founder's fee, 85 to 97 percent of the total facility funding came from residents' fees, and the facility was not required to accept applicants or maintain residents who could not

---

[124]Fla. Stat. Ann. § 196.1975 (West Supp. 1986).

[125]*Mikos v. Plymouth Harbor, Inc.*, 316 So. 2d 627 (Fla. App. 1975).

[126]Hawaii Rev. Stat. §§ 246-32(b)(2), (c)(2) (1985).

[127]*Matter of Tax Appeal of Central Union Church*, 624 P.2d 1346 (Hawaii 1981).

[128]*Appeal of Sunny Ridge Manor, Inc.*, 675 P.2d 813 (Idaho 1984); Idaho Code § 63-105(c) (1976) (general charitable purpose exemption only).

[129]*Clark v. Marian Park*, 400 N.E.2d 661 (1980); Ill. Ann. Stat. ch. 120 § 500.7 (Smith-Hurd 1970) (general charitable purpose).

pay the required fees, even though approximately five percent of the residents were accepted or maintained despite their inability to pay the fees.[130] In Illinois, "all facts are to be construed and all debatable questions are to be resolved in favor of taxation."[131]

(h) Iowa

Iowa has recognized tax exemption for retirement facilities that generate only enough income to stay in operation, do not discriminate against persons unable to pay, and provide some gratuitous or partly gratuitous care.[132] In addition, in a case where residents paid rent sufficient to pay operating costs, but construction costs and some staff services were donated, exemption was granted.[133] However, where a nonprofit home provided no concessions on rent to those unable to pay, there was no basis for tax exemption.[134]

(i) Michigan

Facilities in Michigan that would probably qualify for federal exemption under Revenue Ruling 72-124 are not exempt from state tax where residents must pay substantial entrance fees, pass health and financial examinations, and are provided above average accommodations.[135] Even a facility that provided elderly housing and moved residents to an adjacent nursing unit if they became unable to pay was not exempt, contrary to the federal position in Letter Ruling 8117221 (see § 9.2(b)(7)).[136]

(j) Minnesota

Homes are denied exemption as purely public charities when residents are required to submit financial statements showing the ability to pay entrance

---

[130]*Plymouth Place, Inc. v. Tully*, 370 N.E.2d 56 (1977). *See also Small v. Pangle*, 328 N.E.2d 285 (1975), *cert. den.* 423 U.S. 918 (1975) (facility not exempt as a charitable institution where all residents paid substantial monthly fees, greater source of funds was not from either public or private charity, and home had never had a resident who was unable to pay the substantial monthly charges).

[131]*Methodist Old Peoples Home v. Korzen*, 233 N.E.2d 537, 540 (1968) (facility not exempt where home not obligated to retain residents, amount of founders fees and monthly charges determined location of accomodation, and there were stringent health requirements for admission).

[132]*Twilight Acres v. Board of Rev. of Sac.*, 346 N.W.2d 40 (Iowa App. 1984); Iowa Code § 427.1(9) (West Supp. 1986) (general charitable purpose).

[133]*Hilltop Manor v. Board of Rev. of Marion*, 346 N.W.2d 37 (1984).

[134]*Dow City Senior Housing, Inc. v. Board of Review*, 230 N.W.2d 497 (1975).

[135]*Michigan Baptist Homes v. Ann Arbor*, 223 N.W.2d 324 (1974), *aff'd* 242 N.W.2d 749 (1976); Mich. Comp. Laws Ann. §§ 211.7, 211.7(d) (West 1986) (charitable facilities for the aged and chronically ill and HUD Section 202 and 236 housing for the elderly).

[136]*Retirement Homes of Detroit v. Sylvan Township*, 330 N.W.2d 682 (Mich. 1982).

fees and monthly charges, to undergo physical examinations, and where only one person had been accepted for residency when it appeared he could not meet the monthly payments for at least three-fourths of his lifetime.[137]

(k) Missouri

A Missouri retirement home with residential and medical care facilities was denied a charitable exemption on the grounds that it required a substantial initial endowment by its residents with an equal amount of additional assets remaining in reserve, charged a substantial monthly fee, and retained discretion in determining whether the fee should be waived, thereby effectively denying its services to a large percentage of the elderly based on finances.[138] On the other hand, a facility that operated on a not-for-profit basis, received significant subsidies both from HUD and private charity, and was designed to meet the physical, social, and psychological needs of the elderly, was held to benefit society and lessen the likelihood of burdens on the government, thereby qualifying for a charitable exemption.[139]

(l) Nebraska

Even though a Nebraska home charged residents who could afford fees, it was deemed tax exempt where ability to pay was not a condition of admission and no patient had ever been removed from the home for inability to pay.[140] However, a facility simply operating at cost from rents did not qualify.[141]

(m) New Mexico

A nursing home operated by a nonprofit corporation was exempt from property tax where the substantial and primary use was for charitable purposes, and the residents were largely aged, ill, and indigent.[142]

(n) New York

In New York, a retirement home was found exempt where it provided residential care, 90 percent of the residents received government benefits, and

---

[137]*Petition of United Church Homes*, 195 N.W.2d 411 (1972); Minn. Stat. Ann. § 272.02 (West Supp. 1987) (general charitable purpose).

[138]*Evangelical Ret. Homes v. State Tax Commission*, 669 S.W.2d 548 (Mo. Banc 1984); Mo. Ann. Stat. § 137.100(5) (Vernon Supp. 1987) (general charitable purpose).

[139]*Franciscan Tertiary Prov. v. State Tax Commission*, 566 S.W.2d 213 (Mo. Banc. 1978).

[140]*Bethesda Foundation v. County of Saunders*, 264 N.W.2d 664 (1978); Neb. Rev. Stat. § 77-202(c)(1981) (general charitable purpose).

[141]*Christian Retirement Homes v. Board of Equalization*, 180 N.W.2d 136 (1970).

[142]*Retirement Ranch, Inc. v. Curry Cty. Val. Protest Bd.*, 546 P.2d 1199 (1976); N.M. Const. art. VIII, § 3 (general charitable purpose).

voluntary contributions were required to meet a financial deficit.[143] The fact that a home, in good faith, paid more for its property than it was worth did not disqualify it from exemption.[144]

(o) Ohio

In Ohio, the exemption from real property tax requires that no more than 95 percent of the operating expenses at the facility be paid for by or on behalf of the resident, and that certain services be made available, at or below reasonable cost, for the life of each resident without regard to his or her ability to continue payment for their full cost.[145] On that basis, homes have been denied tax exemption.[146] A congregate housing facility providing below market-rate shelter, food, and minimal care was not eligible for exemption because it provided primarily building maintenance services rather than personal care, residents essentially had to be independent, and no permanent medical facilities existed.[147]

(p) Pennsylvania

An exemption was denied to a retirement community that charged substantial admission and monthly fees, financially screened applicants, had the right to require a resident to vacate for nonpayment of fees, and had only once provided a subsidy to a resident.[148] In a case with similar facts, an exemption was denied because, although the home alleged it had a policy not to terminate residence of those unable to pay, it could point to no instance where a person had become unable to pay.[149] Senior housing adjacent to an exempt home also was not considered a charitable use where the admission fee was calculated to meet the cost of residence, financial and physical screenings were required, and no substantial financial subsidy or benefit was available if a move to the exempt home was required due to financial or health reasons.[150]

---

[143]*Belle Harbor Home v. Tishelman,* 420 N.Y.S.2d 343 (1979), *aff'd* 441 N.Y.S.2d 413 (1981); N.Y. Real Prop. Tax Law § 422 (McKinney 1984) (not-for-profit housing).

[144]*Marino Jeantet Residence for Seniors v. Comm'r of Finance,* 430 N.Y.S.2d 545 (1980), *aff'd* 449 N.Y.S.2d 933 (1982).

[145]Ohio Rev. Code Ann. § 5701.13 (Page 1986).

[146]*Ohio Presbyterian Homes v. Kinney,* 459 N.E.2d 500 (Ohio 1984).

[147]*S.E.M. Villa II v. Kinney,* 419 N.E.2d 879 (1981).

[148]*In Re Marple Newtown School District,* 453 A.2d 68 (1982); Pa. Stat. Ann. tit. 27 § 5020-204(a) (Purdon Supp. 1986) (general charitable purpose). *See also, Lutheran Home at Topton v. Board of Assessment,* 515 A.2d 59 (1986).

[149]*In Re Eastern Dist. Conference,* 455 A.2d 1274 (1983).

[150]*Lutheran Home v. Board of Assessment,* 293 A.2d 888 (Pa. Cmwlth. 1972).

(q) Texas

In Texas, statutory exemptions exist for elderly facilities providing housing, health care, and other services, and for medical care facilities, provided in both cases that services are provided without regard to ability to pay.[151]

Thus, a home that subsidized certain residents from a charitable fund was exempt, even though residents were generally charged fees, and in some years the facility had a profit.[152] Likewise, a nursing home that charged fees, but did not refuse admission or continued occupancy to the indigent, was held to be exempt.[153]

However, where a facility was designed only for those paying with private funds or public welfare monies, and the corporation accumulated large sums over the years, exemption was denied.[154] And where an entrance fee type facility sought to fill one-third of its units with residents in need of charity, but was unsuccessful in doing so except for a very small percentage, exemption was denied.[155]

(r) Washington

An exemption exists in statute for homes for the aging that also meet the general provisions for exemptions for nonprofit corporations.[156] However, for a facility where almost all the income was from resident rents and government rent subsidies, exemption was denied because it was not shown that the organization was supported "in whole or in part by public donations or private charity."[157]

(s) Wisconsin

Wisconsin provides a statutory state tax exemption for "benevolent" nursing homes and retirement homes for the aged.[158] A nursing home that admitted patients without regard to their ability to pay, and that operated at a financial loss was, therefore, found to be exempt.[159]

---

[151]Tex. Tax Code § 11.18(c)(1)(M) (Vernon Supp. 1987).

[152]*Needville Ind. School Dist. v. S.P.J.S.T. Rest Home,* 566 S.W.2d 40 (1978).

[153]*City of McAllen v. Evangelical Lutheran,* 518 S.W.2d 557 (1975), *aff'd* 530 S.W.2d 806 (1976).

[154]*Challenge Homes, Inc. v. County of Lubbock,* 474 S.W.2d 746 (1971).

[155]*Air Force Village v. Northside Ind. School Dist.,* 561 S.W.2d 905 (1978).

[156]Wash. Rev. Code §§ 84.36.040(4), 84.36.805 (West Supp. 1987).

[157]*Yakima First Baptist Homes v. Gray,* 510 P.2d 243 (1973).

[158]Wisc. Stat. Ann. § 70.11(4) (West Supp. 1986).

[159]*Family Hospital Nursing Home v. City of Milwaukee,* 254 N.W.2d 268 (1977).

Five

Joint Ventures

Retirement facilities traditionally have been owned and operated largely by nonprofit organizations. The influx of for profit real estate developers into the retirement housing market, together with the desire of many hospitals and health care institutions to expand into areas of service that are not completely dependent upon reimbursement from government health programs, has caused a heightened interest in the pursuit of joint ventures in the development of retirement facilities. Because the retirement business can entail a combination of several traditionally separate disciplines, such as housing development, hospitality services, delivery of health care, and provision of health insurance, it can make sense for parties from different businesses to join together in the development of a single project.

In this Part, the term *joint ventures* is used loosely,[1] and can include equity pooling in a corporation or partnership, or simply involve contractual arrangements such as leases or management contracts. In either case, it is important to consider the interplay of the respective venturers' abilities, needs, and goals, as well as the possible tax and other regulatory implications of various relationship options.

Although ventures can include two or more parties of any type, this Part concentrates on ventures between nonprofit and for profit entities because these are the most likely type of venture in this field, and also because they raise the most significant business and legal concerns.

---

[1]Technically, joint ventures are treated and taxed as partnerships when certain equity contribution and profit sharing elements are present.

§ 11   VENTURE PARTNER RELATIONSHIPS

§ 11.1   WHAT JOINT VENTURE PARTNERS HAVE TO OFFER

The potential partners who may be available as a resource for the development of a retirement community project are legion, and may include existing owner/operators of for profit or nonprofit facilities, hospitals or nursing home chains, real estate developers, church groups, fraternal or civic organizations, retired persons' affinity groups, such as teachers' or military officers' associations, insurance carriers or health maintenance organizations, hotel operators, physician groups, food service operators, or any others engaged in some service needed for retirement facility development or operation, or with contacts with elderly constituencies.

(a)   Expertise, Staffing, and Resources

Most potential joint venture partners have some area of expertise that is attractive to the other partner and may fill a void in that partner's background. Most commonly, real estate developers seeking to develop and sustain an ongoing interest in a retirement facility with services can use the operational expertise, staff, or other resources of a management company, health care provider, operator of an existing facility, or other person or entity familiar with management of food services, hospitality services, recreational programs, health care, or other services and amenities planned to be offered.

Of course, established facility operators have the most comprehensive and extensive experience. They are likely to have strong convictions about appropriate operating techniques and will probably be less willing than other potential partners to share control over operations. While many hospitals or other health facilities may have significant experience in creating medical model projects, they may have little involvement in the development of residential housing, and may have a tendency toward creation of an institutional type of environment that an experienced developer of housing would know to avoid. However, their familiarity with health facility licensing and operations, and with such complex matters as government reimbursement programs, may be invaluable to a partner inexperienced in such matters. Similarly, those involved in the insurance industry, the delivery of prepaid health services, or of life care or continuing care, are likely to have background in the actuarial and risk-pooling considerations necessary to make a prepaid or endowment type of facility work. The bulk of a facility's day-to-day operations concerns food service, housekeeping, social-recreational programs, transportation, and related hospitality activities with which hotel operators have considerable experience. Although their entrance in the marketplace is recent, they seem particularly well suited to operate facilities, provided sufficient attention is given to planning for health care contingencies.

Real estate developers can offer much more to a venture than their obvious expertise in overseeing construction. Developers often have substantial valuable experience and knowledge in dealing with local zoning and planning agencies, designing structures and amenities that are attractive to consumers, obtaining financing, marketing real estate, and working with leases, restrictions on sales, homeowners association documentation, and related accoutrements of conventional real estate transactions. One concern in entering into an equity joint venture with a developer is to sustain its long-term interest and involvement in operations, as most developers are used to selling their projects after construction or when fully depreciated.

(b) Constituency

Many potential joint venture partners, such as community hospitals, church, fraternal, or civic groups, or established operators of existing retirement facilities, may well have a constituency group, or a following within a given community, that can form the core of the prospective resident population of the planned facility. The marketing advantage of having, for example, a retired military officers' group, a church or religious group, or a respected hospital as a partner in a retirement facility project can be significant. Especially in service-intensive facilities, where residents may be planning to spend the remaining years of their lives, the reputation, trustworthiness, and sense of security imparted by such an affiliation is of great importance. In addition, prospective residents may have a greater assurance that the other retirement facility residents, with whom they may be living on an intimate basis for many years, will share common values and outlooks.

Usually, these affinity groups are formed as nonprofit, tax exempt organizations. In most cases, the benevolent motivations of the group warrant the residents' trust. However, affiliation with such an affinity group is no substitute for a sound financial plan, a quality product, and expert management. Some of the most dramatic retirement facility failures have involved situations where residents placed their faith in affinity groups or individuals who were proceeding without a secure business plan (see § 5.1).

(c) Tax Advantages

Joint ventures between for profit and nonprofit entities can provide certain tax advantages for the project and its residents. Real estate developers faced with problems of substantial income taxation of entrance fees, for example, may work with a nonprofit organization as the operator and recipient of entrance fees on a tax free basis, and still make a profit via property leasing, development fees, or management activities. Facilities owned and operated by nonprofit organizations may also be eligible for local or state property tax exemption. In addition, tax exempt financing may be available to nonprofit facilities. All of these tax savings can make a project more feasible, marketable, and able to generate higher cash flows from operations.

(d) Capital, Land, or Other Assets

Developers may have access to conventional sources of financing and relationships with lenders that are not generally available to church groups or smaller health care institutions. On the other hand, nonprofit organizations generally have greater tax exempt bond financing options under the law (see discussion at § 15.2). Many hospitals or church groups may also have excess land that has been donated to them and remains undeveloped. In addition, health care providers may already have underutilized facilities that could provide nursing care or other services to an adjacent residential complex. Similarly, real estate developers may have completed apartment or condominium units that are not selling or that need to be converted to a more marketable use.

§ 11.2   JOINT VENTURE PARTNER GOALS AND APPROACHES

(a) Hospitals

A major reason for hospitals' increasing interest in the retirement housing market is the combination of pressures directed against the traditional hospital activities of providing acute inpatient care in a large, institutional setting. The Medicare system, which provides for much of the revenues of most acute hospitals, has shifted away from the reimbursement of cost approach, which for many years was the hallmark of the program. Rather than pay whatever the hospitals' costs may be for services delivered to patients, Medicare is now specifying the precise duration and scope of services it will pay for in the hospital setting by dividing virtually all possible hospital procedures into diagnosis related groups (DRGs) (see discussion at § 13.1). In addition, some state Medicaid programs have begun to contract selectively with only the most efficient hospitals, which results in a loss of Medicaid revenues to those hospitals that were not fortunate enough to obtain Medicaid contracts.

DRGs are greatly reducing the ability of hospitals to keep their beds filled with patients for longer occupancy periods, and are encouraging them to discharge patients sooner than they have historically, possibly before medically indicated.[2] As a consequence, many hospitals are interested in being at the receiving end of that transfer as well, and are expanding into the construction of personal care, or nursing or convalescent facilities at an increasingly greater rate.

Moreover, overhead costs involved in maintaining large institutional hospital centers, which include increasingly expensive high technology diagnostic equipment, operating rooms, and other costly support facilities, are helping make hospital charges exceed most people's means, and hospitals

---

[2] See, e.g., J. Sweeney and J. D'Itri, "New Success Factors for Management Under Prospective Payment," Topics In Health Care Financing, Spring 1985, 10.

less cost-efficient places to treat all but the most extreme illnesses or injuries. These pressures have led hospitals to diversify and enter markets that are are less cost-intensive and dependent upon government programs, such as outpatient clinics, ambulatory surgery centers, skilled nursing facilities, freestanding pharmacies, laboratories, or diagnostic centers, and retirement facilities. According to one survey conducted in late 1985, approximately 30 percent of hospitals with 400 or more beds were found to be in some phase of pursuing the development of a continuing care retirement community.[3]

Many hospitals considering development of a retirement facility want to do so within their own communities and at a location that can maximize the benefits to the hospital and make the best use of hospital resources. Sometimes hospitals will have land adjacent to the acute facility that may be available for development as a retirement facility. The retirement facility can serve, to some extent, as a feeder of inpatients to the hospital, and retirement facility residents may also use outpatient services, pharmacy, physical therapy, or other services available at the hospital. Hospitals may also benefit from the retirement community as a source of bequests or volunteers. If nursing facilities are constructed, they may serve as a place for some hospital inpatient transferees to convalesce.

To an extent, hospital staff and facilities may be used on a shared basis to assist in operation of retirement facility services and amenities. The hospital will benefit as well by achieving maximum utilization of its resources and economies of scale in such areas as dining, housekeeping, laundry, pharmacy, shared purchasing, and utilization of nursing, administrative, and other staff. (See discussion of employment issues in § 13.3.) However, developers in joint ventures with hospitals should be cautious to ensure that retirement facility services and amenities such as dining, housekeeping, and interior design do not succumb to the often institutional character typified by many hospitals. The developer should strive to include homelike qualities at the facility and, if necessary, bring in a third party to manage such critical services as dining, especially in upscale, market-rate facilities.

One of the most frequent frustrations voiced by developers in their dealings with hospitals relates to the slow-moving, bureaucratic structure that characterizes many hospitals. Whereas developers tend to want to move quickly, hospitals often spend a good deal of time carefully weighing alternatives. Much of this has to do with the complex structure and politics of most hospitals. The board of trustees is usually composed of civic and health care leaders who may be most concerned with community image and services. The medical staff of physicians has interests that span the hospital, the physicians' patients, and the doctors' own professions and prestige. Finally a business-oriented administration is employed by the board but, in many

---

[3]Survey by Kurt Salmon Associates, Inc. of Atlanta, cited in McMullin, D., "Hospitals and CCRCs: A Growing Alternative," *Contemporary Long Term Care*, November 1985, 43.

respects, is answerable as well to the physicians who are ultimately responsible for bringing patients into the hospital. Many committees, covering hospital departments, medical disciplines, and business functions, further compound the complexities. Because of this byzantine, often politically charged structure, hospitals usually move slowly, considering the impact of the proposed venture upon such diverse issues as profitability, effect on government reimbursement, maintenance of tax exempt status, impact of bond indenture restrictions, community image, effect on physician referral patterns, and competing uses for the hospital's money, land, or other resources, such as creating physician office buildings or freestanding clinics, remodeling or equipping existing facilities, developing health maintenance organizations or home health agencies, and other options. In general, they will want to have substantial controls over projects that bear their name in the role of owner, sponsor, or operator.

(b)   Church Groups and Affiliated Retirement Facilities

Church groups and religiously affiliated retirement communities can cover a broad spectrum, from the very unsophisticated to the extremely well managed business organizations. Most have something in common, however, and that is a constituency group and a sense of mission to serve that group.

In general, individual church congregations should be distinguished from larger, organized church groups, such as a church conference or diocese, or a church-sponsored corporation experienced in developing and operating retirement facilities. Often, an individual congregation has a loosely organized structure composed principally of volunteers. Although individual board members may have expertise in one or more relevant areas, the organization as a whole often cannot be relied upon to take the lead in developing and operating a given facility. If there is a danger in having such smaller groups develop or operate retirement facilities, it is that good intentions, without sufficient business acumen, can lead to financial weakness. They will need to rely heavily upon the leadership of an experienced developer, or a management company involved in formulating the facility's service program. Of course, even with the benefits of a constituency group, careful market and financial feasibility analyses or firm presales are a must.

On the other hand, religiously sponsored retirement facility corporations or hospitals, or regional divisions of major church groups, tend to have professional business management sophisticated in matters of finance, construction, and operations. Those religiously sponsored organizations already in the retirement facility business have invaluable experience in marketing retirement facilities and in the day-to-day operations of a home. Most religiously oriented retirement facility sponsors have a keen interest in operating a facility that is financially sound and not heavily dependent on donations to meet operational expenses. On the other hand, such organizations have an ethical desire, as well as an obligation under the terms of their federal income tax exemptions, to keep operational charges, however luxurious the facilities, reasonably related to the costs of providing services. On balance, these sponsors have demonstrated the ability to operate as successful growth businesses, and still serve their charitable purposes. In working with for profit organizations, they are concerned that their partners are committed for the long term to providing quality services to elderly residents and will not overreach in their pursuit of a return on investment.

Although church groups often have specific congregations or groups of adherents within a community that may form the basis of a retirement facility resident market, most such groups do not limit admissions to persons who are members of the particular denomination. Quite the contrary, most intend to market to all seniors regardless of religious preference. Generally, the signs of religious affiliation, from the consumer's perspective, are limited to the name of the organization and perhaps a chapel where services are regularly held. In some facilities, however, a religious or cultural atmosphere may be more pervasive, including regular religious services and observance of religious holidays, dietary practices, and other traditions.[4]

Religiously affiliated organizations have dominated much of the retirement and health care industries, yet they are not islands without desire to branch out or the need for resources to do so. They are obvious candidates for consideration as joint venture partners.

(c) For Profit Developers

For profit developers are, of course, interested in profit, but it is a mistake to think that profit is their only goal. Most successful developers realize that they must produce the best possible product for the segment of the marketplace they have targeted in order to maintain the kind of reputation necessary for sustained success in housing development.

The need for developers to make a lasting commitment to the ongoing quality of their product is even more crucial in retirement facilities where residents "aging in place" often require increasingly intensive health and service programs in addition to mere shelter. Developers may seek a joint venture partner to help assure that appropriate programs are formulated and can be operated on an essentially permanent basis.

On the whole, developers have a tendency to move much more rapidly than other types of retirement facility sponsors, and may have a greater inclination than others to proceed quickly with marketing and development of the physical facilities and amenities, without sufficient consideration of legal requirements or the details and consequences of service packages. Of course, larger institutional developers and the more sophisticated of the smaller development partnerships moderate their instincts to proceed at breakneck speed with a meticulous study of options. In areas in which many for profit developers are relative newcomers, such as continuing

---

[4]*See* § 23.3 for a discussion of religious discrimination in admissions.

care, many have shown remarkable ability to learn the system and make aggressive strides through determined hard work.

Developer strengths are their ability to move boldly and decisively, quickly and tirelessly in pursuit of a project. They are often lean organizations with few of the bureaucratic burdens of committees or other structures. Smaller developers especially have a strong sense of entrepreneurial independence and have an innate desire to avoid regulation. They use creative means to streamline the development process, reduce costs, and improve the product, but should proceed conservatively and cautiously to ensure compliance with applicable laws. They are strong in conventional finance and marketing abilities, as well as usually very familiar with design, zoning laws and procedures, and all aspects of construction in their particular locale.

National or other large corporate development companies have many of the qualities of smaller developers, but may share some of the institutional characteristics of such organizations as hospitals. Their in-house expertise in an area of development may be so pervasive as to make them disinclined to seek outside consultation when it is advisable to do so for reasons of local land use planning policies, unusual local or state laws, peculiar local market characteristics, or other important issues that may require extensive use of regional expertise.

Developers generally are concerned with the ability to generate and shelter income, depreciate capital investments, deduct losses, minimize governmental regulation, and efficiently produce an appealing product that will sell quickly and enhance the developer's reputation.

(d) Other Possible Partners

Several other types of candidates for coventuring a retirement facility project have emerged in the marketplace. These include those in the hotel or hospitality industry, insurance companies, universities, affinity groups such as military officers, retired teachers, or fraternal organizations, nursing home chains, management companies, and others who can bring a relevant field of expertise or residents to the venture. In any joint venture, it is important to select a partner whose attributes and resources complement your own and with compatible goals and operating style.

§ 11.3   JOINT VENTURE ROLES AND STRUCTURE

(a) Alternative Roles and Relationships and Their Impact on Development Issues

Joint ventures between nonprofit and for profit organizations are a natural result of the need of many for profit developers for operational expertise, health care experience, or resident constituency groups, and the need of nonprofit hospitals or churches for development or marketing expertise and capital. However, the form of the joint venture may vary widely depending on the desires and abilities of the partners and the tax and other legal consequences of mixing taxable and tax exempt entities.

The potential role of a joint venture partner in any retirement center project can be reduced to one or more of three basic functions: development, ownership, or operations. Whether a for profit or nonprofit organization fulfills each of those functions can have a significant effect on, among other things, the facility's marketability, financing, and opportunity to generate profits, on the tax treatment of income, and on property taxation.

Ventures between for profit and nonprofit entities often take one of the following typical forms:

1. A limited or general partnership in which the for profit and nonprofit businesses are cogeneral partners
2. A limited or general partnership in which the nonprofit's for profit subsidiary is partner with another for profit entity
3. A lease of facilities by the for profit developer/owner to the nonprofit operator, perhaps with a share of profits as part of the rent payment
4. A management contract from a for profit facility owner to a nonprofit operator, or from an exempt owner to a for profit operator, either with a share of profits as partial compensation

Each of these circumstances can raise significant taxation issues and other development concerns for both the for profit and nonprofit venturer. (See § 12 for a discussion of taxation concerns.)

Table 11.1 sets forth several possible scenarios of for profit and nonprofit involvement (designated *A* through *G*) in the facility. Its purpose is to present, as a planning guide, some of the alternative roles and relationships and broadly sketch several of the considerations inherent in each format. The notes to the table then offer general commentary on possible issues or consequences of each of the structures as they pertain to marketability, finance, taxation, and related aspects of facility development. These issues are discussed throughout this Part, as well as in Parts III and IV, in greater detail. (See in particular the joint venture example discussed at § 12.3.)

(b)   Formation of New Entities

(1)   Reasons for a New Entity

A joint venture may call for the formation of a new organization to develop, own, or operate the retirement facility, rather than relying upon the existence of the venture partners themselves. Reasons for forming one or more new organizations can include (1) insulation of the joint venturers from liability, (2) the need for a repository for capital or equity contributions of the venturers or third party investors, (3) creation of an organization with specific purposes qualifying it for tax exemption, (4) avoidance of the application of

Table 11.1 Proprietary and Nonprofit Roles and Relationships

	D	E	F
Development	**For Profit**	**For Profit** sale ↓	joint
Ownership	**For Profit** lease ↓	**Nonprofit** contract ↓	joint
Operations	**Nonprofit**	**For Profit**	joint

	G
Development	**For Profit** sale ↓
Ownership	resident contract ↓
Operations	**Nonprofit**

	A	B	C
Development	Nonprofit	For Profit	For Profit sale ↓
Ownership	Nonprofit	For Profit	Nonprofit
Operations	Nonprofit	For Profit	Nonprofit

Table 11.1 *(Continued)*

Notes to Table 11.1

I. Issues

1. Marketability
2. Financing
3. Profit opportunity
4. Tax treatment of fees
5. Tax treatment of property

II. Analysis

A. Nonprofit

1. Perceived trustworthiness, charitable objectives, built-in constituency
2. Additional government financing available: e.g., tax exempt bond issue; state bond programs; HUD § 202
3. No private inurement, but can generate revenues for expansion and improvements
4. a. No tax to operator for entrance fee or unit sales income
   b. Refundable fees may have imputed interest taxable to resident
   c. Resident deduction for medical expense portion of entrance fee and monthly fee
   d. Contributions deductible
5. Exemption from property tax available in some states

B. For Profit

1. New entrants in the market may be suspect, especially where taking large entry fees for future services, unless equipped with excellent reputation and resources
2. May have other capital sources, e.g., syndication
3. Opportunity for profit from operations, resales of units, or life leases
4. a. Entry fees may be taxed as prepaid rent, unless structured as a loan (imputed interest issue) or trust used
   b. Probably does not affect resident medical deduction
   c. No deductions for contributions
5. Probably subject to property tax

C. Developer Sale to Nonprofit

1. a. Credibility and constituency of nonprofit as owner/operator
   b. Developer need not learn health business, but should not build on speculation
   c. Operator should be involved early in development
2. Flexible; can finance through either entity
3. Profit limited to development
4. Favorable tax treatment of nonprofits
5. Same as 4.

D. For Profit Owner, Lease to Nonprofit

1. Most of the marketing attributes of nonprofit ownership, provided lease is long term
2. Nonprofit financing sources probably not available; nonprofit can loan entrance fees or sale proceeds to owner to retire debt
3. Additional profit opportunity in percentage lease
4. Can avoid income tax on entry fees by having operator receive them; percentage lease raises unrelated business income issues

Table 11.1 *(Continued)*

5. Property probably taxable; problem with taking ACRS deduction for tax exempt use property

E. Nonprofit Owner; For Profit Development and Operation

1. Attributes of ultimate nonprofit control over operations
2. Flexibility to finance via developer or owner, but tax exempt finance may be unavailable unless operation contract is limited
3. a. Can profit from development and operation

   b. For profit must have real estate *and* operations expertise

   c. Operation contract can be terminated by owner
4. Possible tax advantages of nonprofit ownership, but mere ownership may not be an exempt activity; percentage contracts with for profits raise a private inurement issue.
5. Same as 4.

F. Joint Undertaking (e.g., Partnership)

1. Marketing attributes of both forms of ownership, but nonprofit control and limited liability are advisable unless for profit subsidiary is formed
2. For profit finance model, syndication opportunities
3. Profit incentive shared with nonprofit party in return for expertise in operations; limits on profit of partners advisable unless nonprofit has formed for profit subsidiary and can take unrelated business income
4. Property and income are taxable; ACRS dilution likely
5. Same as 4.

G. For Profit Development/Resident Ownership/Nonprofit Operation

1. Ownership may have enhanced initial marketability; confidence in nonprofit services; resale market limited; problems of developer/operator control
2. Follows for profit finance model
3. Profit on initial real estate sales, but not necessarily on turnover of units
4. Fees not taxable if paid to nonprofit; exempt status may be questioned if management role only
5. Property taxed, but resident may defer gain on sale of prior residence and apply lifetime exemption on income from resale.

---

venturers' collective bargaining, ERISA, bond indenture, or other strictures upon the new venture, and (5) reimbursement for health care services from government programs such as Medicare.

(2) Pros and Cons of Entity Form

When contemplating the formation of a new entity, thought must be given to the specific form of the entity itself. The primary options are a general or limited partnership or a for profit or nonprofit corporation. In some circumstances, a trust, although not a business entity, may also be used for certain purposes in a retirement facility structure.

A principal advantage of a corporate format is that, if properly capitalized and if corporate formalities (i.e., procedures for operation set forth in articles, bylaws, and state statutes) are observed, the founders and shareholders of the corporation generally will be insulated from liability, and only the corporate assets will be at risk. A major drawback of the corporate form is taxation of earnings at the corporate level in addition to the taxation of shareholders for earnings distributed to them. In addition, corporate formation and continued observance of formalities can make corporate operation more rigid and cumbersome. On the other hand, unlike partnerships, it is relatively simple to transfer ownership interests in corporations through the sale of stock by shareholders.

Nonprofit corporations do not have shareholders as such, but may have members who elect directors and make other important decisions. In some cases, the directors themselves may be the sole members and be self-perpetuating. Nonprofits may be exempt from taxation, except to the extent they receive unrelated business income, but they must adhere strictly to their exempt purpose (see Part IV).

Unlike corporate shareholders, general partners are personally liable for the debts and other obligations of the partnership. However, earnings are not taxed at the partnership level, but are taxed only once upon distribution to partners. Management and operating protocols of partnerships are very flexible and can be informal or spelled out in detail in the partnership agreement. Transfers of partners' interests are cumbersome and may require consent of other partners or even dissolution and reformation of the partnership.

Limited partnerships offer some of the liability-insulating features of the corporate form to limited partners, whose liability is often limited to the amount of their investments. While the general partners of a limited partnership bear the same kind of unlimited liability for partnership debts as partners in a general partnership, many such general partners are themselves corporations, thus limiting the exposure to individual shareholders. Thus, assuming that adequate capitalization and other requirements are met, investor shareholders of the corporate general partner have only their corporate shares at risk, and not other personal assets, in much the same way that the limited partners' liability is limited to the amount of their investments.

§ 12   TAX IMPLICATIONS OF FOR PROFIT/NONPROFIT VENTURES

§ 12.1   PRESERVATION OF TAX EXEMPT STATUS

(a)   In General

Nonprofit hospitals, church groups, and other organizations may be eligible for exemption under section 501(c)(3) of the Internal Revenue Code as organizations "organized and operated exclusively for . . . charitable, scientific . . . or educational purposes" (see Part IV). Tax exempt organizations may not engage in acts that substantially benefit private persons or businesses financially. To the extent a nonprofit organization does not further the specific charitable purposes set forth in its articles of incorporation, there is a threat of generating unrelated business income, which is taxable to the nonprofit corporation. Substantial activity in a nonexempt undertaking may even jeopardize the entire tax exempt status of the organization (see discussion at § 9.10).

The mere fact that an activity of a nonprofit corporation may result in some benefit to a private business or person does not make the activity necessarily inconsistent with the corporation's charitable purposes. Of course, all nonprofit entities, in the course of carrying out their charitable or other exempt purposes, do business with for profit concerns in such matters as purchases of goods or services, leasing of property and related matters. However, the private benefit must be incidental, insubstantial, and not unreasonable in relation to the primary public benefit resulting from the activity.[5] In general, prices paid by nonprofits for goods or services must be reasonable so as not to result in any undue private benefit in excess of value received by the exempt organization in pursuit of its charitable goals.

(b) Equity Joint Ventures

(1) Pursuit of Exempt Purposes

The involvement of a nonprofit organization in the ownership or operation of a for profit business naturally raises concerns about the potential for generation of unrelated business taxable income, or possibly loss of tax exemption (see discussion at § 9.10). While these concerns may not be significant where the exempt organization is merely investing passively in the for profit enterprise as a corporate shareholder,[6] they become more serious where the nonprofit becomes a general partner, placing its assets at risk and actively participating in the business. Although the Internal Revenue Code clearly indicates that an exempt organization may be a partner in an unrelated trade or business,[7] there is virtually no statutory provision, case law, or revenue ruling that amplifies the circumstances under which participation in such a business jeopardizes tax exemption, leading one commentator to call the law on this subject "cryptic."[8] However, some private letter rulings, discussed below, provide guidance on the approach likely to be taken by the IRS in such circumstances.

A nonprofit's participation or limited partnership interest in a joint venture partnership will be analyzed by the IRS to determine whether the activity, if carried on directly by the nonprofit, is related to its exempt

---

[5] See *Plumstead Theatre Society, Inc. v. Comm'r*, 74 T.C. 1324 (1980), *aff'd* 675 F.2d 244 (9th Cir. 1982).

[6] See I.R.C. § 512(b)(1).

[7] See I.R.C. § 512(c).

[8] Hopkins and Beckwith, "The Federal Tax Law of Hospitals: Basic Principles and Current Developments," 24 *Duquesne L. Rev.*, 691, 718 (1986).

purposes. If not, the nonprofit's share of the partnership revenues is subject to unrelated business income tax.[9]

The IRS has found that a hospital may act as a general partner of a limited partnership owning a medical office building without jeopardizing its exempt status or receiving unrelated business income from management fees paid by the partnership. The IRS reasoned that the hospital's general partner interest was related to its tax exempt purpose because physicians would be attracted to the medical office building, which would help the hospital attract a better medical staff and improve patient care.[10] It can similarly be argued that the existence of a retirement facility serves the tax exempt purposes of a hospital either through the provision of health services to the elderly at the retirement facility, or by attracting retirement facility residents, and elderly people in general, to the hospital. Thus hospitals, as well as existing providers of retirement facility services, are logical nonprofit candidates for a joint venture.

In general, the tests of whether a retirement facility is operating for exempt purposes are set forth in the various revenue rulings discussed in Part IV. However, as the letter rulings below demonstrate, these usual tests are not dispositive of the question of whether a nonprofit entity can participate with a for profit enterprise in a retirement facility equity joint venture.

Of course, nonprofit venture partners should also be concerned about whether equity participation with a for profit entity will result in a problem of private inurement. A sharing of profits does not necessarily result in a partnership.[11] In general, however, sharing net profits can lead to unrelated business taxable income for the nonprofit organization.[12] Nevertheless, some sharing of partnership net profits with exempt organizations has been deemed, in letter rulings described below, not to give rise to unrelated business income, even where the nonprofit clearly was a partner.

(2)   Letter Rulings Concerning For Profit/Nonprofit Retirement Facility Partnerships

Several private letter rulings have considered partnerships between nonprofit and for profit organizations in the context of retirement facility projects.

[9]See IRC § 512(c), Rev. Rul. 74-197, 1974-1 C.B. 143; Rev. Rul. 79-222, 1979-2 C.B. 236; *Service Bolt and Nut Company Profit Sharing Trust v. Comm'r*, 78 T.C. 812 (1982), *aff'd* 84-1 USTC ¶ 9127 (6th Cir. 1983).

[10]Priv. Ltr. Rul. 8201072, referencing Rev. Ruls. 69-464, 1969-2 C.B. 132, and 69-463, 1969-2 C.B. 131.

[11]See Reg. § 301.7701-3(a), which describes a lease to a farmer in exchange for a share of crops as not necessarily constituting a partnership. *See also, Herzberg v. U.S.*, 176 F. Supp. 440 (S.D. Ind. 1959).

[12]See § 13.1(d)(2).

RULING 7820058

In Letter Ruling 7820058, the IRS considered whether a nonprofit organization could maintain its tax exemption where it sought to become a general partner, along with two for profit interests, in a limited partnership designed to develop low income senior housing in deteriorated urban renewal areas. The nonprofit would be the managing partner and return on investment would be limited to eight percent. The IRS ruled that such an arrangement would jeopardize the nonprofit's exempt status because the organization:

> Would be a direct participant in an arrangement for sharing the *net profits* of an income producing venture with private individuals and organizations of a noncharitable nature. By agreeing to serve as the general partner of the proposed housing project, [the nonprofit] would take on an obligation to further the private financial interests of the other partners. This would create a *conflict of interest* that is legally incompatible with [the nonprofit] being operated exclusively for charitable purposes. (Emphasis added.)

Despite the serious concerns about profit sharing raised by Letter Ruling 7820058, several later IRS pronouncements have concluded that some forms of for profit and nonprofit equity partnerships are permitted and will not affect the exempt status of the nonprofit, nor result in taxable income to it. In General Counsel Memorandum 37852 (1979), the IRS's General Counsel acknowledged that private benefit or inurement from the earnings of a nonprofit organization does not necessarily result merely from the organization's involvement in a joint venture or partnership with a for profit business.

RULING 8417054

In Letter Ruling 8417054, the IRS reviewed a request from a nonprofit organization intending to enter into a limited partnership as a cogeneral partner along with a for profit entity that was totally independent from the nonprofit organization. All dealings between the general partners were at arm's length. The nonprofit organization proposed to sell an existing retirement facility project operated by the nonprofit to the limited partnership at fair market value. Limited partnership interests would then be sold to independent investors. The nonprofit organization was to participate actively in managing the project and receive a one percent allocation *of profit* or loss in the limited partnership, plus a standard management fee pursuant to a HUD-approved management contract, as well as reimbursement for expenses incurred. The limited partnership agreement would state that the nonprofit would not be responsible for any operating losses. The project was subject to HUD mortgage insurance requirements and operated for the benefit of low and moderate income elderly persons. Part of the nonprofit's management duties was to insure that the to-be-formed for profit facility would be operated to serve the special needs of the elderly, and would comply with HUD policies and procedures.

The IRS noted that:

An exempt organization's participation in a partnership arrangement as a general partner will not *per se* result in loss of status under Section 501(c)(3) of the Code. Each partnership arrangement must be examined closely to determine that the statutorily-imposed obligations on the general partner do not conflict with the exempt organization's ability to pursue its charitable goals.

The IRS examined first whether the nonprofit organization was serving a charitable purpose, noting that *charitable* includes "relief of the poor and distressed,"[13] and that the term also includes caring for the "special needs of the aged."[14] The IRS determined that the management functions of the nonprofit organization of insuring compliance with HUD policies and procedures and implementation of various tenant grievance systems and social programs would serve the special needs of the elderly and constitute sufficient charitable activities.

The IRS then reviewed the partnership arrangement itself to determine if it "permits the exempt organization to act exclusively in furtherance of the purposes for which exemption was granted and not for the benefit of limited partners." The IRS concluded that the partnership did not, to a substantial extent, further private interests, in that the nonprofit organization was insulated from loss due to the HUD-insured mortgage, and was further protected by the partnership agreement's provision that the nonprofit would not be responsible for operating losses. The government concluded that the nonprofit's tax exempt status would not be adversely affected, and that management fees received from the partnership would not be considered unrelated business income.

Although letter rulings are not to be relied on as precedent, this 1984 ruling is indicative of the approach that the IRS may take in reviewing the implications upon tax exempt status of a retirement facility joint venture partnership between for profit and nonprofit entities. While, in Ruling 7820058, the IRS seemed concerned with (1) the sharing of net profits, and (2) the obligation of a nonprofit general partner to further the for profit limited partners' interests, the 1984 Ruling appeared more concerned with the ongoing charitable nature of the nonprofit manager's role and its insulation from liability.

RULING 8449070

In another 1984 Letter Ruling regarding a retirement facility (No. 8449070), the government determined that a nonprofit organization acting as a managing general partner in a limited partnership with a one percent interest in profits and losses, and receiving a fee of six percent of *gross* rentals, was not jeopardizing its exempt status or receiving unrelated business income. Again, the IRS appeared concerned not with the sharing of profits so much as the "charitable goals" of managing and maintaining the

---

[13]Reg. § 1.501(c)(3)-1(d)(2).
[14]Rev. Rul. 72-124, 1972-1 C.B. 145.

elderly housing complex and the "limited responsibility" of the nonprofit under the partnership agreement.

RULING 8425129

Yet another 1984 Ruling (No. 8425129) involving senior housing permitted a nonprofit organization to enter into an arrangement where it would act as the general partner, contributing a 20 percent share of capital, and having a 10 percent share of profit. In addition, a for profit management company was to be treated as a special limited partner entitled to a 10 percent share of profits in return for making a 10 percent capital contribution, *and* would receive a five percent management fee for managing the project. In response to the IRS's concerns about the payments to the management company constituting a private benefit, the applicant convinced the IRS that the transaction was exempt by showing that the nonprofit general partner could not be removed without its consent, and the five percent management fee was reasonable. Here, even for profit management appeared acceptable provided it was for a reasonable fee and did not disempower the nonprofit entity of control.

RULING 8545063

In Letter Ruling 8545063, the Internal Revenue Service considered the exempt status of a nonprofit corporation acting as the general partner in limited partnerships established to invest in low income housing and eventually sell the properties to tenant cooperatives. Although the limited partnership was to have a "standby general partner" required to maintain a minimum net worth in the event the nonprofit's net worth decreased, it was the nonprofit entity that was to manage the entire partnership. Importantly, however, the nonprofit's liability for partnership obligations, unlike most general partners, was to be limited to the amount of its capital investment, which equaled 10 percent of project cost. In addition, general and limited partners were to receive a return on investment of only about four percent per year from rental payments made after the coop reserved for capital improvements and operations expenses.

The IRS noted that the participation of a nonprofit organization in a partnership arrangement does not per se result in denial of exempt status, but that if a charitable purpose is established, the partnership arrangement will be examined to determine if it "permits the exempt organization to act exclusively in furtherance of the purposes for which the exemption may be granted and not for the benefit of the limited partners."

After finding the cooperative housing purpose to be exempt as "combating community deterioration" (see § 9.4), the IRS listed several factors supporting its conclusion that the joint arrangement was exempt and the income was not subject to tax:

1. The nonprofit made nominal contributions to capital;
2. Its liability was limited to its investment, and it had no responsibility to repay limited partners from its account;

3. The obligations to provide additional working capital were shared with the standby partner;
4. The for profit limited partners had no voice in management, and the standby general partner had no managerial control absent a severe deficit or mismanagement;
5. Leases to low and moderate income tenants were required by the terms of construction loans; and
6. Income to limited partners was limited due to the requirements for reserves, and the cap on return on investment.

While private letter rulings cannot be relied upon as precedent,[15] the pattern of rulings relating to the role of a nonprofit general partner in a senior housing limited partnership indicates an IRS position permitting such transactions where the nonprofit maintains control over the charitably oriented operations and does not put its assets at unlimited risk for partnership liabilities. In other words, where the nonprofit has the management and control attributes of a general partner, but has limited liability more akin to that of a limited partner, the nonprofit can, at least in these circumstances, venture with for profit investors on an equity contributing, profit sharing basis, without jeopardizing its exempt status or generating unrelated business income. However, the parties to any contemplated joint venture partnership between nonprofit and for profit entities should give careful consideration to obtaining a private letter ruling in advance of formation.

MEDICAL OFFICE BUILDING RULINGS

Although rulings related directly to retirement facilities have largely concerned nonprofits in the role of general partner of a limited partnership, several other permutations of involvement have been reviewed by the IRS in the context of medical office buildings, in which exempt hospitals joint venture with private physicians. In general, medical office buildings have been found to promote the general exempt purposes of the nonprofit hospital by attracting physicians and their patients to use the hospital and its services. Various IRS letter rulings have approved joint ventures between exempt hospitals and physicians where the hospital's nonprofit subsidiary is a general partner in the limited partnership,[16] where the hospital itself was the general partner,[17] where the hospital's for profit subsidiary was the general partner in a limited partnership,[18] where the hospital forms a general partnership directly with a for profit entity,[19] and where it enters into various lease relationships with the profit entity.[20]

---

[15] I.R.C. § 6110(j)(3).
[16] Priv. Ltr. Rul. 8226146.
[17] Priv. Ltr. Rul. 8201072.
[18] Priv. Ltr. Rul. 8243212.
[19] Priv. Ltr. Rul. 8206093.
[20] See, e.g., Priv. Ltr. Rul. 8134021, 8232035.

(c) Use of a Subsidiary Corporation

While it is possible for a nonprofit to engage directly in a partnership or other equity joint venture with a for profit organization or individual investors, required limitations upon the financial commitment of the nonprofit entity, and upon the opportunity for sharing control with profit-motivated investors, may dictate a different structure. Therefore, nonprofit organizations often form a for profit subsidiary corporation to act as the joint venture partner with the coventuring for profit organization. In addition, a for profit subsidiary, although subject to taxation, may create less risk of jeopardy to the nonprofit's exempt status than a more direct coventure.

The IRS has generally permitted exempt organizations to perform unrelated business activities through for profit subsidiary corporations. The government has viewed the situation as a permissible investment by the nonprofit parent, which results in no taxation of dividends paid to the parent, and no attribution of the subsidiary's income to the parent, even though the parent and subsidiary share office space and management (but not financial accounts).[21] Note, however, that if the subsidiary's corporate identity is ignored, due to undercapitalization or other defect, dividends would likely be treated as interest income and taxed to the parent.[22]

In GCM 39326, IRS counsel opined that where the taxable subsidiary of a nonprofit exempt organization was formed for a bona fide business purpose, and not as a mere agent of the parent, the parent's exemption would not be jeopardized. The analysis considered, among other things, the degree of involvement of the parent in the management structure and in day-to-day activities. Despite the fact that the parent owned all the stock of the subsidiary and received dividends, appointed the subsidiary's board of directors, and had the same executive director as the subsidiary, the subsidiary was found not to be a mere instrumentality of the parent.

For reasons such as insulation from liability, or health care reimbursement advantages, nonprofit parent organizations may wish to create a nonprofit subsidiary to participate in the venture. In addition to issues related to the relationship between the joint venturers, there is in that case the question of whether the joint activity is itself charitable or otherwise eligible for exemption (see, generally, Part IV). Even if a subsidiary organization engaged in a nonexempt activity turns over all its profits to its tax exempt parent, that organization will still be subject to taxation as a "feeder organization."[23] For example, laundries or other shared service organizations controlled by tax exempt hospitals have been found not to be eligible for exemption.[24] One exception that may be applicable in the retirement

---

[21]Priv. Ltr. Ruls. 8111030, 8116121, 8303019. *See, generally,* Hopkins & Beckwith, note 8, above, at 736.

[22]*See* I.R.C. §§ 482, 512(b)(13).

[23]*See* I.R.C. § 502.

[24]*See Associated Hospital Services, Inc.* 74 T.C. 213 (1980).

facility context is for organizations engaged in deriving rents, where the rents qualify as income exempt from unrelated business income taxation.[25] Thus, a nonprofit's subsidiary whose sole purpose is collecting rents and turning them over to the parent could still qualify for exemption.[26]

However, most nonprofits that joint venture with for profit entities resort to the use of for profit subsidiaries. Formation of a for profit subsidiary amounts to acquiescence that the joint venture activity is unrelated to the parent corporation's exempt purpose and that the income from the venture is taxable. Nevertheless, it is a desirable option for the venturers where the benefits of the venture are not limited to tax considerations, and provided the nonprofit parent's exempt status is not jeopardized.

(d) Nonprofit Vendor Contracts

Equity joint venture relationships between for profits and nonprofits may pose significant concerns for both parties about their tax treatment. While these problems can be overcome with careful planning to the mutual benefit of the joint venturers, it is often easier to structure a relationship that involves a simple management contract or development agreement.

(1) Unrelated Business Taxable Income

Nonprofit organizations with contracts to provide goods, facilities, or services to for profit entities normally receive income from the for profit organizations. An exempt corporation's receipt of payments from for profit organizations does not necessarily lead to receipt of unrelated business taxable income. For example, under Internal Revenue Code Section 512 (b)(1), interest received by a tax exempt corporation as a result of a loan to a for profit venture is exempt. Similarly, rents received by an exempt organization as the result of a lease of real or personal property to a for profit business are exempt from unrelated business income tax, unless significant services are provided to the lessee under the rental agreement,[27] rent is based on a percentage of income or profits derived from the leased property (unless based on a fixed percentage of gross receipts or sales),[28] or substantial personal property is leased with the real property.[29] The tax exempt organization can also receive income from the sale of real property to the venture without substantial fear of taxation.[30] However, the exempt organization is subject to tax on rents or interest received

---

[25]I.R.C. §§ 502(b)(1); 512(b)(3). *See, generally,* discussion at § 9.10(b), above.
[26]*See also* I.R.C. §§ 501(c)(2), (c)(25) regarding tax exempt title holding corporations and trusts.
[27]Reg. § 1.512(b)-1(c)(5).
[28]Reg. § 1.512(b)-1(c)(2)(iii)(b).
[29]Reg. § 1.512(b)-1(c)(2)(iii)(a).
[30]*See* I.R.C. § 512(b)(5).

from a for profit entity that it controls (i.e., owns 80 percent or more of the shares).[31]

Where a tax exempt hospital and its tax exempt subsidiary leased land to a limited partnership for the construction of a medical office building and parking lot, the IRS found that the hospital's receipt of fair market value rent for the land on which the for profit medical office building was to be constructed, plus a percentage of receipts from the parking lot, was passive income and not taxable as unrelated business income.[32] However, rental income based on a percentage of the lessee's net profits, rather than gross receipts, is subject to tax on unrelated business income.[33]

Passive involvement on the part of the exempt entity simply may not be a sufficient incentive for either party to proceed with the venture. Nonprofit organizations are often approached by developers of retirement facilities because of their experience in operations and delivery of services. Nonprofits are a natural choice, especially for the delivery of health care services. However, in situations where the nonprofit is acting as the retirement facility manager, it should be noted that mere management of elderly housing (even tax exempt elderly housing) may not be deemed consistent with its charitable purposes, and may lead to the realization of unrelated business taxable income, or even loss of tax exemption if pursued to a substantial degree.[34] One solution may be for the managing nonprofit to have some form of equity interest in the venture.

(2)   Private Inurement

A major tax exemption concern for nonprofits contemplating contractual relationships with for profit organizations is private inurement. In general, the exempt organization must receive adequate compensation for its services, for rental of its property, or for loans of its money to a for profit organization.

Gifts or transfers of assets have been found to result in private inurement,[35] as have rentals or sales of the nonprofit's property at less than fair market value,[36] as well as loans at below market rates, or loans insufficiently secured.[37]

Nevertheless, some arrangements appearing on the surface to be for less than full value have been upheld. For example, in Private Letter Ruling 8134021, the leasing by a nonprofit hospital of its land to a for profit corporation for one dollar per year was deemed not to constitute private inurement, where the corporation was to develop a medical office building on

---

[31]I.R.C. §§ 512(b)(13), 368(c).

[32]Priv. Ltr. Rul. 8138024. *See also* Priv. Ltr. Ruls. 8232035, 8134021.

[33]*Ohio County & Independent Agricultural Societies*, 43 T.C.M. 1126, T.C.M. 1982-210.

[34]See Rev. Rul. 70-535 and discussion at § 9.7, above.

[35]*Maynard Hospital, Inc. v. Comm'r*, 52 T.C. 1006 (1969).

[36]*Harding Hospital, Inc. v. U.S.*, 505 F.2d 1068 (6th Cir. 1974).

[37]*Lowry Hospital Ass'n v. Comm'r*, 66 T.C. 850 (1976).

the site for the hospital's benefit and the building would revert to the non-profit at the end of a 40 year lease term. A key to the ruling was a finding that the value of the building at the end of the 40 years was over double the fair market rental value of the land during the same period.

In general, if contract prices are negotiated at arm's length and represent fair market values when the entire transaction is viewed in context, private inurement problems should be easily avoided.

(e)   For Profit Vendor Contracts

Many nonprofit organizations, such as smaller church groups or congregations, may have little or no experience in the operation of a complex business such as a retirement facility. Many for profit management companies in the marketplace specialize in comprehensive retirement facility operations, food service, or health care services delivery. Nonprofits may maintain a tax exempt status for their retirement facility while contracting with a for profit organization to manage and operate the entire facility, provided all the prerequisites of the applicable revenue rulings are met (see § 9), the nonprofit organization maintains sufficient control over the operations of the facility, and compensation to the for profit does not result in private inurement.

If absolute discretion in management is given to the for profit management company, a question arises as to whether the nonprofit organization retains sufficient control over the retirement facility to assure that exclusively charitable purposes are pursued. Revenue Ruling 72-124, and successive rulings, tended to focus on retirement facilities that are owned and operated by the tax exempt organization, and have not dealt with the issue of for profit management of a facility owned by an exempt organization. However, in at least one General Counsel Memorandum,[38] the fact that a retirement facility lost control over its no eviction policy, by permitting uncontrolled banks to hold mortgages against units sold as condominiums, was enough to result in loss of exempt status for the facility. Therefore, it is important for the tax exempt owner to retain sufficient control over operations, such as by restrictions in the for profit manager's contract, to ensure that the charitable activities are carried out.

In addition to retaining control, the exempt entity must be sure that its activities do not benefit private interests except to the extent necessary to pursue its exempt goals. A nonprofit, in its contractual dealings with the for profit entity, therefore, cannot pay more than is reasonable when purchasing goods or services, borrowing money, or leasing property.

Although it has been held that compensation paid by a nonprofit corporation based on a percentage of its revenues resulted in private inurement,[39] such compensation is permissible where it is reasonable and negotiated at

---

[38] GCM 38478, Aug. 6, 1985.

[39] See, e.g., Sonora Community Hospital v. Comm'r, 46 T.C. 519 (1966), aff'd 397 F.2d 814 (9th Cir. 1968).

arm's length, where the income base bears some relation to the services being performed, and where the arrangement does not result in undue control over the exempt entity's activities.[40] A retirement facility venture between a non-profit and for profit entity, resulting in payment of a management fee to the for profit of five percent of gross rents, plus 10 percent of profits (in return for an equity contribution) was approved by the IRS as reasonable compensation.[41]

If the nonprofit organization has obtained tax exempt financing for the project, certain limitations on for profit management contracts are imposed by Revenue Procedures 82-14 and 82-15.[42] The Tax Reform Act of 1986 directs the Treasury Department to liberalize the contract guidelines contained in Revenue Procedures 82-14 and 82-15.[43] The new guidelines provide that in order to preserve the tax exempt status of the financing, the for profit manager may have a contract of no more than five years' duration, including renewal options, with an option on the part of the nonprofit facility owner to terminate the contract every three years. In addition, at least 50 percent of the annual compensation of the for profit manager must be based on a periodic fixed fee, and any portion of the compensation based on a percentage of revenues must be based on gross revenue, rather than net profits. If the governing body of the exempt organization has five or more members, one member, other than the chief executive officer, may be an employee or officer of the manager.[44]

§ 12.2   PRESERVING FOR PROFIT TAX ADVANTAGES

(a)   ACRS after the Tax Reform Act of 1986

The accelerated cost recovery system (ACRS) permits an owner to depreciate real property, equipment, and improvements on real property, such as buildings, at an accelerated rate, depending on the class in which the Internal Revenue Code places the particular property. Prior to the Tax Reform Act of 1986, real property could be depreciated over a 19 year recovery period using 175 percent accelerated depreciation.[45] Low income housing could be depreciated by using a 200 percent acceleration factor.[46] For residential rental property, the excess of accelerated depreciation over the straight line method is recaptured on its disposition, that is, treated as ordinary income.[47] For commercial property, the entire depreciation is recaptured.[48]

---

[40]*University of Maryland Physicians v. Comm'r*, 41 T.C.M. 732 (1981).

[41]Priv. Ltr. Rul. 8425129.

[42]1982-2 C.B. 459, 460.

[43]P.L. 99-514 § 1301(e); *see also* I.R.C. §§ 145(a) and 141(b)(1)–(2).

[44]Rev. Proc. 82-14, 1982-2 C.B. 459.

[45]I.R.C. § 168(b)(2)(A) as it existed prior to the Tax Reform Act of 1986.

[46]I.R.C. § 168(b)(4)(A) as it existed prior to the Tax Reform Act of 1986.

[47]I.R.C. §§ 1245(a)(5) and 1250 as they existed prior to the Tax Reform Act of 1986.

[48]I.R.C. § 1245(a).

The 1986 Tax Reform Act retains a modified ACRS system, but requires that residential real property be depreciated using the straight line method, over a 27.5 year period. There is no recapture of depreciation for residential or commercial property under the new rules. However, the difference between the amount allowable under this method and the ADR system (see § 12.2(b)) is treated as a tax preference item. The 1986 Act's changes are generally effective for property placed in service after December 31, 1986.

Certain exceptions are available for property acquired or constructed under a contract binding as of March 1, 1986, not subject to substantial modification, and placed in service prior to 1991. A contract is deemed binding only if it is legally enforceable and does not contain a provision limiting damages for breach to less than five percent of the contract price. A binding contract includes a contract subject to a condition, provided neither party has control over the condition.[49] It also includes an irrevocable put, but not an option to purchase the property.[50] A disqualifying substantial modification does not include design changes made for reasons of technical or economic efficiencies that do not significantly increase project costs.

Relief from the new rules is also available for certain property constructed or reconstructed by the taxpayer if (1) the lesser of $1 million or four percent of the property cost was incurred or committed by March 1, 1986, (2) significant work on the property had been commenced by that date, and (3) the property is placed in service by January 1, 1991. Qualifying property is also eligible for this exemption if it is sold and leased back within three months of being placed in service by the buyer.

Prior to the 1986 Act, low income housing had a special ACRS status as 15 year real property, as compared with the 19 year depreciation classification of other residential real property. The favored treatment of low income housing in this regard has now been eliminated, and it is treated, along with all other residential rental structures, as 27.5 year property.

Nonresidential real property is subject to a 31.5 year ACRS depreciation schedule.[51]

(b) Tax Exempt Use Property

(1) In General

An alternative to the 27.5 year depreciation schedule outlined above is based on asset depreciation range (ADR) midpoints. Under this methodology, real property depreciation is based on a straight line method over a 40 year recov-

---

[49]P.L. 99-514 § 203(b)(1)(A), 203(b)(2); Rep. of the Comm. of Conf. on H.R. 3838, at II-53, reprinted in 1986 U.S.C. Cong. & Admin. News No. 9B, at II-53.

[50]Rep. of the Comm. of Conf. on H.R. 3838, at II-55, reprinted in 1986 U.S.C. Cong. & Admin. News No. 9B, at II-55.

[51]I.R.C. § 168(c).

ery period. No tax preference income is attributable to use of the ADR depreciation system. While use of the ADR system is always an option for real property owners, its use in lieu of the 27.5 year ACRS system is mandatory for "tax exempt use property" and tax exempt bond financed property.[52]

Tax exempt use property includes residential rental property that is leased to a tax exempt entity, and where any one of the following circumstances applies: (1) the lease is for a term of more than 20 years, (2) any part of the property was financed by the exempt corporation or a related entity using tax exempt financing under Code Section 103, (3) the exempt entity retains an option allowing it or a related entity to purchase the property at a fixed or calculable price, or (4) the property has previously been used by the tax exempt corporation or a related entity and the property is then sold and leased back to the tax exempt organization.[53] Tax exempt use property must be depreciated over a term of 40 years or 125 percent of the lease term, whichever is greater, using the straight line method.[54]

Low and moderate income housing projects financed with tax exempt bonds are not subject to the 40 year depreciation schedule used for other forms of tax exempt use property, but may qualify for an alternative 27.5 year schedule.[55]

The restrictions of the 1986 Act do not apply to exempt bond financed property placed in service after December 31, 1986, to the extent that the issue was prior to March 2, 1986.[56] In addition, the new rules do not apply to projects with binding construction contracts in place prior to March 1, 1986.[57] However, pre-1986 law also placed similar 40 year depreciation schedules upon tax exempt use property, and the 1986 Act does not represent a significant departure from prior law.[58]

A nonprofit organization cannot avoid tax exempt use rules simply by creating a new for profit organization to, for example, lease property in its stead, due to a five year "look back" rule, which characterizes the transaction as one with the parent exempt entity.[59]

(2) Service Contracts

Another attempted method of avoiding tax exempt use property rules has been to structure transactions as service agreements rather than leases.[60]

---

[52] I.R.C. § 168(g)(1)(B), (C).

[53] *See* I.R.C. § 168(h)(1)(B).

[54] I.R.C. § 168(g)(2), (3).

[55] I.R.C. §§ 168(g)(5)(C), 142(a)(7), 142(d).

[56] P.L. 99-514, § 203(c).

[57] P.L. 99-514, § 203(b).

[58] *See* I.R.C. § 168(j) prior to amendment by the Tax Reform Act of 1986.

[59] I.R.C. § 168(h)(2)(E).

[60] See I.R.C. § 7701(e)(1).

However, the IRS may recharacterize the transaction as a lease, based on such factors as whether:

(1) The service recipient is in physical possession of the property;

(2) The service recipient controls the property;

(3) The service recipient has a significant economic or possessory interest in the property;

(4) The service provider does not bear any risk of substantially diminished receipts or substantially increased expenditures if there is nonperformance under the contract;

(5) The service provider does not use the property concurrently to provide significant services to entities unrelated to the service recipient; and

(6) The total contract price does not substantially exceed the rental value of the property for the contract period.

In the context of retirement housing, for example, a contract for more than 20 years in which a for profit facility owner purports to deliver operational or other services to a nonprofit organization may be recharacterized as a lease where the exempt organization has possession or control of the property, pays service fees approximately equal to the property's rental value, and has no right to withhold payments or terminate the contract in the event of the for profit's nonperformance of services. A more typical service agreement is one in which a nonprofit organization is the provider of services to a for profit retirement facility owner and, in the course of managing the facility, it takes possession or control of the premises. Such an arrangement should not be subject to recharacterization as a lease, assuming the nonprofit service provider receives reasonable payment for the services, and is not in effect performing them as some form of in-kind payment of rent to the for profit owner.[61]

Low income housing operated by a 501(c)(3) or 501(c)(4) organization, 80 percent or more of the units of which are leased to low income tenants, is exempt from the service contract rules.[62]

§ 12.3   EXAMPLE OF A FOR PROFIT/NONPROFIT JOINT VENTURE

(a)   Benefits of the Venture

One possible joint venture scenario between a for profit developer and a nonprofit operating entity involves a lease of the premises from the developer to

---

[61] *See, e.g., Federal Tax Coordinator,* 2d, RIA, ¶ L-8090, at 34,652 K, citing S. Rep., P.L. 98-369, 7/18/84, at 140.

[62] I.R.C. § 7701(e)(5).

the nonprofit entity. In projects where entrance fees or other substantial sums are to be received by the retirement facility from residents, for profit facility operators are justifiably concerned about the considerable tax consequences of receiving such fees as income.[63] Although the use of a loan of entrance fees from the resident to the facility can solve the problem of taxable income to the for profit operator, it can also create an imputed interest problem for the resident-lender, unless market rate interest is paid to the resident.[64]

A lease arrangement between a for profit and nonprofit entity permits the retirement facility to receive entrance fee proceeds via the nonprofit organization, without taxation, and also allows the for profit owner to take advantage of the accelerated depreciation deductions available to real property owners. Of course, to avoid characterization as tax exempt use property, the lease must be for 20 years or less, cannot contain a fixed or calculable price purchase option, and cannot be part of a sale-leaseback transaction, and the project cannot be financed by tax exempt bonds.[65] The facility will not be eligible for exemption from real property tax because the nonprofit organization has the status of lessee, without any ownership interest.[66]

Depreciation and rental incomes may be sufficient economic reward and motivation for developers in many real estate transactions. However, some developers may want to receive the benefits and bear the responsibilities of ongoing operation of the project. Lease payments to a for profit business based on revenues of a tax exempt organization may raise significant concerns about private inurement.[67] However, sharing profits as a form of lease payment may be justifiable if commercially reasonable. For example, periodic rents initially set at a below market rate may justify the later payment of a bonus to the developer once the facility has sold out and is generating positive cash flows on a consistent basis. A further potential reason for sharing net revenues from the nonprofit operation may include unusual risks taken or benefits offered by the lessor/developer in the development process, such as delivering a turnkey, sold-out project, or covering tenant operating deficits pending sell out of the project.

In the context of a continuing care facility, where substantial entrance fees may be paid to the nonprofit corporation by residents at the outset of facility operations, the developer may also be interested in obtaining some use of those entrance fees to help retire construction debt. It may be possible, therefore, for the nonprofit organization to loan some or all of the entrance fees received from residents to the developer. To some extent, interest on the loan received by the nonprofit may be used to fund the cost of monthly lease payments.

---

[63] *See* discussion at § 6.1(b), above.

[64] *See* § 6.2(b), above.

[65] *See* § 12.2(b), above.

[66] *See* discussion at § 10, above.

[67] *See* discussion at § 12.1(e), above.

Figure 12.1 illustrates a structure[68] where a for profit owner-developer leases a retirement facility to a nonprofit operating organization, which sells transferable memberships to residents for a substantial price. The nonprofit loans the entrance fees, less amounts needed for reserves and operations, to the for profit at a market rate of interest. Whenever a resident sells a membership to another person at an appreciated value, the resident is required to turn over a portion of the appreciation to the nonprofit. Rent payable by the nonprofit lessee includes a bonus payment consisting of a share of any appreciation received by the nonprofit from residents.

The goals and possible benefits of this structure include the following:

1. The resident, nonprofit operator, and for profit developer all benefit by sharing in the appreciated value of memberships when resold, and thus all retain a long-term interest in the success of the project.
2. The development experience of the for profit and the operational experience of the nonprofit are each utilized for the benefit of the overall project.

FIGURE 12.1 SAMPLE NONPROFIT/FOR PROFIT JOINT VENTURE

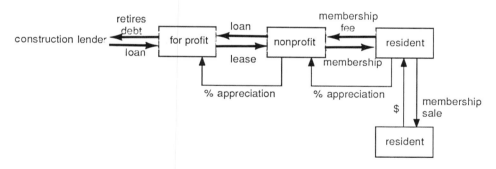

For Profit

1. Borrows construction financing
2. Owns and develops property
3. Leases building to nonprofit
4. Borrows membership fees from nonprofit to repay construction lender

Nonprofit

1. Rents building from for profit
2. Obtains license to operate facility and collects resident fees
3. Loans membership fee proceeds to for profit owner
4. Collects share of appreciated membership values and pays portion as rent

[68]This structure is presented for purposes of illustrating business considerations and legal issues that may be present in a for profit-nonprofit coventure. It is not meant to describe any particular transaction or facility structure in the marketplace. Its presentation and the discussion do not purport to represent the position that the IRS or the courts would take respecting such a structure.

3. Lump sum fees paid by residents reach the developer, via a loan from the nonprofit, for use in retiring construction debt, without taxation of the fees as income to the developer.

4. Residents have the opportunity to recover some or all of their payments through resale of the memberships, as do residents of refundable entrance fee facilities, but they are not subject to tax on imputed interest because the transaction is fashioned as a sale, rather than as a loan.

5. The nonprofit organization is able to fund at least part of its lease payment obligation from interest income received from the loan to the developer.

6. The developer, as owner, can depreciate the property.

(b) Venture Legal Issues

Any complex structure such as this example can raise a host of legal questions, related primarily to the tax consequences of the transaction. Among the issues[69] raised by the illustration are:

(1) Whether the tax exempt status of the nonprofit organization is jeopardized because:
   (a) The payment of bonus rent from appreciation in membership values results in private inurement or gain from the exempt organization's activities; or
   (b) The transaction is tantamount to an equity joint venture in which the nonprofit has significant liability exposure and insufficient operational control, or other factors exist that compromise pursuit of its charitable purposes.

(2) Whether the loan from the lessee to the lessor will result in treatment of the transaction as a sale rather than a true lease, or characterization of the loan as prepaid rent.

The lease/loan structure has many advantages for both parties, but the transaction must be approached with caution. The nonprofit corporation should not be created or controlled by the for profit organization so that there is less risk of its being considered a mere instrumentality or alter ego of the for profit,[70] resulting in possible loss of the organization's tax exempt status. The transaction between the nonprofit and for profit must be at arm's length, and lease payments and interest rates must be set at fair

---

[69]These issues are also discussed generally elsewhere in this book, *e.g.*, private inurement (§§ 9.1(b), 12.1), equity joint ventures (§ 12.1(b)), loans versus sales (§ 6.2(a)).

[70]*See, e.g., Vaughn v. U.S.*, 740 F.2d 941 (Fed. Cir. 1984) for a discussion of agency for federal tax purposes.

market values. It is also important, if the nonprofit corporation is to avoid being characterized as a passive agent or nominee for the for profit entity, that it have broad functions and business purposes not solely limited to improving the tax consequences of the retirement facility transaction for the for profit entity.[71] If the nonprofit corporation has been created solely for the purpose of engaging in the lease and loan transactions with the for profit owner, or if the nonprofit has no business or economic purpose other than tax avoidance for the for profit owner, its exempt status, or very existence, may be ignored and the transaction subjected to taxation as a sale directly from the for profit entity to the resident. On the other hand, where the nonprofit has significant management functions and control over its charitable activities, its separate status should be recognized.

A further concern with a for profit/nonprofit lease and loan arrangement is to ensure that the for profit owner of the property is treated as the owner by the IRS, so that depreciation deductions may be taken. In addition, if viewed as a sale, the loan proceeds could be viewed as the sale price and taxable income received by the developer.

In *Sun Oil v. Commissioner*,[72] the federal Third Circuit Court of Appeals pointed to several factors in a lessee-financed sale-leaseback transaction[73] that tended to jeopardize the status of the lessor as owner, including: (1) the correlation between the lessee's rental payments and the lessor's interest and principal payments on the loan, (2) the lessee's option to purchase the property at the end of the lease term for less than fair market value, (3) the right of the lessee to renew the lease for a cumulative term of 90 years, with reduced rental payments during the later renewal periods, (4) the right of the lessee to terminate the lease by purchasing the property in certain situations, and (5) the right of the lessee to receive all appreciation value of the property in the event of a taking by eminent domain. The court found that in that case the seller/lessee had not relinquished ownership of the property.

In another sale-leaseback case, *Frank Lyon Co. v. United States*,[74] the Supreme Court found that because, among other things, the lessor/owner financed the purchase of the building through a third party lender and was personally liable for the debt, the lessor was the true owner, despite the fact that the rental payments were equivalent to the loan payments due, that the lessee had purchase options designed to return a calculable profit on the lessor's investment, and that the lease term exceeded the useful life of the building.

---

[71] *See, generally, Stringfellow v. U.S.*, 246 F. Supp. 474 (D.C. Wash. 1965), *Niagara County Savings Bank v. Comm'r*, T.C.M. 1984-247.

[72] 562 F.2d 258 (3d Cir. 1977), *cert. den.* 436 U.S. 944 (1978).

[73] In a sale-leaseback transaction, the property owner sells the property and then leases it back from the buyer. The issue analogous to this example is whether the lease terms in actuality give the lessee an ownership interest in the property.

[74] 435 U.S. 561 (1978).

However, in *Hilton v. Commissioner*,[75] a sale-leaseback was found to lack economic substance where lessee's rents and lessor's debt service were correlated, the lessee had options to renew the lease, rental payments were not tied to fair market value, and investors had made no significant investment in the property and could realize no significant gain from their participation in the transaction. Likewise, the Tax Court has construed as advance rental payments, loan proceeds from a lessee where the lease and loan payments were identical, each was due at the same time, no money changed hands, and the loan was neither interest bearing nor secured.[76]

A lessee-financed or leveraged lease from a for profit to a nonprofit entity is less likely to be recharacterized as a sale or prepaid lease if (1) the obligations of the loan and lease are severable and not contingent upon each other, (2) the financial obligations of the parties to each other under the lease and loan do not exactly offset each other and payments are actually made, (3) the lease is for a term substantially less than the property's useful life, (4) the loan bears interest and is secured, (5) rental payments, interest, and purchase options are at fair market value and the purchase option price is not fixed or calculable at the beginning of the lease term, (6) the lessee does not have substantial ownership rights (see discussion below), and (7) the lessor retains some of the risks and benefits of ownership. In addition, the existence at least of initial third party recourse financing arranged by the lessor, to be taken out by the loan of entrance fee proceeds, can aid in a determination that the lessor is the owner.

One of the incidents of ownership in a retirement facility operation may be the right to benefit from appreciation in the value of units upon resale. For reasons noted earlier, it may well be in the interest of both parties to structure the transaction so that any appreciation resulting from the resale of a unit is shared by the owner and lessee. In a service-oriented facility, sharing appreciation in value with the lessee should be justifiable on the basis that the lessee, as operator of the facility's services, contributes substantially to the appreciation in value of a given unit. To that extent, receipt of a portion of the appreciated value of that unit is not necessarily an indicator that real property ownership is being retained by the lessee, and the owner's relinquishment of a portion of the appreciation should not eliminate the owner's ability to take advantage of ownership tax benefits.

Although sharing appreciation of unit values is a form of profit sharing, which is a characteristic of a partnership, the transaction should not be characterized as such. The central feature of a joint venture that will be treated as a partnership for tax purposes is "a proprietary interest in the net profits of the enterprise coupled with an obligation to share its losses."[77] In this example, a portion of gross profit is divided by contractual arrangement, any of

---

[75]74 T.C. 305 (1980), *aff'd* 671 F.2d 16 (9th Cir. 1982), *cert. den.* 459 U.S. 907 (1982).

[76]*Blue Flame Gas Co.*, 54 T.C. 584 (1970). *See also* Rev. Proc. 75-21, 1975-1 C.B. 715.

[77]*Federal Bulk Carriers, Inc.*, 66 T.C. 283, 293 (1976).

the nonprofit's losses from business operations are not shared by the owner, and the owner's losses, if any, as a result of a decline in real estate values are not shared by the lessee.

§ 13 OTHER JOINT VENTURE CONSIDERATIONS

Numerous other legal and business structure issues may be present in any joint venture retirement facility transaction. These may include such matters as the antitrust consequences of the creation of a new joint venture entity or of the venture parties' dealings with it, Medicare reimbursement implications to one or more of the venturing parties, or the effect on their pension plans or collective bargaining agreements.[78] Although these are matters that may not arise until operations are well under way, they should be considered at least in general terms during the project's planning and development.

§ 13.1 MEDICARE/MEDICAID ISSUES

(a) Reimbursement

Medicare reimbursement considerations can be extremely complicated, particularly for institutional coventurers such as hospitals. Historically, Medicare has reimbursed almost all covered health care services on the basis of the lesser of the provider's cost, or reasonable charges.[79] Normally, this means, for example, that a nursing facility purchasing a service, such as laundering, from another entity would be reimbursed for the percentage of cost of the service, based on Medicare utilization, to the nursing facility, which would include a profit margin charged by the laundry service. However, when a provider receives facilities, goods, or services from another organization related to it by common ownership or control, Medicare limits the purchasing provider's reimbursement to the related seller's cost or the market price, whichever is less.[80] There is, therefore, little reimbursement advantage in a joint venture context for parent organizations to lease facilities or sell services or goods to a subsidiary joint venture entity (which can be reimbursed only for the seller's cost) when a sale to an unrelated provider can be reimbursed in the amount of the seller's cost plus a reasonable margin of profit or return on investment.[81]

The adoption in 1983 of the prospective payment system (PPS) for Medicare reimbursement of inpatient hospital services has provided a strong

---

[78] See, generally, Roble & Mason, "The Legal Aspects of Health Care Joint Ventures," 24 Duquesne L. Rev. 455 (1985).

[79] See, generally, 42 C.F.R. §§ 405.402, et seq.

[80] 42 C.F.R. § 405.427.

[81] See, e.g., 42 C.F.R. § 405.429.

incentive for hospitals to become involved in other activities where more favorable Medicare or Medicaid reimbursement is available. Under PPS, hospital inpatient services are not reimbursed retroactively on the basis of costs, but according to a schedule of rates prospectively determined for each hospital discharge, according to diagnosis related groups (DRGs).[82] The PPS system is designed essentially to reduce overall expenditures by the Medicare program. Even if related party rules could be circumvented, PPS eliminates the incentive to maximize reimbursement for inpatient services by creating multiple cost-reimbursed profit centers. The prospective payment is the total payment for the service, even if portions are supplied by other entities.[83] Thus, hospitals may be looking for joint venture opportunities involving health services other than inpatient hospital care that are reimbursable directly by Medicare on the more favorable basis of cost.

Retirement facilities present opportunities for provision of Medicare cost-reimbursable health services such as skilled nursing,[84] home health,[85] rehabilitation,[86] and health maintenance.[87] Hospitals or other health providers may benefit from the more favorable reimbursement principally by having an equity interest in the nursing facility or other cost-reimbursed provider.[88] In addition, if the hospital furnishes facilities, goods, or services to the cost-reimbursed provider, the buyer, even if a subsidiary or controlled entity subject to the related party rules discussed above, can pay and be reimbursed for the hospital's cost of providing the services.[89] Even this cost reimbursement for the hospital's services or resources (without any profit) may be more remunerative than if the same resources were used to provide inpatient services subject to DRG limitations. Therefore, parent hospitals can indirectly subsidize with cost based reimbursement some of their existing in-house activities, such as laundry, dining, or pharmacy, that

---

[82]See 42 C.F.R. §§ 412.1, et seq.

[83]42 C.F.R. § 412.50.

[84]Unlike most other cost-reimbursed services under Medicare, skilled nursing services may be limited to a maximum per diem rate, which corresponds with the per diem rate for nursing services paid by states under their Medicaid programs. The federal government must satisfy itself that the state Medicaid rate fairly reflects costs and in some cases may pay a higher daily rate for Medicare skilled nursing services than does the state Medicaid program. See CCH, Medicare and Medicaid Guide, ¶ 6081. It should be noted that Medicare coverage for skilled nursing care is quite limited in scope. See discussion at § 26.1(b), below.

[85]See discussion at § 20.4, below.

[86]See 42 C.F.R. §§ 485.50, et seq. regarding Comprehensive Outpatient Rehabilitation Facilities (CORF).

[87]See 42 C.F.R. §§ 417.530, et seq.

[88]Skilled nursing facilities that are distinct parts of hospitals or are directly operated by them may be eligible for reimbursement on a cost basis in the same manner as other hospital services not subject to the prospective payment system. See CCH, note 84, above, at ¶ 6081.

[89]See, generally, Medicare Prov. Reimb. Man., Part 1, § 2135, CCH, Medicare and Medicaid Guide, ¶ 5995.

might be used to service a controlled rehabilitation, nursing, or other facility, or to provide services to a home health agency or health maintenance organization. Of course, using existing in-house departments to service outside enterprises also can promote desirable efficiencies and economies of scale.

(b)   Fraud and Abuse

(1)   Bed Reserve Agreements

Often, coventuring nursing facilities and hospitals contract to hold beds open or reserve other facilities or services for use when needed by the other venture party. For example, hospitals may be induced by Medicare or Medicaid reimbursement restrictions to discharge patients to a lower level of care sooner than if full reimbursement were available for a longer hospital stay. Hospitals may therefore desire to have an arrangement with a retirement facility that has excess bed capacity in its nursing unit to hold beds open and available to receive transfers from the hospital on a moment's notice. Similarly, a residential retirement facility can benefit from an arrangement with a nursing home or hospital to hold beds or otherwise grant priority admission, reduced fees, or favored treatment to retirement facility residents whenever health services are needed.

One Medicare/Medicaid issue inherent in such relationships concerns the payment received by a provider in exchange for its agreement to hold beds or bestow other favored treatment upon the other contracting party. Medicare and Medicaid providers are prohibited by regulatory fraud and abuse provisions from charging an individual for its agreement to admit the individual at a specified future date for inpatient services covered by the program.[90] In addition, there are criminal sanctions against requiring any payment from a Medicaid recipient or his family for covered services as a condition of admission or continued stay at the facility.[91]

Bed reserve agreements in which, for example, a hospital agrees to pay the difference between the nursing facility's private pay charges and the lower payment made by Medicaid for patients referred from the hospital, violate the nursing facility's provider agreement.[92] It is also a violation for the hospital to agree to provide personnel to the nursing facility whenever Medicare covered patients referred by the hospital occupy a reserved bed.[93] However, the hospital may pay a fee to the nursing facility for each day a bed is held open, or may agree to provide personnel or services to the

---

[90] 42 C.F.R. § 489.22(d).

[91] Social Security Act § 1909(d); 42 U.S.C. § 1396h(d); *see* discussion at § 9.2(b)(4), above.

[92] *See* note 89, above, ¶ 5875B.

[93] *Id.*

nursing facility without regard to whether the reserved beds are filled with Medicare patients, so long as the payment of consideration for holding beds open is not dependent on admission of or service to a Medicare or Medicaid patient.[94] Because the payment for reserving beds is not related to the care of patients, it is not an allowable cost to the payor, nor need the revenue be offset by the payee against its reimbursable costs.[95]

(2) Referral Payments

Solicitation, offering, payment, or receipt of remuneration for referring a person for the furnishing of goods or services reimbursed by Medicare or Medicaid or for participating in or recommending a sale, lease, or order of any reimbursable item is a federal felony.[96] An exception is made for discounts or price reductions if disclosed and properly reflected in cost reports, and for payments to employees for provision of covered items or services.[97]

A principal concern underlying this prohibition appears to be that a person in a position to control or direct the delivery of federally funded goods or services can be compensated for that exercise of discretion.[98] In one case, a medical laboratory was convicted for an arrangement in which it gave shares of its corporate stock to a medical clinic and a percentage of profits to the clinic director, and in return was permitted to set up its laboratory in the clinic at no cost to the clinic or its owners and with no real administrative duties required of the clinic director.[99] The court viewed the arrangement as one clearly involving remuneration for arranging for the purchase of Medicaid reimbursable lab services. Even where a provider performs a service for the party making the incentive payment, criminal conduct has been found where the purpose of the payment is to induce future referrals.[100]

Health care providers participating in retirement facility coventures must be cautious where there is an expectation that the retirement facility will serve as a source of referrals of patients or services to the health facility, or where the retirement home receives referrals from the other provider. If the entity making the referral of a Medicare or Medicaid patient or reimbursable product or service has a financial interest in the referee, the parties should have a strong independent basis for the referral. However, if the two entities are so closely related as to be considered a single entity, for example, equity partners, there is arguably less danger of

---

[94] *See id.*

[95] *Id.*

[96] 42 U.S.C. §§ 1395nn(b)(1)–(2), and 1396h(b)(1)–(2).

[97] 42 U.S.C. §§ 1395nn(b)(3), 1396h(b)(3).

[98] *See, generally,* Roble and Mason, note 78, above, at 463ff.

[99] *U.S. v. Universal Trade and Industries, Inc.,* 695 F.2d 1151 (9th Cir. 1983).

[100] *U.S. v. Greber,* 760 F.2d 68 (3d Cir. 1968).

a violation.[101] Exclusive transfer agreements or bonus payment arrangements generally should be avoided.[102]

§ 13.2 ANTITRUST ISSUES

Any joint venture may raise antitrust or restraint of trade issues, including the Sherman Act violations of participation in a contract, combination, or conspiracy in restraint of trade,[103] or creation of a monopoly.[104] Automatic or *per se* violations can occur where competitors contract or otherwise join forces to fix prices, or to divide markets, or where a party with sufficient economic power over the sale of one product or service establishes a tying arrangement that requires the buyer to purchase a second product or service in order to obtain access to the first.[105] In addition, exclusive dealing arrangements can be deemed *per se* violations where a significant number of competitors is excluded from the marketplace as a consequence.[106]

Another area of antitrust concern is price discrimination between purchasers in the sale of like commodities (not services), where the effect is to restrain competition.[107] An exemption exists for sales to nonprofit institutions purchasing the products for their own use in pursuit of their operations.[108]

Retirement facility coventurers must carefully analyze the antitrust implications of such practices or arrangements as:

1. Agreeing to make certain coventurer goods or services available only to the joint venture entity or to purchase certain goods or services exclusively from it (exclusive dealing problem);

2. Agreeing not to enter into other ventures or operations, or to go into other territories, that may compete with the other coventurer or with the joint venture entity (market division problem);

3. Requiring patients who use, for example, a coventurer's hospital services to accept a discharge to the joint venture nursing facility (tying arrangement problem);[109]

---

[101] *See* Roble and Mason, note 78, above, at 469.

[102] *Id.*

[103] Sherman Act, Section 1; 15 U.S.C. § 1.

[104] Sherman Act, Section 2; 15 U.S.C. § 2.

[105] *See, generally*, Roble and Mason, note 78, above, and discussion regarding tying arrangements at § 7.1(c), above and § 22.5(d), below.

[106] *See Jefferson Parish Hosp. Dist. No. 2 v. Hyde*, 466 U.S. 2 (1984) for a discussion of exclusive dealing arrangements (no violation found).

[107] Robinson-Patman Act, 15 U.S.C. §§ 13-13b, 21a.

[108] *See* 15 U.S.C. § 13c and *Abbott Laboratories v. Portland Retail Druggists Ass'n.*, 425 U.S. 1 (1976).

[109] An exception may exist where a unifying dimension to the arrangement, such as a life care contract or comprehensive health insurance policy, makes the hospital and nursing service part of a unified, single product.

4. Where a nonprofit hospital co-venturer uses pharmaceuticals that it received at a discount for patients of a for profit venture entity (price discrimination issue);

5. Where a co-venturer, with 50 percent or less ownership of the venture, agrees with the venture to set the price of a product or service they both sell (price fixing issue).

The presence of any significant market power on the part of a coventurer or the joint venture entity exacerbates the potential antitrust problems associated with any of the foregoing activities.

For those violations, such as price fixing and market division, that require a combination or conspiracy, at least two parties must be involved before a violation occurs. Independent joint venturers, of course, will be found to engage in such a prohibited agreement or understanding, but very closely related parties, such as a parent corporation and its wholly owned subsidiary, may be viewed as a single entity incapable of conspiring as a matter of law.[110] Similarly, competitors who combine as equity-contributing, risk-sharing partners in a joint venture business are treated as a single entity and may set the price that business will charge.[111]

§ 13.3   EMPLOYMENT RELATED ISSUES

(a)   ERISA

The principal employment related issue in a joint venture is whether the venture results in creation of a separate employer or will instead be treated as a mere extension of one or both of its founders.

Employee benefit plans under ERISA[112] must not unduly discriminate in favor of shareholders, managerial employees, or others similarly situated,[113] and top heavy plans where officers and shareholder employees earn more than 60 percent of the benefits must meet special tests regarding contributions and vesting.[114] When two entities are affiliated, they may be considered as a single employer for purposes of aggregating top-heavy benefit calculations and for review of discrimination.[115] The ostensible purpose of this law is to prevent employers from shifting higher level employees or shareholder-employees to related or controlled entities in order to permit favored treatment or avoidance of top-heavy rules.

[110]*Copperweld v. Independence Tube Co.*, 467 U.S. 752 (1984).

[111]See *Arizona v. Maricopa County Medical Society*, 457 U.S. 332, 356 (1982).

[112]Employee Retirement Income Security Act, I.R.C. §§ 401, *et seq.*

[113]*See, e.g.*, I.R.C. §§ 105(h), 125, 401, 410, and 505.

[114]I.R.C. § 416.

[115]*See* I.R.C. §§ 414(c), 416(c)(2).

Common vertical control is deemed to exist where one organization (the parent) owns at least 80 percent of another (the subsidiary).[116] Horizontally, an affiliation exists where five or fewer individuals, estates, or trusts, in aggregate own at least 80 percent of two or more organizations, or where the smallest of each such owner's interests, taken together, exceeds 50 percent of the organizations' ownership. In addition, affiliated service groups, which can include, among other things, an entity whose principal business is performing management services for another organization and the managed organization, are treated as a single employer.[117]

Joint venturers, such as hospitals, often loan employees to the joint venture retirement facility for reasons of economic efficiency and maximum utilization of existing resources. However, such practices could also be used to circumvent the intent of ERISA by employing only managerial or upper level employees at the retirement home, and using leased hospital employees to perform all other functions. ERISA addresses this problem by treating the leased employee as the employee of the recipient of the employee's services where (1) the services are performed pursuant to an agreement between the service recipient and the leasing organization, (2) the person has performed the services for the recipient or a related organization on a substantially full time basis for at least one year, and (3) the service is of a type historically performed by employees in the recipient's business field.[118] An exception to this rule exists for employees covered by certain pension plans that vest immediately, require an employer contribution of at least 7.5 percent of the employee's earnings, and are not dependent on employer profit.[119]

(b) Labor Laws

Minimum wage and overtime (time-and-a-half) pay requirements for work weeks of more than 40 hours are mandated by the Fair Labor Standards Act.[120] Again, the principal issue for joint ventures is whether an employee is working for one or more employers when his or her services are received by more than one of the entities involved in, or resulting from, the venture. Federal regulations state that a joint employment relationship, requiring aggregation of work hours and wages for overtime and minimum wage calculations, generally will be considered to exist in situations such as: (1) arrangements among employers to share or interchange employees, (2) where one employer acts, in relation to the employee, in the interest of the other employer, or (3) where the employers are not disassociated and can

---

[116]I.R.C. § 414(c).
[117]I.R.C. § 414(m)(5).
[118]I.R.C. § 414(n)(2).
[119]I.R.C. § 414(n)(5).
[120]29 U.S.C. §§ 201, *et seq.*

be deemed to share control over the employee by reason of the fact that one employer controls the other or both share common ownership.[121]

Similarly, for purposes of determining appropriate collective bargaining units under the National Labor Relations Act,[122] the National Labor Relations Board (NLRB) will look to such factors as centralized control of labor relations, functional interrelation of operations, and common ownership, control, or management, to determine if multiple entities should be treated as a single employer.[123] If treated as a single employer, the employees of all the related businesses may be aggregated for purposes of union elections and collective bargaining.[124]

[121] 29 C.F.R. § 791.2.

[122] 29 U.S.C. §§ 151, et seq.

[123] See Radio & Television Broadcast Technicians Local 1264 v. Broadcast Services of Mobile, Inc., 380 U.S. 255, 256 (1965).

[124] See, e.g., Blumenfeld Theatres Circuit, 240 N.L.R.B. 206, 216 (1979).

Six

Financing Retirement Facilities

By Stephen L. Taber*

§ 14 HUD FINANCING PROGRAMS**

The U.S. Department of Housing and Urban Development (HUD) offers three basic types of housing finance programs: mortgage insurance, direct loans, and grants to local government bodies.[1] The mortgage insurance program is today the most active of these three approaches. Over the past few years, there has been a significant amount of activity in creating new mortgage insurance and financing alternatives for retirement facilities that combine housing and services, including care. These efforts increasingly involve the private sector as both a coinsurer and processor of HUD-backed mortgage insurance (see, §§ 22.1, 22.2).

The applicability of HUD-financing vehicles to retirement housing depends largely on the kinds of architectural amenities (e.g., private kitchens or common dining areas) and services packages (e.g., medical care, meal programs) intended to be offered by the facility. (See § 22 for a detailed discussion of HUD operational requirements.) In addition, the income level of residents, the area in which the development is proposed, and the facility's financial relationship with the resident (e.g., rental or entrance fee) have a bearing on the availability of government funding or loan insurance.

*Stephen L. Taber is a partner at the law offices of Hanson, Bridgett, Marcus, Vlahos & Rudy, San Francisco, and specializes in the financing of retirement facilities.

**Special thanks to John P. Hays for preparing the HUD Financing section.

[1] See, generally, Programs of HUD (U.S. Department of Housing and Urban Development, 1984).

In addition to the numerous conditions on eligibility imposed by HUD that affect the structure and operations of the facility, a variety of financial requirements is imposed by the federal government as conditions of receiving either direct loans or mortgage insurance for the construction of eligible retirement facilities. Section 14.1 first discusses the detailed HUD procedures for obtaining mortgage insurance or direct loans. It then outlines some of the specific characteristics and requirements for the individual HUD mortgage insurance and secondary financing programs. Section 14.2 covers HUD's direct loan programs, and Section 14.3 explains the general grant programs for local development.

In addition to the financial provisions discussed in this section, HUD mortgagors and facilities are subject to a number of general operational requirements (outlined in detail in § 22) that concern such things as the type of structure that may be built, the services that can be made available, escrows, rent coltrols, eviction procedures, and related topics. A project is also subject to various federal and state antidiscrimination provisions in providing housing (see § 23).

§ 14.1   MORTGAGE INSURANCE

(a)   General Procedural Requirements

HUD prescribes extremely detailed procedures for applying for mortgage insurance under its housing finance programs. While the following sections provide a broad overview of these general procedures and some of the specifics for each program, developers are advised to consult the local HUD field office and the relevant HUD regulations, handbooks, and notices (see Table 22.1, page 309).[2]

HUD mortgage insurance applications involve several parties. The mortgagor (borrower) is the organization or entity that owns the property that is the security for the mortgage insured by HUD. The sponsor is the organization or entity that initiates and promotes the development of the facility. That sponsor, if it meets HUD requirements, may qualify as the mortgagor or it may set up a separate entity for the purpose of qualifying as a mortgagor. The sponsor, if different from the mortgagor, must also be a bona fide entity. Most mortgagors under HUD programs must be single asset mortgagors; that is, they may not own more than one major asset that is the subject of a HUD mortgage.[3]

The sponsor or mortgagor is responsible for locating a source for the required mortgage funds. HUD may not recommend a specific source of

---

[2]HUD Handbook 4561.1, which is designed for participants in the § 221(d) multifamily co-insurance program (*see* § 22.1(a), below) provides one of the clearest examples of the overall HUD processing requirements.

[3]*See, e.g.,* Notice H86-20 (HUD) at 3 (issued Aug. 11, 1986) (on § 232 mortgage insurance for board & care homes).

mortgage funds, although its local offices may assist sponsors to the extent of providing lists of approved mortgagees (lenders) in the area who make loans of the type and amount desired. These approved lenders include national banks, state banks, mortgage banking companies, insurance companies, savings and loan associations, and savings banks.[4]

The procedures set out below cover the three stages of processing: feasibility, conditional commitment, and firm commitment. Processing may require only one or two stages, depending on the level of experience of the sponsor. The total HUD-processing procedure is as follows:

The sponsor makes the first contact with the HUD Field Office on the proposal, which may include a preapplication conference.

The sponsor prepares the application with related exhibits that outlines the proposal.

HUD makes a feasibility analysis of the proposal.

A Feasibility Conference is held. If HUD and the sponsor are in substantial agreement, at the conclusion of the conference, a Feasibility Letter is prepared. The Letter is signed by the Field Office Director and presented to the sponsor.

The sponsor prepares forms, exhibits, and brief specifications, and pays his application fee if he files an application for conditional commitment.

HUD reviews the sponsor's exhibits and issues a conditional commitment to the mortgagee.

The sponsor's architect prepares complete architectural drawings and specifications on the project.

The mortgagee makes application for firm commitment and pays the application fee (unless already paid) and the commitment fee. HUD reviews the contract drawings and documents and issues the firm commitment.

The Preconstruction Conference is held.

Initial closing is held and the original credit instrument is endorsed ("initial endorsement").

The project is constructed.

Cost Certification is made.

Final Closing is held ("final endorsement").[5]

(b) HUD Evaluations

The procedural stages involve a number of different analyses and evaluations by HUD, summarized below, to determine whether the project is eligible for HUD-backed mortgage insurance.[6] Other conditions cover such

---

[4]HUD Handbook 4600.1, ch. 1–6 (§ 232 board & care homes).

[5]*Id.* at ch. 2. Processing for new construction is known as "Site Area Market Analysis" (SAMA).

[6]*See, generally,* HUD Handbook 4561.1 (§ 221(d) multifamily coinsurance).

concerns as displacement of existing tenants in rehabilitation projects, construction in flood hazard areas, historic site concerns, and the payment of Davis-Bacon prevailing wages during construction.

(1) Architectural Analysis

Architectural review is required to determine the acceptability of the physical improvements, provide architectural consultation essential to minimize mortgage risk, and improve housing. The scope of the analysis includes the buildings and their attachments, parking facilities and their adaptation to the site, land improvements (such as water supply, sanitary sewage disposal systems, gas mains, and heating tunnels) and all other elements of design or construction. A site analysis is also required to alert the lender to any soil faults, drainage problems, zoning ordinances, and other possible problems affecting design.

(2) Architectural Inspection

The stated purpose of the architectural inspection is to protect the interests of the lender and HUD, evaluate the performance of the contractor and architect responsible for administration of the construction contract, see that construction is according to contract documents, and report on conformance with prevailing wage and other contract requirements. The lender and HUD must have access to the property at all times and the right to inspect all work performed and materials furnished to complete the project.

(3) Cost Estimation and Processing

A further requirement is the provision and evaluation of cost estimates for the project to be insured. These estimates include on-site land improvements, structures, major movable equipment, minor equipment, supplies, general overhead expenses, architect's fees, carrying and financing charges, organizational and audit expenses, and a profit and risk allowance for either the builder, the sponsor, or both (where there is an identity of interest between the two).

(4) Valuation Analysis

Conclusions with respect to feasibility, suitability of improvements, the extent, quality, and duration of earning capacity, and other factors related to the acceptability of insurance risk or the economic soundness of the property must be developed. The analysis must show a reasonable expectation that project income will, for the duration of the mortgage term, be adequate to:

Properly maintain the property.

Pay all required project expenses.

Meet debt service requirements and provide a reasonable return on the owner's equity investment.

This procedure involves estimating annual project expenses and net income before mortgage payments, figuring the tentative mortgage amount, determining the maximum allowable rents and operating deficit, and figuring the replacement cost of the facility.

(5)   Mortgage Credit Analysis

Mortgage credit analysis involves credit investigation, review of the amount and amortization period of the loan, determination of estimated requirements for completion of the project, determination of the mortgagor's ability to close the transaction, insurance of advances, review of possible construction changes, and cost certification. Among the mortgage credit risks reviewed by HUD are the probability of the failure of the mortgagor to satisfactorily complete the construction of the project, or to provide competent management for operation of the facility, and the likelihood that income will not provide for all operating expenses, liquidation of the mortgage, and all other debts. The credit determination thus involves analysis of the character and reputation of the project sponsors, the financial capacity of the mortgagor, and the anticipated net income of the facility.

(c)   Closing and Funding Procedures

Once the mortgage insurance has been approved, a variety of documents is required by HUD both at the initial and at the final closing, including an assurance of completion by the mortgagor in the form of either a performance bond, a completion assurance agreement, or a personal undertaking.[7] At initial endorsement, all mortgagors, other than nonprofit, must set up an escrow of at least two percent of the face amount of the mortgage by either cash, letter of credit, U.S. bearer bonds, or excess mortgage proceeds, if any.[8] The deposit is used to defray the initial marketing and rent-up, set up accruals for items due during the first operating year that project income is not expected to cover, and cover shortfalls in mortgage insurance premiums, taxes, interest, and other items. The lender controls disbursements from the escrow, which must be fully documented by the mortgagor. If the mortgage is not in default, the balance of the working capital escrow is generally released one year after the construction completion date.

---

[7]*Id.* at ch. 12.

[8]For a discussion of the special escrow and operating deficit requirements for ReSC projects under §§ 221(d)(4) and 223(f), *see* § 22.1, below.

Escrows from projects in poor financial condition are held until the problems are resolved.

Advances on the mortgage are made by HUD and the lender in three stages. The first advance, usually made at initial closing, covers the mortgagor's early expenditures (e.g., design architect fees, bond fees, insurance premiums, building fee permits, etc.). Unless there was an early start of construction,[9] no construction funds may be advanced at this point. Subsequent advances of the insured mortgage proceeds are based on the construction progress documented in inspections. The final balance is made at final endorsement. For each advance, there is a 10 percent hold-back requirement as an incentive to the mortgagor and general contractor to see that the job is completed promptly, to submit cost certification, and to reach final endorsement. After all the required contractor cost certification documents are approved, the contractor (through the mortgagor) is entitled to the balance of the holdback (less certain escrows) and the balance of the mortgage proceeds are insured.[10]

(d) Specific HUD Mortgage Insurance Programs

(1) Retirement Service Centers under Section 221(d)(4)

The U.S. Department of Housing and Urban Development has recently developed regulations to provide for a new housing insurance program within the current Section 221(d)(4) program[11] to cover the gap between the totally independent living arrangements of noncongregate housing for the elderly and the health-care-oriented nursing home.[12] The Section 221(d)(4) program is designed to assist in financing the construction or substantial rehabilitation of rental housing for low- and moderate-income families.[13] Under this program, HUD and the FHA insure mortgages made by approved lenders, which is intended to increase the mortgage credit available from private lenders. The Retirement Service Center (ReSC) program builds on the existing Section 221(d)(4) mortgage insurance to provide meals, services, and an amenities package that exceeds that normally submitted under this program. All mortgage insurance proposals under this program must be processed under both the general Section 221(d)(4) and the ReSC procedures.

The maximum insurable loan for a ReSC facility is limited to the lesser of:

---

[9]Construction may not begin before the initial closing and recording of the coinsured mortgage, except under certain conditions where a construction delay could seriously jeopardize the project. HUD Handbook 4561.1, ch. 7–12.

[10]*Id.* at ch. 13.

[11]For the operational requirements of this program, *see* § 22.1(a), below.

[12]*See* Notices H85-33, 84-41, 83-58 (HUD).

[13]*See, generally,* 24 C.F.R. § 251; HUD Handbook 4560.1.

Statutory dollar limits

Ninety percent of the estimated replacement cost

Ninety percent of the project's estimated value, assuming that no more than 90 percent of the net operating income will be required for debt service, or

If the property is owned by the sponsor and subject to existing financing, 90 percent of the lender's estimate of value prior to rehabilitation plus the full cost of rehabilitation.

Property is considered to be undergoing substantial rehabilitation if:

The cost of repairs exceeds the greater of:

Fifteen percent of the property's value after repair, or

$6500 per dwelling unit (adjusted by applicable high-cost area factor), or

Repairs involve the replacement of more than one major building component.

Under the ReSC procedures, nonprofit sponsors are subject to the same maximum insurable limitations as any other type of mortgagor. The term of the mortgage may be up to 40 years, with the interest rate negotiated by lender and mortgagor. No secondary financing is permitted. The mortgagor may also obtain an insured construction loan, with insured advances administered by the insurer.

Because of what HUD perceives as the extremely narrow market band for ReSCs (which results in slow initial rent-up), limited market comparables, and industry experience, substantial reserves are required in the program. ReSC projects require one of the following: (1) an operating deficit escrow funded at 200 percent of HUD's determination of the initial operating deficit, (2) a six-month debt service reserve, or (3) an operating deficit escrow and a six-month debt service reserve.

The reserve requirements for ReSC projects are determined by calculating the initial operating deficit and a six-month debt service reserve amount. If the operating deficit is less than the six-month debt service reserve amount, the amount of reserve funds required will be the greater of two times the operating deficit calculation or the six-month debt service reserve amount. If the anticipated operating deficit equals or exceeds the debt service reserve amount, both an operating deficit escrow and debt service reserve are required. Funds remaining in the operating deficit escrow and/or debt service reserve can be released after sustaining occupancy has been maintained for 90 days.

All rents and other receipts of the project must be deposited in the project's name in accounts that are fully insured by an agency of the federal government. Project funds may only be used for payment of mortgage obligations, payment of reasonable expenses necessary to the proper operation and maintenance of the project, and certain distributions of surplus cash as specified in HUD procedures.

The general HUD processing procedures described above are subject to a few additional requirements for ReSC projects. First, in figuring the replacement cost of the facility, both major movable equipment for congregate dining facilities and furniture in common areas may be included. Minor movable equipment is not included. Moreover, no leasing or lease purchase agreements are permitted for these items.

Secondly, in calculating the debt service limitation under the valuation analysis, the cost of shelter services must be separated from the fees and costs of nonshelter services and amenities. Only the gross income from the shelter income factor is used in calculating the debt service limitation. The intent is for HUD to process elderly proposals and determine project feasibility where a mortgage amount attributable to shelter or realty only is established and reflects an acceptable degree of risk. In addition, special market analysis is required to determine whether the demand exists among ReSC's target group (fragile elderly of 70 years and up) to support the project (see also § 22.1(a)).

(2)   Retirement Service Centers under Section 223(f)

HUD also permits the financing of existing structures as Retirement Service Centers under the Section 223(f) program.[14] Section 223(f) authorizes HUD to insure mortgages in connection with the purchase or refinancing of existing multifamily projects without requiring a program of substantial rehabilitation.[15] Substantial rehabilitation projects for ReSCs must be insured under the Section 221(d)(4) program, outlined above.

No more than one major building component may be replaced for Section 223(f) projects, and the cost of repairs cannot exceed the greater of:

Fifteen percent of the property's value after repairs, or

$6500 per dwelling unit (adjusted by applicable high-cost area factor), plus equipment.

The term of the mortgage may be up to 75 percent of the estimated remaining economic life of the structure, but may not exceed 35 years. The interest rate is negotiated by lender and mortgagor. For acquisition loans, the mortgage amount cannot exceed the lower of:

Statutory limits

Eighty-five percent of the project's estimated value, or

---

[14]For operational requirements of the 223(f) program, *see* § 22.1(b), below.

[15]24 C.F.R. § 255; HUD Handbook 4561.1; HUD Fact Sheet.

Eighty-five percent of the costs of acquisition, repairs, architectural, legal, title, and organizational costs, discounts, and the initial deposit to the reserve for replacements.

For refinancing loans, the mortgage amount cannot exceed the lower of:

Statutory limits, or

The greater of 70 percent of the project's estimated value or 100 percent of costs (not to exceed 85 percent of value).

In no event can debt service exceed 85 percent of net operating income. Section 223(f) applications must also meet the financial reserve, marketing, and sponsor criteria required for ReSC financing under Section 221(d)(4). However, no insurance of construction advances is available.

HUD will permit a second mortgage on the property, but it may not exceed seven and one-half percent of the property's value (if an acquisition) or half the difference between the cost to refinance and the maximum mortgage amount (if a refinance). The second mortgage may only be a promissory note approved by HUD. The note shall not be due before the maturity date of the mortgage, but may be paid from surplus cash. Nonpayment of the note cannot trigger a default on the first mortgage. The note may be recorded to protect the noteholder in the event of a sale or refinancing of the project.

(3)   Coinsurance Programs

HUD has recently initiated a coinsurance program for the Section 221(d)(4) and 223(f) programs.[16] Under this program, the HUD-FHA mortgagee assumes approximately 20 percent of the loan loss if a loan defaults, and no longer assumes a strictly processing role. This program is designed to increase the amount of mortgage credit available from the private market for HUD-approved projects. In return, the private coinsurer retains a portion of the mortgage insurance premiums and fees otherwise payable to HUD.

Participants in the coinsurance program must be approved by HUD. The coinsurer assumes all processing functions that were previously performed by HUD, including review of plans and specifications, cost analysis, appraisal of the projects, mortgage credit review, and management review. The coinsurer may contract out the technical reviews or perform them in-house, but it retains full liability under the coinsurance contract. The program is designed to give the approved lenders maximum oversight and servicing responsibility and autonomy. Only a few documents must still be submitted to HUD for review and approval.

---

[16]HUD Handbook 4561.1.

(4)   Section 232 Board and Care Homes

The Housing and Urban-Rural Recovery Act of 1983 amended the Section 232 program[17] to permit federal mortgage insurance to help finance the construction or improvement of board and care homes.[18] Section 232 had previously been limited to nursing homes and intermediate care facilities (ICFs). Board and care homes are known by many different names in different states, such as domiciliary care, shelter care, adult congregate living, personal care, and residential care.[19] This type of facility provides living arrangements for individuals who cannot live independently but who do not require the more extensive care offered by ICFs or nursing homes.

Board and care homes may be privately owned and operated for profit, or owned by a private nonprofit corporation or association, to qualify for FHA financing. A proprietary mortgagor may be a corporation, partnership, trust, individual, or any other qualified legal entity. A nonprofit mortgagor must be a nonprofit corporation or association. The law specifically requires that no part of the net earnings of the nonprofit mortgagor shall inure to the benefit of any private shareholder or individual. Public bodies wishing to sponsor a project must create a separate private nonprofit corporation or association to be the mortgagor.

The maximum mortgage amount is governed by a loan-to-value limitation of 90 percent of the HUD-FHA estimate of the value of the property, including major movable equipment, covered by the mortgage; and statutory dollar limitations for different project types:

1. *New Construction.* All projects not involving rehabilitation or reconstruction of existing structures are considered new construction. The insurable mortgage amount for new construction may not exceed the lowest of:

The statutory dollar limitation,

Ninety percent of the HUD-FHA estimated value of the property or project in fee when the proposed improvements are completed,

An amount that entails a debt service not in excess of 90 percent of estimated net earnings attributable to the realty and nonrealty (major movable) equipment, or

When the mortgagor is a private nonprofit corporation or association, HUD-FHA's estimated total replacement cost of the project, including land, furnishings, and mortgageable equipment, plus nonmortgageable

[17]For operational requirements of the 232 program, *see* § 22.2, below.
[18]P.L. 98-181; 24 C.F.R. § 232, Notice 86-20 (HUD).
[19]*See* discussion at § 20.3, below.

items (to be covered by grants) minus the amount of gifts (including land) from other sources that are intended to offset cost and mortgage financing.

2. *Rehabilitation.* Rehabilitation includes substantial upgrading of an existing facility. Additions may be included as part of the rehabilitation of the facility, but an addition without other upgrading of the existing facility is not eligible as rehabilitation. The rehabilitation must affect, materially, the livability, marketability, and competitive position of the project. The project must have been completed for more than one year.

The insurable mortgage amount for rehabilitation may not exceed the lowest of:

The amounts set forth for new construction.

For Owned Property[20]: The HUD-FHA estimated current cost of rehabilitation plus the lesser of:

> The principal amount of existing indebtedness secured by the property, if any, or
>
> Ninety percent of the HUD-FHA estimate of the fair market value (as is) of the property before rehabilitation.

For Property to Be Acquired: Ninety percent of the HUD-FHA estimated cost of rehabilitation plus the lesser of:

> Ninety percent of the actual purchase price of the property; or
>
> Ninety percent of the HUD-FHA estimate of fair market value (as is) of property before rehabilitation.

Where there is an identity of interest, regardless of how slight, between the seller(s) of the existing property and the sponsors, the proposal will be considered as a refinancing transaction rather than a purchase for the purpose of determining the mortgage amount. The limitation for Property Owned will apply in lieu of the limitation for Property to Be Acquired.

The maximum mortgage term for 232 projects is 40 years, and the mortgage may not bear interest at a rate greater than the maximum prescribed by HUD-FHA regulations. In addition to making monthly payments covering the principal, interest, and mortgage insurance premium under the mortgage, the mortgagor will be required to include in the monthly payment an amount sufficient to provide for the payment of taxes, property insurance, special assessments (if any), and ground rents.

---

[20]If the properties owned were acquired within a 12 month period, prior to the date of the original application, the limitation for "Property to be Acquired" will apply in lieu of the limitation for "Property Owned."

(5) Cooperatives

The Department of Housing and Urban Development insures project mortgages on cooperative housing projects under Sections 213 and 221(d)(3).[21] HUD insures mortgages made by private lending institutions on cooperative housing projects of five or more dwelling units to be occupied by members of nonprofit cooperative ownership housing corporations. These loans may finance new construction, rehabilitation, acquisition, improvement or repair of a project already owned, and resale of individual memberships; construction of projects composed of individual family dwellings to be bought by individual members with separate insured mortgages; and construction or rehabilitation of projects that the owners intend to sell to nonprofit cooperatives.

Legislation establishing this program was enacted in 1950. Nonprofit corporations or trusts organized to construct homes for members of the corporation or beneficiaries of the trust, and qualified sponsors who intend to sell the project to a nonprofit corporation or trust are eligible under this program.

For Section 213 projects, the mortgage amount cannot exceed the lesser of an amount equal to 98 percent of the HUD estimated replacement cost of the project or a statutory limitation. The mortgage amount is 100 percent of estimated cost for Section 221(d)(3) projects. If the project is to be rehabilitated, further limits apply.

The term of the mortgage in these management type cooperatives cannot exceed 40 years. Interest is paid monthly on the principal outstanding. The HUD mortgage insurance premium is one-half of one percent.

(6) Condominium Housing

HUD insures mortgages made by private lending institutions for the purchase of individual family units in multifamily housing projects under Section 234(c).[22] Sponsors may also obtain FHA-insured mortgages to finance the construction or rehabilitation of housing projects that they intend to sell as individual condominium units under Section 234(d). A project must contain at least four dwelling units in detached, semidetached, row, walkup, or elevator structures. Recent changes in legislation permit insuring mortgages on individual units in existing condominiums.

A condominium is defined as joint ownership of common areas and facilities by the separate owners of single dwelling units in the project. Legislation establishing this program was enacted in 1961. Any qualified profit-motivated or nonprofit sponsor may apply for a blanket mortgage

---

[21] 24 C.F.R. § 213, HUD Handbook 4550.1 (§ 213); 24 C.F.R. § 251, HUD Handbook 4560.1 (§ 221(d)(3)).

[22] 12 U.S.C. § 1715y; 24 C.F.R. § 234.

covering the project after conferring with his local HUD-FHA Field Office, and any creditworthy person may apply for a mortgage of individual units in a project.

(e)   Secondary Financing

(1)   Purpose of the Secondary Market

Residential mortgages are marketable commodities to be sold either individually or pooled with other similar mortgages to back the sale of a mortgage security. Although savings and loan associations and other institutions involved in home lending originate mortgage loans for their own portfolios, many mortgages are originated specifically to be sold on the secondary mortgage market.

Perhaps the most basic purpose of the secondary mortgage is to improve lender liquidity. Given a finite amount of lendable proceeds, a lender is limited in the number of mortgages it can have outstanding at a given time. However, by having a market to sell its mortgages, a lender can maintain a cash position enabling it to originate new mortgage loans.

Traditionally, the secondary market existed to correct national imbalances of mortgage funds. That is, lenders in a geographic region in which the mortgage lending capacity exceeded the local demand could purchase existing mortgages from lenders in areas where the demand for mortgage money outstripped its local availability. This flow of capital maintains an equilibrium throughout the country, inhibiting sharp regional differences in interest rates.

The federal agencies' entry into the secondary mortgage market was intended specifically to serve as a countercyclical market force—to buy mortgages when lenders run short of funds and to sell loans as money for mortgages becomes more plentiful. Theoretically, the national outreach of the secondary market should prevent the boom and bust cycles in the housing industry by maintaining an overall balance between mortgage credit demand and its availability. The secondary market has developed methods to maintain this countercyclical function by providing a constant nationwide availability of mortgage financing.

(2)   Federal National Mortgage Association

The Federal National Mortgage Association (FNMA), also known as Fannie Mae, is the nation's largest investor in residential mortgages. The corporation, which is chartered by Congress, is publicly owned, with its shares traded on the New York Stock Exchange.[23] It invests in mortgages originated by others, thereby providing an added degree of liquidity for mortgage

[23] 12 U.S.C. § 1717.

lenders and improving the distribution of investment capital available for financing the construction and sale of housing.

The types of mortgages covered in its programs include conventional, HUD/FHA insured, and VA guaranteed mortgages on one- to four-family properties, including condominiums and Planned Unit Developments, second mortgages on residential properties, HUD/FHA project mortgages, conventional multifamily mortgages, and cooperative blanket and share loans. Supportive living and nursing homes are not covered.

Today, virtually all of Fannie Mae's mortgage purchases are conventional mortgages, although FHA/VA mortgages still account for a significant part of the corporation's mortgage portfolio.

(3) GNMA Mortgage-Backed Securities

The Government National Mortgage Association (GNMA or "Ginnie Mae") guarantees the timely payment of principal and interest on securities issued by private lenders and backed by pools of government-underwritten residential mortgages. The program's purpose is to attract nontraditional investors into the residential mortgage market by offering them a high-yield, risk-free government-guaranteed security that has none of the servicing obligations associated with a mortgage loan portfolio. It will issue securities backed by Section 221(d)(4) and 232 insured project mortgages.

Legislation establishing this program was enacted in 1968.[24] Applicants must be FHA-approved mortgagees in good standing and have a net worth that meets GNMA's minimum requirements. Since its inception, GNMA has guaranteed more than $200 billion in mortgage-backed securities, and the program has helped finance more than five million housing units. For fiscal year (FY) 1987, the mortgage guarantee limit for GNMA is set at $150 billion, $25 billion below the FY1986 cap.[25]

The newer GNMA II mortgage-backed securities program provides a more efficient means of channeling funds from security markets. The program provides a comprehensive menu of new GNMA securities that take advantage of technological improvements that have emerged since GNMA's introduction. GNMA II supplements, rather than replaces, the original mortgage-backed securities program.

The new program, which began August 1, 1983, has a central paying agent that makes consolidated payments to investors, offers larger, geographically dispersed multiple-issuer pools, as well as custom pools, and provides for a mix of interest rates among mortgages within a pool. Securities are privately issued and are backed by pools of FHA, VA, and FmHA

[24] 12 U.S.C. § 1721(g).

[25] Department of HUD-Independent Agencies Appropriations Bill, 1987, H.R. Rep. No. 977, 99th Cong., 2nd Sess. at 9 (1986) (Conference Report).

mortgages. They are guaranteed by GNMA to ensure investors timely and accurate monthly payments. They provide for pools of single-family level payment, graduated payment mortgage,[26] growing equity mortgage,[27] and manufactured housing loans.

A firm must first be approved as an issuer based on net worth, staffing, and experience criteria. An approved issuer then applies for a commitment for the guaranty of securities. The issuer originates or acquires mortgage loans and assembles them into a pool or package of mortgages. The issuer selects the securities funding method and submits the documents to Chemical Bank, the central paying agent. Chemical Bank prepares and delivers securities to investors. Issuers are responsible for marketing the securities and servicing the mortgages that back the securities. Issuers provide the paying agent with monthly payments due investors. The paying agent makes consolidated payments to security holders and provides GNMA with activity and control reports.

(4) Federal Home Loan Mortgage Corporation

The Federal Home Loan Mortgage Corporation (FHLMC), commonly referred to as Freddie Mac, was created by Congress in 1970, under Title III of the Emergency Home Finance Act of 1970, Public Law 91-351.[28]

Freddie Mac was established as a new secondary mortgage market within the Federal Home Loan Bank system, with the 12 Federal Home Loan Banks as its sole stockholders. Its original purpose was to provide a secondary market for mortgages originated by federally insured savings and loan associations and other federally insured financial institutions. Section 321 of the Housing and Community Development Amendments of 1978 (Public Law 95-557) permits Freddie Mac to expand its operations to include HUD-approved mortgage bankers.

Freddie Mac, unlike Fannie Mae, prefers not to hold mortgages for its own portfolio. Rather, most of the mortgages it purchases are resold in the form of guaranteed mortgage securities, primarily as mortgage Participation Certificates (PCs) or Collateralized Mortgage Obligations (CMOs).

Freddie Mac purchases a variety of fixed-rate, adjustable-rate, and graduated-payment first mortgages. The corporation buys both whole loans and participations (i.e., 50 to 95 percent) on one- to four-family properties. In addition, Freddie Mac purchases second mortgages on single-family homes and conventional mortgages on multifamily (five or more units) properties. Supportive living and nursing home projects are not considered.

---

[26] 24 C.F.R. §§ 203.45, 203.46.
[27] 24 C.F.R. § 203.49.
[28] 12 U.S.C. § 1451.

§ 14.2   DIRECT LOANS

(a)   Section 202/8 Program

The HUD Section 202/8 program[29] provides loans at reduced interest rates to nonprofit sponsors for the development cost of new or substantially rehabilitated housing for the elderly or handicapped.[30] Section 202 provides 40 year loans at below-market interest rates for up to 100 percent of the total development costs of the project. Rental subsidies are offered through the Section 8 program to qualifying low income families and individuals living in approved residential facilities. With the consolidation of the application requirements of both the Section 202 and the Section 8 programs, projects that meet the requirements of the Section 202 program are deemed by HUD to have met the requirements for housing assistance payments under Section 8. Accordingly, a separate application for Section 8 assistance is not necessary.

(1)   Financial Requirements

The Housing and Community Development Act of 1974 amended the Section 202 program to permit construction loans and direct 40 year permanent financing to nonprofit sponsors for the construction or substantial rehabilitation of housing projects for the elderly, handicapped, or disabled. Because the Section 202 program is one of direct loans, availability of federal funding is dependent on annual appropriations by Congress. The actual level of recent HUD funding for Section 202 has been relatively low, making it difficult to get money even for projects deemed worthy by HUD. In FY1987, for example, approximately $593 million was appropriated for Section 202 loans, to provide some 12,000 housing units.[31] The Administration has repeatedly requested that no further funding be provided for the Section 202 program, but this recommendation has been rejected by Congress.[32]

Funds are also allocated on a geographical basis among the 10 HUD regions, and further between metropolitan and nonmetropolitan areas based on a needs formula. This geographical distribution takes into account the number of elderly households in each region, those households lacking some or all plumbing facilities, and those with incomes below regionally adjusted poverty levels. Of the total amount of Section 202 assistance, 20 to 25 percent must be allocated to nonmetropolitan areas. Moreover, approximately

---

[29]For operational requirements of the 202/8 program, *see* § 22.3, below.

[30]24 C.F.R. §§ 880, 885; HUD Handbook 4571.1 REV-2, 7420.1 REV-1.

[31]HUD Appropriations Bill, 1987, H.R. Rep. No. 731, 99th Cong., 2nd Sess., at 9 (1986) (House Committee Report). *See also* note 39, below, for FY 1988 levels.

[32]*Id.*

15 percent of the total funding must be set aside for the development of facilities specifically designed to meet the needs of the nonelderly handicapped. These restrictions further limit the availability of Section 202 funds to interested borrowers.

(2)   Eligible Applicants

Only private nonprofit corporations, including incorporated nonprofit consumer cooperatives, are eligible under the regulations to apply for Section 202 loans. Such an applicant is defined as the borrower in the program regulations and handbook. The borrower is responsible for the construction, rehabilitation, ownership, and operation of the project.

Frequently, the borrower will be a local nonprofit corporation established by a national organization, such as a religious group or a labor union. This organization, defined as the sponsor, does not have to be incorporated, but it does have to be a private nonprofit group.

When a sponsor sets up a nonprofit corporation to act as the 202 borrower, HUD will look to the sponsor for the financial strength and experience needed to successfully carry out the project. The sponsor is expected to pledge its support to the borrower for the full 40 year term of the 202 loan. The relationship between the sponsor and borrower should be spelled out in detail in the application.

Actually, the law creating the Section 202 program allows public agencies and private profit-motivated entities to be project developers, as well as nonprofit corporations. However, HUD regulations and annual appropriations bills have restricted the program to nonprofits.[33] The program handbook makes it clear that even indirect participation by public agencies or profit-motivated groups is prohibited. A profit-motivated entity may not sponsor a nonprofit borrower, and a public agency may not set up an agency or instrumentality to participate in the 202 program.[34]

(3)   Amount and Terms of Financing

Projects may be new construction or substantial rehabilitation. They must be designed in accordance with the appropriate HUD minimum property standards, and must include only units that are designed for elderly or handicapped persons. The total amount of the loan approved under Section 202 shall not exceed the lesser of:

The total development cost of the project as determined by the HUD field office;

[33]*Id.*
[34]HUD Handbook 4571.1 REV-2, ch. 2–7.

An amount that entails a debt service of no more than 97 percent of anticipated net project income; or

The sum of:

The cost of exterior land improvements;

The cost of improvements not attributable to dwelling use, such as
game rooms, central kitchens and dining rooms, and commercial
space; and

A statutory amount per unit for the part of the property attributable to
dwelling use.

The following additional limitations apply to rehabilitation projects:

For property held by the borrower in fee simple, the maximum loan
amount is 100 percent of the cost of rehabilitation.

For property subject to an existing mortgage, the limit is the cost of rehabilitation plus such portion of the outstanding debt that does not exceed the fair market value of the property prior to rehabilitation.

For property to be acquired and rehabilitated through Section 202 financing, the loan is limited to the cost of rehabilitation plus such portion of the purchase price that does not exceed the fair market value
prior to rehabilitation.

The loans are made at a rate based on the average interest of all interest-
bearing obligations of the United States that form a part of the public debt,
plus an amount to cover administrative costs. As of FY1987, the interest
rate was frozen by statute at 9.25 percent.[35]

(4) Procedural Requirements

1. *Invitations for Applications.* After determining the amount of loan
authority to be allocated to each field office, the assistant secretary for
housing publishes an Announcement of Fund Availability in the *Federal
Register*. This announcement indicates the amount of loan authority (and
approximate number of units) made available to each field office, the date
by which the field offices will publish invitations for applications in news-
papers of general circulation and notify the minority media, minority organizations, and groups with special interest in housing for the elderly or
handicapped.

No organization can participate as a sponsor, cosponsor, or borrower in
applications for more than 300 units in a single region in a single fiscal
year. Affiliated entities are treated as a single organization for purposes of
this limit.

---

[35] HUD Appropriations, note 31, above, at 9.

2. *Contents of Applications.* The application must provide detailed information on the project proposal and on the borrower and sponsor.

Required information on the proposal includes:

Number of 202 units and dollar amount of the loan requested.

Number of units for which Section 8 assistance is requested. This must be at least 20 percent of the units. If fewer than 100 percent of the units are to receive Section 8, the application must demonstrate that there is sufficient market demand for the unsubsidized units to assure the financial feasibility of the project.

Narrative description of the proposed housing, including type of structure, bedroom mix, and special features.

Narrative description of the anticipated occupancy (elderly and/or handicapped; what type of handicap).

In the case of projects for the elderly, information on the site and neighborhood, including a statement on displacement and plans for relocation.

Information on the borrower and sponsor must include:

Ties to the community and support from local community groups.

Satisfactory evidence of the legal authority to finance, construct, or substantially rehabilitate and maintain the project and to apply for the loan.

Evidence of previous participation in HUD programs, if any.

Description of all rental housing projects and medical facilities owned and operated by borrower or sponsor during the previous five years. A shorter period is accepted if information for five years is not available.

Evidence of management capabilities.

Estimate of startup expenses and the source of funds to meet those expenses.

Financial records, including a description of any default or other problem incurred during the previous three years.

3. *Approval of Applications.* Borrowers whose applications are approved receive a notice of Section 202 fund reservation specifying the 202 loan amount, number and mix of units, project location (or locality, in the case of projects for the nonelderly handicapped), and the amount of Section 8 contract authority reserved. The 202 funds reserved cannot be transferred to another borrower, and they cannot be used for a project submitted in response to a separate Section 8 invitation.

A 202 fund reservation is subject to cancelation at any time if the borrower is not making satisfactory progress toward the start of construction, and it will be canceled if work is not started within 18 months after issuance of the notice of reservation. This deadline can be extended for up to six months by the field office director.

(5)   Direct Loan Financing Procedures

1. *Request for Conditional Commitment.* A borrower whose project involves substantial rehabilitation must submit a request for a conditional commitment. The conditional commitment stage is optional for a new construction, though the HUD field office must approve a borrower's request to skip it.

HUD's processing of a request for a conditional commitment includes an evaluation of contract rents, affirmative marketing plans, and financial feasibility. If the evaluation is favorable, the conditional commitment is issued. It includes the estimated cost of the project, value of the site (both "as is" and fully improved), detailed estimates of operating expenses and taxes, supportable cost, financial requirements, loan amount, and approved contract rents. If the contract rents are lower than the rents proposed by the borrower, the reason for the reduction is given.

The conditional commitment also sets a time limit for submission of a request for a firm commitment.

2. *Loan Disbursement Procedures.* After the mortgage has been recorded and all initial closing requirements have been satisfied, the field office releases the initial disbursement of loan funds to the borrower.

Disbursal of the loan amount is made directly from HUD to or for the account of the borrower. The payments may be made through an approved lender, mortgage servicer, title insurance company, or other agent satisfactory to HUD and the borrower.

The payments are made on a periodic basis, in amounts not exceeding the HUD-approved cost of portions of the construction or rehab work completed and in place, minus any appropriate hold-back or retainage determined by the field office.

(b)   Section 312 Rehabilitation Loans

Section 312 loans are designed to assist rehabilitation in federally aided Community Development Block Grant and Urban Homesteading areas.[36] Direct federal loans finance rehabilitation of single-family and multifamily residential, mixed use, and nonresidential properties in the above areas certified by the local government. By financing rehabilitation to bring the property up to applicable local code, project, or plan standards, the loans prevent unnecessary demolition of basically sound structures. A loan may also provide for insulation and the installation of weatherization materials. Loans may not exceed $27,000 per dwelling unit, or $100,000 for nonresidential properties, although the actual amount of a loan may be less, depending on certain factors. Loans are repayable over 20 years, at interest rates of three percent or nine percent based on family income for single-family loans, and five percent or nine percent for multifamily properties (five or more units) based on the level of private dollars being leveraged.

[36]42 U.S.C. § 1452b; 24 C.F.R. 510; *see also* discussion of CDBGs, § 14.3(b), below.

Legislation establishing this program was enacted in 1964. Property owners in the aforementioned federally aided areas, and business tenants of such property whose leases have at least as long to run as the terms of the loan, are eligible for the program. The applicant must evidence the capacity to repay the loan. Priority is given to low and moderate income applicants, and Section 202/8 projects have historically used such loans.

For FY1987, $91 million from repayments and other income sources is estimated to be available for new loans and other expenses.[37] No new funds have been allocated to the program, and the amount available from repayments has been steadily declining.

§ 14.3 GRANTS TO LOCALITIES

(a) Urban Development Action Grants

Urban Development Action Grants (UDAGs) assist cities and urban counties that are experiencing severe economic distress to help stimulate economic development activity needed to aid in local economic recovery.[38] This is done through a combination of public and private investments in economic development projects. The private sector's financial commitment must be secured by the community prior to the preliminary approval of an Action Grant project.

The program is intended to help revitalize cities and urban counties that have a combination of characteristics used to measure economic distress, such as aged housing, low per capita income change, high percentage of poverty, loss of population and jobs, unemployment, and designation as a labor surplus area. A minimum ratio or 2.5 private dollars to every Action Grant dollar is required. Generally, projects should take no more than four years to complete. No additional funding will be available for a project following the execution of a Grant agreement, although additional Action Grants may be available to a city to support different projects during the life of the program. Legislation establishing this program was enacted in 1977.

Eligible applicants are cities including those participating in the Community Development Block Grant program in cooperation with urban counties; and urban counties, provided that they have (1) met minimum criteria that indicate severe economic distress; and (2) demonstrated results in providing housing for low and moderate income persons and equal opportunity in housing and employment for low and moderate income persons and members of minority groups. Communities that do not meet the distress criteria may qualify for Action Grants if they contain distressed areas defined as Pockets of Poverty. The city must meet special eligibility criteria and plan to target the Action Grant assistance and benefits to the

[37]HUD Appropriations, note 31, above, at 15.
[38]42 U.S.C. §§ 5318, 5320.

residents of the Pocket area. Interested communities must request a deter-mination of eligibility from the HUD Field Offices before applications can be submitted. Retirement facilities may use funds for off-site costs.

From each year's appropriation, at least 25 percent will be set aside for small communities with populations of less than 50,000. Up to, but not more than, 20 percent of each year's appropriation may be used to fund projects in Pockets of Poverty communities. Action Grant funding is not based on entitlement. Each calendar quarter, HUD reviews all new applica-tions received and all applications held over for further consideration, and determines which projects are fundable. Each application must compete against all of the applications under review that quarter for the funds avail-able. Many criteria, as specified in the regulations, are considered in the selection of projects for funding. The primary criterion is the comparative degree of economic distress among all applicants. Applications are ac-cepted on a quarterly basis for large and small cities throughout the year, and awards are announced approximately 60 days after receipt.

For FY1987, $225 million has been allocated for the UDAG program. While Congress has rejected the Reagan Administration's repeated proposals to ter-minate the program, funding levels have continued to decline.[39] The FY1987 level, for example, is some $91 million below the FY1986 expenditure level.

(b) Community Development Block Grants

(1) Entitlement

The Community Development Block Grant (CDBG) program provides an-nual grants on a formula basis to entitled communities to carry out a wide range of community development activities directed toward neighbor-hood revitalization, economic development, and improved community fa-cilities and services.[40] Grants are useful for non-FHA-eligible development costs.

Entitlement communities develop their own programs and funding prior-ities and consult with local residents before making final decisions. All CDBG activities must either benefit low and moderate income persons, aid in the prevention or elimination of slums and blight, or address other com-munity development needs that present a serious and immediate threat to the health or welfare of the community. Some of the activities that can be carried out with community development funds include the acquisition of real property, rehabilitation of residential and nonresidential properties, provision of public facilities and improvements, such as water and sewer,

---

[39]HUD Appropriations, note 31, above, at 14–15. Congress recently approved a budget preclud-ing cuts for FY 1988 for the UDAG and CDBG programs, and maintaining Section 202 funding levels. *Housing & Development Reporter*, 15:6 (July 29, 1987) 101.

[40]42 U.S.C. §§ 5301 *et seq.*; 24 C.F.R. § 570.

streets, and neighborhood centers, and assistance to profit-motivated businesses to help with economic development activities.

No less than 51 percent of the funds must be used for activities that benefit low and moderate income persons, over a period specified by the grantee, but not to exceed three years.

Metropolitan cities and urban counties are entitled to receive annual grants. Metropolitan cities are central cities of Metropolitan Statistical Areas (MSAs) or other cities within MSAs that have populations of at least 50,000. Urban counties are those within MSAs that are authorized to undertake community development and housing activities and that meet certain population requirements.

From each year's appropriation, excluding the amounts provided for the UDAG program and the Secretary's Discretionary Fund, 70 percent is allocated to metropolitan cities and urban counties. The amount of each entitlement grant is determined by a statutory formula that uses several objective measures of community need, including poverty, population, housing overcrowding, age of housing, and growth lag.

Congress has allocated some $3 billion to the CDBG program for FY1987. This program has been level-funded by Congress in recent years, although the current appropriations represent approximately a 14 percent decline in funding below historical program appropriations.[41]

(2)   Nonentitlement for States and Small Cities

The Nonentitlement CDBG program for states and small cities provides grants to carry out a wide range of community development activities directed toward neighborhood revitalization, economic development, improved community facilities, and services. As with the entitlement program, applicants must give maximum feasible priority to activities that will benefit low and moderate income families, aid in the prevention or elimination of slums and blight, or address other community development needs that present a serious and immediate threat to the health or welfare of the community. No less than 51 percent of the funds must be used for activities that benefit low and moderate income persons over a period specified by the State, but not to exceed three years.

Under the 1981 amendments to the CDBG legislation, each State has the option to administer the block grant funds provided for its nonentitlement areas.

If this option is exercised, the block grant funds are provided to the states, which distribute them as grants to the eligible units of general local government. The states' objectives and methods of distributing the funds are determined in consultation with affected citizens and local elected officials, and must be made available to citizens and units of general local

[41]HUD Appropriations, note 31, above, at 13–14. *See also* note 39, for FY 1988 funding levels.

government throughout the State. States are required to report annually the use of funds.

If the self-administration option is not exercised, HUD continues as administrator and awards funds in a competition on the basis of selection criteria established by the Department.

Legislation establishing this program was enacted in 1974. Nonentitlement units of government are generally those under 50,000 in population, which are not metropolitan cities or part of an urban county.

From each year's CDBG appropriation, excluding the amounts provided for the Urban Development Action Grant program and the Secretary's Discretionary Fund, 30 percent is allocated to nonentitlement areas. This amount is then allocated among the states on a formula basis. Each state's allocation is distributed to units of general local government by either the State or HUD under the option described above.

(c) Housing Development Grants

The Housing Development Grant (HODAG) program is intended to increase the availability of rental housing for lower income people in areas where there is a severe shortage of housing. Development grants are used to help private developers construct or substantially rehabilitate rental housing in those areas.[42] They are useful for off-site retirement facility improvements in rural areas.

All projects assisted by development grants must reserve at least 20 percent of the units for families with incomes at or below 80 percent of the median income of the area. Owners of projects must agree to keep the assisted units available for occupancy by lower income tenants for 20 years, and must agree not to convert the units to condominiums during the 20 year period.

Development grants cannot exceed 50 percent of the total cost, less acquisition, of rehabilitating or developing the building. Once selected, the projects must be under construction within 24 months of HUD approval. When construction or rehabilitation of a project has been completed and the project reaches a certain level of occupancy, it is closed out by HUD. At that time, the city, urban county, or state becomes responsible for monitoring project operations and approving rent increases.

Like the Urban Development Action Grant program, funds for housing development grants are awarded to cities, urban counties, and states, acting on behalf of units of government, through national competition.

Eligible areas are cities designated in the June 30, 1984, *Federal Register*, or urban counties that are determined to be experiencing severe housing shortages as defined in accordance with the statutory criteria. Other areas may apply if they can demonstrate a special housing need or if they have a particular neighborhood preservation purpose.

[42] 42 U.S.C. § 1437o; 24 C.F.R. § 850.

Selection criteria include, but are not limited to, the severity of shortage of decent rental housing, the availability of public-private funding, and the provision of the maximum number of units for the least cost to the federal government. No project will be approved without proof of firm financial commitments. A total of $99.55 million was allocated for the HODAG program for FY1987, to provide approximately 4500 rental units.[43]

(d) Rental Rehabilitation

The Rental Rehabilitation program provides grants to cities and states to encourage rental housing rehabilitation, and rental subsidies to help lower income tenants remain in the building or relocate to other suitable housing. It is designed to attract private financing to rehabilitation.[44]

Grants are awarded on a formula basis to communities with 50,000 or greater population, urban counties, and states. Rental Rehab funds (generally not more than an average of $5000 per unit) may be used for up to one-half the total eligible rehabilitation costs of the project. An average minimum rehabilitation of $600 per unit is required to assure that a certain level of rehabilitation is necessary before public subsidies are provided.

Eligible rehabilitation activities are limited by the Act to those necessary to correct substandard conditions, make essential improvements, and repair major systems in danger of failure. Energy related repairs considered necessary by the grantee, as well as those repairs necessary to make rental units accessible to the handicapped, are also eligible.

After rehabilitation, 70 to 100 percent of the units in the local program must be occupied by low income families. In addition, an equitable share of grant funds must be used to aid large families. Rents after rehabilitation must be at market rates and not limited by rent controls.

Grants may be used only in neighborhoods where the median income does not exceed 80 percent of the area median, and where rents are not likely to increase more rapidly than the market area.

Metropolitan cities and urban counties are entitled to funds if their minimum grant under the HUD formula is at least $50,000. States also receive funds based on the formula for distribution to nonentitled areas (excluding those rural areas eligible for assistance from the Farmers Home Administration under Title V of the Housing Act of 1949).

For metropolitan cities, urban counties, and states, HUD awards funds based on a formula that considers three specific factors:

1. Rental units where the income of rental households is at or below the poverty level;
2. Rental units built before 1940, where the income of the household is at or below the poverty level; and

---

[43]HUD Appropriations (Conference Report), note 31, above, at 6.
[44]42 U.S.C. § 1437o; 24 C.F.R. § 511.

3. Rental units with at least one of four housing problems: overcrowding, high rent costs, incomplete kitchen facilities, or incomplete plumbing. This factor is weighted double in the formula.

In order to allow a reasonable program level, the lowest amount HUD grants to a city or urban county under the formula is $50,000 each fiscal year. Lesser amounts are added to the appropriate state's formula amount for distribution to eligible units of general local government.

In any state that does not elect to administer its share of Rental Rehab funds, HUD awards funds to eligible grantees through a competitive program.

A total of $200 million for approximately 28,000 rental rehabilitation units was allocated in FY1987.[45] Each of these units is available for use in conjunction with the Housing Voucher Demonstration Program. This voucher program, which is similar to the Section 8 Existing Housing Program, provides families with monthly housing assistance payments but permits them to use the vouchers in renting units with higher than the HUD Fair Market rents. The monthly payments are based on the difference between a payment standard for the area (not the actual rent) and 30 percent of their monthly income.[46]

§ 15   TAX EXEMPT FINANCING

§ 15.1   GENERALLY

Tax exempt bond financing has long been an attractive option for financing public facilities. Pursuant to Section 103 of the Internal Revenue Code, as a general rule, private individuals and corporations are not required to include in gross income for purposes of federal income tax interest received with respect to governmental obligations. Consequently, an issuer can pay a lower interest rate on its obligations and yet produce after tax earnings to bondholders equivalent to a taxable investment.

While tax exempt financing had been used extensively for financing purely governmental facilities, it was only in the 1970s that it began to be used extensively for various private activities. In order to comply with the terms of the exemption, public agencies issued revenue bonds and either lent the proceeds to private companies or used the proceeds to construct facilities for lease to private companies. The use of tax-exempt financing was available only for public purposes, but such a finding was not difficult, and ranged from the provision of health or educational services to the community by nonprofit institutions to the general economic benefits conferred upon the community by for profit businesses.

[45] HUD Appropriations (Conference Report), note 31, above, at 6.
[46] 42 U.S.C. § 1437f(o).

Tax exempt financing began to be used by cities, counties, and special authorities as a means to compete against each other for new business enterprises or to retain existing businesses. Congress was alarmed by the prospect of a substantial amount of the capital financing of the nation being done on a tax exempt basis, thereby resulting in a serious revenue drain for the Treasury. Therefore, beginning in 1968 Congress enacted legislation greatly restricting the use of tax exempt "industrial revenue bonds," a term that was defined in Section 103(b) of the Internal Revenue Code to include bonds issued to finance the trade or business of a nonexempt person.[47] The 1986 revision to the Code imposes even greater restrictions, as described below.

While tax exempt financing has been restricted over the years for for-profit activities, it has been retained virtually without restriction for most nonprofit ventures. Thus, hospitals, universities, and homes for the aged operated by nonprofit organizations that are exempt from taxation under Section 501(c)(3) of the Internal Revenue Code are able to finance their projects using a governmental agency as a conduit with few restrictions that do not apply to the governmental agency itself.

§ 15.2   NONPROFIT ORGANIZATIONS

Despite early proposals to the contrary, the 1986 Internal Revenue Code revisions are very favorable to tax exempt financing for organizations described in Section 501(c)(3) of the Code. The Code now includes special provisions for Qualified 501(c)(3) Bonds[48] and, for the most part, treats those bonds the same as it does bonds issued for governmental agencies. However, Section 145 of the Code applies to these bonds and imposes the following qualifications:

All property provided by the net proceeds of the issue must be owned by a 501(c)(3) organization or a governmental unit.

Not more than 5 percent of the net proceeds may be expended on property used in a private business and not more than 5 percent of the security for the bonds may be used in a private business.

No individual borrower or group of related borrowers may have outstanding at any time debt derived from Qualified 501(c)(3) bonds (including defeased bonds that have not yet been redeemed) exceeding $150 million except that portion of any bond issue devoted to hospital purposes (not including skilled nursing facilities).[49]

None of the foregoing limits apply if an election is made for the bond issue not to be governed by Section 145 but, rather, to come within another

[47]P.L. 90-364.
[48]I.R.C. § 145.
[49]I.R.C. § 145(b).

exemption category, such as those for residential rental project bonds or redevelopment bonds (see § 15.3).

For this type of financing to be used, the bond proceeds must be used only for operations that qualify the organization for 501(c)(3) status. Thus, this type of tax exempt financing could not be used for a project that does not provide low income housing, provide the elements of security set forth in Revenue Procedure 72-124, or otherwise constitute a charitable activity.[50]

Because the regulations have been tightened significantly by the 1986 amendments, limitations on the use of proceeds of qualified 501(c)(3) bonds for any nonexempt purpose may be problematic. The law provides that no more than 5 percent of the net proceeds of the bond issue may be used for a nonexempt purpose. Because the law deems that the costs of issuance are not an exempt purpose, that expense (capped at 2 percent; see below) must be deducted from the 5 percent, leaving 3 percent maximum private business activity permitted to be financed by net proceeds of or to secure the bonds. The following are some general guidelines as to the treatment of typical retirement home activities as nonexempt businesses:

1. In general, property made available to a private business enterprise on a preferential or exclusive basis is considered a nonexempt business. Thus, if the facility contains retail stores, a beauty parlor, or a private physician's office, rented to a private person or subject to a concession agreement, this portion of the facility would be considered a nonexempt business.

2. A component of the housing may be considered a nonexempt business, depending on the basis of the organization's exemption. For example, if an organization's exemption is based on the provision of low income housing, and it develops a project in which 50 percent of the units are low income and 50 percent are market rate, the operation of the market rate housing may be a nonexempt business because it does not advance the charitable purpose of providing low income housing. Because the unrelated business component is more than three percent, expenditure of bond proceeds on this component of the project could endanger the tax exempt status of the entire issue. A solution to this problem is to use tax exempt bond proceeds only for the low income units and finance the market rate component using taxable financing or equity.

3. Management contracts with for profit managers are also considered nonexempt businesses unless they meet certain tests, including a term not exceeding five years, the owner's right to terminate without cause at the end of any three-year period, at least 50 percent of the compensation based on a periodic fixed fee, and no amount of compensation based on a share of net profits.[51] A nonqualifying management contract for the entire facility

---

[50]For a discussion of the standards for determination that a retirement home activity is related to an organization's 501(c)(3) status, see § 9.

[51]Rev. Proc. 82-14, 1982-1 C.B. 459. Tax Reform Bill of 1986, Statement of the Managers, at ¶¶ 688–689.

disqualifies the entire facility from tax exempt financing, while a nonqualifying contract with respect to a particular portion of the facility (e.g., food service), relates only to the facilities managed, resulting in these facilities being deemed a private business.

4. There are special rules[52] with respect to physician contracts, counting such contracts as nonexempt businesses unless the following tests related to compensation termination date and early termination without cause are met:

A contract which provides for compensation based on a periodic flat fee must not exceed a term of five years. In addition, the owner must have the right to cancel the contract at the end of each two-year period of the contract term. Compensation must be reasonable and any automatic increases in compensation must be based on an agreed upon external standard, such as the percentage increases in the Consumer Price Index.

A contract providing for compensation based on a percentage of fees charged for services rendered by the physician must be reasonable and may not exceed a term of two years and the owner must have the right to cancel the contract without penalty or cause by giving 90 days' notice. The compensation must be reasonable and the percentage may not be based on a percentage of net profits of the owner or one of its divisions. It could, however, be a percentage of gross fees or modified gross fees. A contract that permits the physician to retain 100 percent of the professional fee is generally treated by bond counsel as a percentage contract, subject to these standards.

There are occasions in which it is desirable for a facility to contain private business activity in excess of the limit set forth in the Code—as, for example, where street-level commercial spaces would be desirable to generate income and to provide shops for the convenience of residents. In such a case, the space devoted to private business activity could be financed by a separate taxable loan, which is secured on a parity basis with the tax exempt loan, or the space could be developed as a separate condominium until pledged separately as security for a taxable loan.

§ 15.3 RESIDENTIAL RENTAL PROJECTS

Section 142(d) of the Internal Revenue Code of 1986 provides that governmental bonds issued for residential rental projects developed by either for profit or nonprofit owners are tax exempt if, at all times during the qualified project period, one of the following tests is met (at the election of the issuer):

[52]Rev. Proc. 82-15, 1982-1 C.B. 46.

Twenty percent or more of the residential units are occupied by individuals whose income is 50 percent or less of area median gross income; or

Forty percent or more of the residential units are occupied by individuals whose income is 60 percent or less of area median gross income.

The qualified project period commences on the first day on which 10 percent of the units are occupied and terminates either (1) 15 years after 50 percent are occupied, (2) upon repayment of the bonds, or (3) at termination of a federal Section 8 rental assistance contract.

Determination of median area income is made in accordance with existing HUD guidelines and is adjusted by family size. The Code permits residents to qualify if their income increases during residency up to 140 percent of the qualifying income; above that amount, the project does not cease to qualify so long as the next available unit of comparable or smaller size is made available to a qualified resident.[53]

Residential rental project bonds can be used in cases in which 501(c)(3) bonds cannot be used, such as where the sponsor is not a 501(c)(3) organization, a long-term management contract with a for profit organization is desired, or the project is an unrelated trade or business of a 501(c)(3) organization. However, because interest on the bonds is includable as preference income for the alternative minimum tax, residential rental project bonds will sell at a somewhat higher interest rate than 501(c)(3) bonds and should be used only where 501(c)(3) bonds are not available.

§ 15.4   LIMITATIONS ON ALL TAX EXEMPT BONDS

The following limitations apply to all types of tax exempt bonds described above.

(a)   Arbitrage

The Internal Revenue Code defines an *arbitrage bond* as any bond that is part of an issue, any portion of the proceeds of which are reasonably expected, at the time of issuance of the bond, to be used directly or indirectly to acquire higher yielding investments or to replace funds that were used for that purpose.[54] This type of investment is disfavored because it permits a borrower to profit at the expense of the federal treasury and, therefore, interest on arbitrage bonds is generally taxable.[55] The Code makes certain exceptions to the definition, including:

---

[53]I.R.C. § 142(d)(3).
[54]I.R.C. § 148(a).
[55]I.R.C. § 103(b)(2).

1. The Code permits unlimited yield during a "reasonable temporary period until such proceeds are needed for the purpose for which [the bond] issue was issued."[56] In general, the period may not exceed three years. However, with respect to pooled bond issues, the higher yield may be retained only during a six month period prior to being loaned to the ultimate borrower. That borrower may then take advantage of the remainder of the three year temporary period.[57]

2. The Code permits unlimited yield on a reasonably required reserve or replacement fund, not to exceed 10 percent of the proceeds of the bond issue unless the Secretary of the Treasury is satisfied that a higher amount is necessary.[58] Typically, a tax exempt amortized bond issue has included a debt service reserve fund equal to maximum annual debt service (principal, interest, and credit enhancement fee, if any). If interest rates return again to the levels that prevailed in the early 1980s, this traditional formula will result in a debt service reserve in excess of that permitted in the Code.[59] However, because it is no longer possible to earn arbitrage on such a reserve bond, it may become less common.

The foregoing exceptions are subject to the requirement that excess earnings be rebated to the federal government every five years.[60] Therefore, while these exceptions allow arbitrage gains and losses to be averaged over the five year period, they do not permit retention of any net arbitrage profits.

For the purpose of calculating arbitrage, the issue price of the bonds is used, rather than the net proceeds to the borrower. Therefore, it is no longer permissible to use arbitrage earnings to pay for the costs of issuance. However, in calculating arbitrage, it is permissible to count as interest expense the cost of credit enhancement, such as bond insurance premiums and letter of credit fees.

(b) Relationship of Bond Maturity to Life of Assets

The Internal Revenue Code prohibits the average maturity of tax exempt bonds from exceeding 120 percent of the average reasonably expected economic life of the facilities being financed with the net proceeds of the bond issue.[61] Land is not taken into account unless it represents 25 percent or

---

[56]I.R.C. § 148(c)(1).

[57]I.R.C. § 148(c)(2).

[58]I.R.C. § 148(d).

[59]The pre-1986 Code permitted a 15 percent reserve, which was adequate for even the highest interest rates prevailing during that period.

[60]I.R.C. § 148(f).

[61]I.R.C. § 147(b).

more of the bond issue, in which case it is treated as having a life of 30 years.[62]

(c) Public Approval Requirement

The Code also requires that tax exempt bonds issued for private activities be approved either by the electorate or by the applicable governmental representatives of the governmental unit having jurisdiction, after notice and a public hearing.[63]

(d) Restriction on Issuance Costs

Issuance costs financed by the bond issue cannot exceed two percent of the aggregate face amount of the issue.[64] Issuance costs include underwriting discounts, attorneys fees, commitment fees, and other fees incidental to issuance of the bonds. Issuance costs do not include credit enhancement fees and prepaid interest. Issuance costs may, and often will, exceed the two percent limit but, to the extent they do, must be paid from a source other than bond proceeds. For established institutions, corporate equity can be used. Where corporate equity is not available, as with a start-up corporation, a supplemental taxable borrowing may be necessary to meet these costs.

(e) Advance Refundings

A typical fixed rate long-term bond issue provides call protection[65] for a specified period (e.g., 10 years) and thereafter will provide the right of redemption with a declining premium for a further specified period (e.g., 2 percent, declining at one-half percent per year for four years). During the call protection period, the borrower may wish to refinance the debt. The borrower may do this in order to obtain new debt at lower interest rates or to modify certain covenants or conditions in the underlying debt instruments that would otherwise require bondholder consent. Typically, refinancing occurs through an advance refunding. In an advance refunding, new bonds are issued and the proceeds are used to purchase United States Government securities in such denominations and maturities as will discharge the old bonds at the first permissible call date or a specified later date. These securities are then placed in trust for the benefit of the old bondholders, and the existing indenture or other security instrument is thereby released, permitting the security instrument for the new bonds to be installed in its place.

---

[62]*Id.*

[63]I.R.C. § 147(f).

[64]I.R.C. § 147(g).

[65]That is, a prohibition against calling the bonds for repayment, *see* § 18.4.

The result of an advance refunding is that there are, for some period of time, two bond issues outstanding where previously there was one and tax exempt interest is paid on principal representing approximately twice the borrower's capital requirement. If the second bond issue is refunded, likewise, there could be three issues outstanding. Potentially, any number of refundings could occur prior to the first bonds being redeemed. Out of concern about the resulting revenue loss to the United States Treasury, Congress in 1986 provided that tax exempt bonds issued for governmental or 501(c)(3) organizations generally can be advance refunded only once, and all other tax exempt bonds may not be advance refunded at all.[66] Generally, the Code defines *advance refunding* as a transaction in which the refunding bond is issued more than 90 days before the redemption of the refunded bond.[67] Prior to the 1986 Act, the standard was 180 days. This is significant in that many debt instruments provide for redemption of bonds to occur on only one of the semiannual interest payment dates. In order to assure maximum flexibility, provision for redemption at least quarterly should be provided.

The Code additionally requires that refunded bonds be redeemed on the earliest date on which the bond may be redeemed. For bonds issued after 1985, there is no exception related to the premium that must be paid on that date and, therefore, there is no opportunity to time the redemption to avoid paying a high premium.[68] Furthermore, an advance refunding may be undertaken only "if the issuer may realize present value debt service savings (determined without regard to administrative expenses) in connection with the issue of which the refunding bond is a part."[69] However, the Conference Committee Report indicates that Congress did not intend to prohibit low to high refundings to avoid adverse covenants or to restructure debt, so long as it does not constitute a device to obtain a material financial advantage based on arbitrage.[70]

§ 15.5   USE OF BOND PROCEEDS FOR RELIGIOUS PURPOSES

Because many retirement communities are developed by organizations affiliated with religious denominations, it is important to consider the implications of the First Amendment prohibition against the establishment of religion in the context of tax exempt financing.[71] The First Amendment does

[66] I.R.C. § 149(d).

[67] I.R.C. § 149(d).

[68] I.R.C. § 149(d)(3)(A).

[69] I.R.C. § 149(d)(3)(B)(i).

[70] Tax Report Bill of 1986 (H.R. 3838) Statement of the Managers, pp. II–758.

[71] Regarding the historical origin and application of the Establishment Clause, see Note, *Establishment Clause Analysis of Legislative and Administrative Aid to Religion*, 74 Colum. L. Rev. 1175 (1974).

not preclude the lending of proceeds of tax exempt bonds to religious institutions merely because they are religious but it does preclude the use of such funds for purposes that are solely for religious purposes, such as the construction of a chapel used solely for religious services, and the construction of housing exclusively for members of a religious order. However, a multipurpose assembly facility can be financed, even if it will be expected to be used, among other purposes, for religious services.

§ 15.6   THE ISSUER AND FORM OF TAX EXEMPT BONDS

As noted above, while the proceeds of tax exempt bonds may be used to finance the activities of a nongovernmental entity, tax exemption is granted only if the bonds constitute an obligation of a state or a political subdivision of the state, such as a city, county, or special district. Thus, it is essential that a public agency be willing to act as a conduit for the transaction. As the term implies, a conduit is merely an instrumentality through which bond proceeds flow on their way from the bond purchasers to the ultimate borrower, for the sole purpose of rendering the bonds tax exempt. The conduit has no liability for repayment of the bonds other than from the debt service payments made by the borrower and is, in many cases, a thoroughly disinterested party. However, in some cases, especially where a state authority is used, the conduit imposes various requirements on the borrower and monitors its activities for both programmatic reasons reasons and in order to protect its reputation or carry out legislatively mandated policy.[72]

Occasionally, location of a suitable and willing conduit is difficult. The following lists possible candidates and explains factors to consider in making the selection.

(a) State Authorities

Most states have established separate units of state government, known as authorities. They operate under legislative enabling acts that set out their power to issue bonds, limitations on bonding capacity, and often other rules and regulations connected with their operations. State authorities are usually limited to specific purposes (e.g., health care, housing, education, pollution control) or combinations of purposes, and most states have several authorities. Most appropriate to retirement homes are state housing financing authorities and state health facility financing authorities. The advantages of these agencies are that they are well established, have sufficient legislative authority, and often sponsor pooled programs, which can help spread the costs of smaller projects. The disadvantages are that

---

[72]For example, the California Health Facilities Financing Authority imposes, pursuant to its enabling act, a "community service obligation," requiring financed facilities to provide services to a population representative of the community served, including Medicaid patients. Cal. Gov. Code § 15459.

they may have rigid program requirements, require borrowers to use pre-
selected investment bankers and other consultants, may have a maximum
aggregate debt authorization, and may have politicized project selection
processes.

(b)   Local Authorities

In many localities, state law allows cities and counties to establish independent financing authorities. These function like the state authorities, but
are controlled at the local level. Examples of these authorities include local
health facility financing authorities, housing authorities, and redevelopment agencies. They have the advantage of greater flexibility, since most of
these authorities are less bureaucratic and more open to borrower initiative than are the state authorities. A disadvantage is that they may be overly
influenced by local politics, and they may lack sufficient legislative authority for certain types of projects.

(c)   City or County Bonds

Often, cities and counties can issue revenue bonds and loan the proceeds to
private borrowers in order to accomplish ends that are to the benefit of
their residents. Authority for such bonds must be either specifically granted
by the state legislature or provided pursuant to a city's charter under its
constitutional home rule authority.[73] As a general rule, cities are vested
with more extensive authority than counties. As with the foregoing options,
these bonds do not constitute a debt or obligation of the public agency but
are issued entirely on the strength of the private borrower. A city or county
may offer more flexibility than an authority, but smaller governments especially may suffer from lack of experience with conduit financing. Additionally, they may be overly influenced by local politics and may charge excessive fees.

(d)   Certificates of Participation

A relatively new vehicle has been developed in recent years to permit a
local governmental entity to serve as a conduit even if it does not have the
authority to issue bonds. Internal Revenue Code Section 103, grants tax
exemption for interest on obligations, generally, rather than bonds, specifically, and therefore the Internal Revenue Service has found that it extends
also to interest components of a public agency's obligation to make payments under a lease or a contract of sale.[74] Because public agencies, usually

---

[73]Generally, municipal corporations can exercise only those powers granted, in express
words, by either an authorizing statute or a charter. 56 Am. Jur. 2d, *Municipal Corporations*,
§ 194.

[74]*Marsh Monument Co, Inc. v. U.S.*, 301 F. Supp. 1316 (E.D. Mich. 1969).

cities, have been given broad authority to buy and sell or lease property to effectuate public purposes, they can contract to buy property from the owner and sell it back to the owner and the interest component of the entity's obligation under the purchase contract will be exempt from taxation. The seller's right to receive these payments are assigned to a trustee, and the trustee then sells participations in the right to receive the payments. These participations, (called certificates of participation) are marketed in conventional bond denominations and are treated by the market as though they were bonds.

(e) 63-20 Bonds

One arrangement permits a nonprofit organization to directly issue tax exempt bonds without the use of a governmental conduit. Under Internal Revenue Service Revenue Ruling 63-20,[75] a nonprofit corporation can directly issue tax exempt bonds for the benefit of a public agency. This form of debt, which is becoming less popular, is burdened with some very stringent conditions:

The public agency on whose behalf the bonds are issued must approve the transaction.

A deed, conveying the property from the nonprofit corporation to the public agency, must be placed in escrow, to be delivered on the date on which the debt is repaid; the property may not be encumbered with other debt when conveyed.

The public agency must be given the option to purchase the property at any time by repaying the debt.

Once the property is conveyed to the public agency, it may not be reconveyed back to the borrower for at least 90 days.[76]

Because the property may not be further encumbered beyond the term of the bonds, refinancings can be accomplished only for shorter and shorter periods as time goes on, making expansions and renewals less and less feasible. Use of this method requires a great deal of trust between the nonprofit borrower and the public agency, since there is no guarantee that the public agency will not decide to acquire the property for the amount of the debt and oust the nonprofit borrower, and undoing the transaction is difficult. Therefore, this method is generally looked upon as a last resort.

§ 15.7   PARTICIPANTS AND DOCUMENTS IN A TAX EXEMPT BOND ISSUE

Because tax exempt bond issues are usually carried out as conduit transactions, they are more complex and involve more parties than a conventional

---

[75] 1963-1 C.B. 24.

[76] Rev. Proc. 82-26, 1982-1 C.B. 476.

loan transaction. This section discusses the structure of a tax exempt bond issue, describes the parties who are involved in structuring and administering it, and notes the duties and particular considerations applicable to these parties.

(a) Structure and Participants

In a typical tax exempt conduit financing (see Figure 15.1), bonds are issued by a public agency issuer and are sold at a discount to an underwriter, which resells them to individual bondholders at a price that usually (but not always) equals par. The underwriter's discount is its compensation for structuring the transaction and selling the bonds. The issuer then lends the bond proceeds to the borrower, a nonprofit organization, for a qualified project. The issuer assigns to a trustee its obligation to the bondholders and its rights against the borrower, and thereafter, since it is only a conduit, the issuer has little if any rights or obligations. If the bonds are credit-enhanced, the credit enhancer (such as an insurance company or a bank) enters into an agreement with the borrower for the benefit of the bondholders, usually naming the issuer and the trustee as beneficiaries. The borrower then grants a security interest (such as a deed of trust) for the benefit of the credit enhancer.

The following is a list of the participants in a tax-exempt bond issue, together with a brief description of their functions:

1. *The Borrower.* The borrower is the organization that develops the project and, for that purpose, borrows the proceeds of the bond issue.

2. *Borrower's Counsel.* The borrower is represented by legal counsel, who is responsible for reviewing and negotiating the documents to see that they meet the borrower's needs. Borrower's counsel also drafts documents related to the borrower, such as resolutions, certificates, and various contracts and, at closing, delivers an opinion relating to the borrower's participation in the transaction.

3. *Financial Consultant.* The borrower often engages the services of a financial consultant, whose role it is to analyze the capital needs of the borrower and recommend a course of action. The role of the financial consultant may be combined with that of the underwriter, although some borrowers desire to obtain independent advice, fearing that the underwriting firm may tend to structure the transaction more to facilitate sale of the bonds than meet the needs of the borrower and may not explore alternatives outside the transactions with which the firm is familiar.

4. *The Underwriter.* The underwriter is an investment banking firm that structures the transaction and agrees to purchase the bonds for resale to the ultimate purchasers. The underwriter's role is the key to making the financing work, since it coordinates the demands of the market with the needs of the borrower. The underwriter also frequently functions as the leader of the financing team, coordinating the activities of the other participants.

5. *Underwriter's Counsel.* Underwriter's counsel is an attorney who advises the underwriter with respect to the structuring of the transaction. In addition, underwriter's counsel usually drafts the official statement and the bond purchase agreement as well as any remarketing agreement, tender agent agreement or paying agent agreement required as part of a variable rate transaction. Underwriter's counsel is responsible for advising the underwriter with respect to compliance with securities laws, giving an opinion with respect to exemption from registration with the Securities and Exchange Commission and qualification of the bonds with the securities commissioners in the various states in which it is expected that the bonds will be sold.

6. *Bond Counsel.* Bond counsel drafts the principal legal documents setting forth the form of the bonds and the terms and conditions on which they are issued. In addition, bond counsel gives an opinion for the benefit of the bondholders to the effect that the bonds have been legally issued and that interest on the bonds is exempt from federal income tax. Bond counsel usually orchestrates the issue and assists the underwriter in coordinating the performance by the other parties.

7. *Issuer.* The issuer, which is a public agency, takes those actions necessary to issue the bonds, but otherwise has a fairly passive role.

8. *Issuer's Counsel.* The issuer usually has an attorney who reviews the documents and issues an opinion at closing. As this opinion is usually narrowly drawn, relating largely to the due existence and organization of the issuer and its approval of the transaction, the issuer's attorney usually plays a fairly passive role.

9. *Trustee.* The trustee under the indenture is responsible for maintaining funds, authenticating bonds, paying principal and interest payments and, in the event of a default, protecting the interests of the bondholders through foreclosure or other remedies. The trustee is concerned that its duties be provided for in a manner with which it is comfortable and that it be indemnified with respect to the acts of other parties.

10. *Trustee's Counsel.* Trustee's counsel advises the trustee with respect to matters of concern to it and may render an opinion at closing.

11. *Credit Enhancer.* The credit enhancer, which may be a bank, insurance company, or other guarantor, agrees to make payments in the event of a default by the borrower. It is concerned that its obligation be set forth clearly and that the transaction as a whole be structured so as to give it adequate security prior to and following any default.

12. *Credit Enhancer's Counsel.* The credit enhancer's attorney drafts the principal credit enhancement documents such as the letter of credit, reimbursement agreement or insurance contract and negotiates other documents affecting the security or obligations of the credit enhancer. This attorney also gives an opinion at closing to the effect that the credit enhancer has legitimately entered into the transaction.

13. *Accountants.* The accountants for the borrower are asked to present audited financial statements and comfort letters, as described below.

14. *Feasibility Consultants.* A feasibility consultant is engaged with respect to a new or expanded facility, in order to assure the bondholders that the revenue generated by the new project will be sufficient to service the debt. The feasibility consultant's report is usually included in the closing documents and may be included in the official statement or made available to prospective bondholders upon request.

15. *Rating Agencies.* Rating Agencies must approve all documents prior to giving their ratings and, therefore, they receive copies of draft documents and comment on provisions which they do not find acceptable.

(b)   Basic Bond Documents

The issuer—a governmental agency such as a state or local authority or a city or county government—issues the bonds. The issuer usually evidences its determination to do so by means of two resolutions: the first, often called an inducement resolution, is adopted before the transaction is structured in order to let the parties know that the issuer will look favorably on the bond issue and that they can expend time and money in structuring the transaction. The final resolution is adopted after the documents are in substantially final form and the principal amount and other terms are substantially established.

The bonds are issued in accordance with the terms of an Indenture, which is a trust agreement between the issuer and a trustee, usually a substantial bank or trust company. The Indenture governs the terms of the bonds, setting forth such matters as the actual text of the bonds, the establishment of various funds to be held and administered by the trustee, restrictions on and conditions of parity debt and additional bonds, repayment and defeasance provisions, and other matters. The Indenture usually does not contain particular covenants of the ultimate borrower, but pledges as security the borrower's payments to the issuer.

The actual bonds are held by the trustee and, once the transaction is closed, they are authenticated by the trustee pursuant to the provisions of the Indenture and are delivered to the purchaser, usually one or more investment bankers, pursuant to the terms of a Purchase Agreement. The Purchase Agreement is an agreement between the issuer, the purchaser, and the borrower and governs the terms under which the purchaser will purchase the bonds. This agreement has numerous terms and conditions, which are described in great detail, since it obligates the purchaser to a multimillion dollar expenditure for securities, which the purchaser will sell in the securities markets; therefore, the purchaser is concerned that the bonds conform to the standards of that market. Typically, the Purchase Agreement conditions the purchaser's obligation to purchase the bonds on the following:

The issuance of a letter of representation by the borrower, making certain factual statements regarding the borrower and its operations.

The receipt of opinions of counsel, in substantially the form set forth in the Purchase Agreement, from:

Counsel to the borrower, who will opine that the borrower is duly incorporated and in good standing, that it has authorized, executed, and delivered the documents required by the transaction and that such documents are valid and binding against the borrower in accordance with their terms, that the borrower holds title to its property, which is not subject to any nonpermitted encumbrances (in many states, counsel relies on a policy of title insurance), that the transaction does not violate law, the organizational documents of the borrower, or contracts to which the borrower is a party and that there is no litigation pending which materially affects the borrower other than that which has been disclosed.

Counsel to the issuer, who will opine that the issuer is a duly organized public agency and has authorized, executed, and delivered the transaction documents, and that such documents are valid and binding against the issuer.

Counsel to the underwriter (purchaser), who will opine that the bonds are exempt from registration under federal securities laws and that the applicable state securities laws have been complied with.

Bond counsel, who will opine that the transaction documents have been properly entered into and are valid and enforceable, and that interest on the bonds is tax exempt under federal tax laws. Following the 1986 Tax Reform Act, this opinion has been expanded to note certain exceptions to the general rule related to tax exempt status in the case of the environmental superfund tax on corporations and other similar exceptions. In the case of bonds other than 501(c)(3) bonds, this tax opinion is further qualified by references to the alternative minimum tax.

Counsel to the credit enhancer, who will opine that the credit enhancement documents have been properly executed and delivered and are enforceable against the credit enhancer.

The receipt of a comfort letter from the borrower's auditors, which brings down the audit to within an acceptable period prior to the closing (usually five days). This is often referred to as a cold comfort letter, because it states only that nothing has come to the attention of the auditor that indicates that a substantial change has occurred since the date of the audit.

Usually the purchaser has purchased the bonds for resale in the public market. It may sell the bonds using entirely its own personnel, especially if demand for the bonds is good and the aggregate principal amount is not large. However, often the purchaser consists of a syndicate of investment bankers, with one as the manager. The manager structures the transaction and receives a fee for that service and the other investment bankers agree, pursuant to an agreement among underwriters, to take a certain portion of the issue and to sell it using their own retail facilities.

The purchaser is usually compensated by means of a discount. That is, if the face amount is $10 million and the underwriters' discount is 2 percent, the issuer sells the bonds to the purchaser for $9.8 million and the purchaser sells them to investors at par, retaining $200,000 to compensate it for its services.

In connection with the transaction, the issuer issues an Official Statement. This document consists of an explanation of the terms of the bond issue, the covenants to which the borrower is subject, the credit enhancement, certain facts about the issuer, the borrower, the credit enhancer, and the project being financed, and risks involved in the transaction. The Official Statement is similar to a prospectus included in a registration statement filed with respect to a public offering of securities under federal securities laws. However, tax exempt obligations are exempt from registration requirements of a prospectus. Nonetheless, because Rule 10b-5 promulgated under Section 10(b) of the Securities Act of 1934 applies to all offers or sales of securities and prohibits dissemination of inadequate, false or misleading information to prospective investors, the Official Statement is the conventional means of providing disclosure in compliance with that law. Investors are accustomed to seeing information disseminated by means of the prospectus format, and, therefore, that format is used for the Official Statement. However, there are no explicit federal guidelines or approval processes for this document and generally the extent and style of disclosure in any Official Statement is greatly influenced by what appears to be the practice of the investment banking community in recent comparable transactions.

The Official Statement is usually first distributed in preliminary form prior to the pricing of the bonds. This is called the "red herring" because it has red printing on the cover warning readers that it is preliminary and subject to change. On the basis of this document, which explains the bond issue but leaves blank the interest rate and certain other key terms, the investment banker tests the market and then, when it knows on what terms it can sell the bonds, the bonds are priced. Once the terms are established, a final Official Statement is prepared and disseminated. If there are only insubstantial differences between the preliminary and final Official Statement, there is no need for further explanation. However, in exceptional cases, there may be a substantial change, and then it is necessary to call attention to the change on the cover of the Official Statement by means of a sticker.

The purchaser, at closing, pays for the bonds by delivering funds to the trustee, which deposits those funds in trust accounts established under

FIGURE 15.1

EXAMPLE OF A SUMMARY OF PROPOSED TERMS FOR A PUBLICLY OFFERED TAX EXEMPT BOND ISSUE

Principal Amount:	$40,000,000
Maturity:	No principal payments for first 3 years. Serial bonds due May 1 of 1991 through 2002. Term bond due 2021, with mandatory sinking fund.
Issuer:	_____ Health Facilities Authority
Borrower:	
Closing:	Closing date to be November 25, 1987, or such other date mutually agreed to.
Dated:	Bonds will be dated November 1, 1987
Interest Rate (estimated):	Serial bonds - 4.5%–6.6% Term bonds - 7%
Rating:	AAA Standard & Poors Aaa Moody's
Credit Enhancement:	California health facility construction loan insurance program
Security:	(1) First deed of trust on the project; (2) Pledge of gross revenues of the borrower
Project:	Construction of a life care facility with 300 residential units, 30 personal care units and a 50 bed skilled nursing facility
Presales:	60% of the units to be sold prior to closing with non-refundable deposits of not less than $10,000
Rate Covenant:	Maintain rates to produce debt service coverage ratio of at least 1.10. Covenant is met if ratio is at least 1.0 and a report of a management consultant is obtained and followed
Additional Debt:	Additional parity debt, either by issuance of additional bonds or otherwise, may be issued if the debt service coverage ratio for the most recent fiscal year (adjusted to include the proposed debt service) is at least 1.25 or if the report of a management consultant projects a debt service coverage ratio of at least 1.30 for the next three fiscal years
Call Provisions:	No call permitted prior to November 1, 1997. The bonds may be called at the borrower's option on any interest payment date on or after November 1, 1997, at a premium of 3% declining one percent per annum until the percentage equals par.

the Indenture. Occasionally, funds are transferred outside of the Indenture, as in the case in which prior indebtedness is paid off directly, with a receipt delivered to the trustee. The trustee uses the bond proceeds, as provided in the indenture, to repay prior indebtedness, pay the cost of issuance, pay the credit enhancement fee, and to advance proceeds to the borrower.

Proceeds advanced to the borrower are advanced pursuant to an agreement between the issuer and the borrower. While this document is usually a Loan Agreement, it could be an Installment Purchase Agreement or a Lease, depending how the transaction has been structured. These latter arrangements are used in situations in which the issuer is not permitted by law to make a direct loan but is permitted to purchase and sell or lease and sublease property. In the Loan Agreement, the borrower obtains the funds from the loan, agrees to repay the bonds, and agrees to abide by certain restrictive covenants imposed pursuant to the transaction, and is subject to certain default provisions. (See § 18.3) In the case of a transaction involving a Master Indenture, there are few restrictive covenants in the Loan Agreement, but the borrower's obligation under the Loan Agreement constitutes an obligation under the Master Indenture.

The Loan Agreement usually contains a cross default provision, which provides that a default under the loan constitutes a default under the Indenture and vice versa and that the borrower has ultimate responsibility for all performance under the transaction except in the case of malfeasance by one of the other parties. The reason for this provision is that the other parties (such as the issuer) are in the transaction for the benefit of the borrower and, ultimately, only the borrower is responsible for the debt. Thus, the loan from the bondholders to the issuer and the loan from the issuer to the borrower are essentially collapsed into one obligation. The only exception to the rule is encountered in certain HUD-financed conduit transactions in which HUD insures the loan from the issuer to the borrower and refuses to permit a default under the bond issue to adversely affect its insured mortgage.

§ 16   CONVENTIONAL FINANCING

The foregoing discussion has involved different forms of governmentally-assisted debt financing, involving government loans, guarantees, or bond issuance. Completely private financing is an option which should be considered for the following reasons:

It involves no approval by a public agency.
It may permit greater flexibility in structuring the terms and covenants.
Certain fees and expenses may be avoided.

On the other hand, public financing programs usually confer substantial benefits where they are available and feasible for a particular project.

These benefits include lower interest cost, less expensive credit enhance-ment, and greater access to the capital markets. The decision as to whether to use conventional financing or governmental assistance should be made on a case-by-case basis.

A full discussion of conventional financing (or the conventional aspects of government-assisted financing) would take more space than is available here. Therefore, the following is a brief discussion of certain aspects that are of particular concern to retirement home developments.

§ 16.1 SOURCES OF CONVENTIONAL FINANCING

The sources of conventional financing have typically consisted of banks and insurance companies, although the variety of sources that are poten-tially available is virtually limitless, including conventional business cor-. porations, individuals, and mutual funds. This discussion will, however, focus on banks and insurance companies. Both of those types of institu-tions lend substantial amounts of money and, since they are in the busi-ness of doing so, have established standard policies and criteria that must be met.

Approaching a bank or insurance company for a loan may be done di-rectly, especially if there is a preexisting business relationship that can facilitate the contact. Often, the use of a mortgage broker or other profes-sional is advantageous, since many lenders, especially insurance compa-nies, rely on a broker for their loans, and the broker has contacts that are used to place debt. Often, larger loans are placed with a consortium of lenders that has been structured by a broker.

§ 16.2 STRUCTURE OF THE TRANSACTION

A conventional financing transaction involves, in its simplest terms, a loan of money from the lender to the borrower and a promise to repay. Usually, the parties execute a document that is called a Loan Agreement if the lender is a bank, and a Note Purchase Agreement if the lender is an in-surance company. The distinction in these titles is historical. Banks con-ceive of their business as that of making loans and insurance companies as that of purchasing investments. References here to Loan Agreement encom-pass both.

The Loan Agreement contains a recital of the nature of the transaction and attaches a form of the promissory note. It establishes the terms and conditions of the closing, including the closing date and location, responsi-bility for payment of expenses, representations and warranties of the bor-rower, and the conditions of closing, which include opinions of counsel and certifications that the warranties and representations recited in the Loan Agreement remain true as of the date of closing. If the transaction uses a short form promissory note, the Loan Agreement includes the terms and conditions of repayment of the note, including interest rates, restrictions on prepayment, and other such terms. The Loan Agreement contains restrictive covenants relating to'the borrower, unless such covenants are contained in some other document, such as a deed of trust.

The Promissory Note, if in the short form, contains a basic promise to pay, the interest rate, and some additional terms, but refers back to the Loan Agreement with respect to the detailed terms. If in the long form, it contains all the promises to the noteholder without reference to the Loan Agreement. Even with a long form note, additional promises, especially including the business covenants, are found in security instruments such as a deed of trust.

A loan may be a general unsecured promise to pay. This form, especially if coupled with negative covenants precluding the borrower from pledging security to anyone else, may be sufficient. However, usually a security arrangement is necessary, involving a pledge of an asset or stream of revenue. The most common form of security is that of a deed of trust or mortgage on the facility. The deed of trust pledges the facility for the benefit of the lender and, in addition, restricts the borrowers by requiring maintenance and upkeep of the facility and restrictions on its use, and imposes other covenants on the borrower to protect the security of the lender. Other security devices, such as a pledge of personal property and a pledge of funds and accounts, may be required. In a life care facility, a pledge of the escrowed entrance fees may be requested.

§ 16.3 COOPERATIVES AND CONDOMINIUMS

Cooperatives and condominiums are methods whereby individual ownership of units within a retirement home can be effected. Permanent financing of such a development involves the sale of units to residents, who are directly or indirectly responsible for debt service. The advantages of this type of arrangement are that qualification for financing is based on the financial condition of the resident rather than an owner of the development, and residents may be entitled to certain tax benefits such as the principal residence interest deduction and the deferral of capital gains on the sale of a previous residence. Condominiums and cooperatives differ substantially in how they are financed, as follows:

1. A condominium consists of a common ownership of the underlying ground and the sole and exclusive ownership of the air rights that the dwelling unit occupies. The resident is the sole owner of a particular space and the portion of the building contained within it. That separate unit may be purchased and sold, and it may be pledged as security for a loan. Condominiums are usually financed by means of a mortgage or deed of trust on each individual unit. In the event of a foreclosure, the unit itself may be foreclosed and sold.

FIGURE 16.1

EXAMPLE OF A SUMMARY OF PROPOSED TERMS FOR A PRIVATELY PLACED TAXABLE DEBT ISSUE
$6,000,000 10% SECURED NOTES DUE 2010
THE ("SECURED NOTES")

Amount:	$3,500,000	*Maturity:*	2010
Rate:	10%, payable monthly	*Closing:*	January, 1988

Repayment: Interest only, payable semiannually, until 1990. Starting January 1, 1990, equal amortized semiannual principal and interest payments of $343,668.97.

Prepayment: The Secured Notes are nonrefundable for life; otherwise callable after year seven at a premium equal to the coupon, declining to par at maturity.

Collateral: The Secured Notes will be collateralized by: (i) a first mortgage lien on the _____ Health Center; (ii) a second mortgage lien (junior only to an existing first mortgage lien securing no more than $1,000,000 of debt due 1991 owing to _____, which lien will not be extended) on the _____ retirement residence; and (iii) an assignment, subject only to the prior lien, if any, of _____ as in (ii) above, of Owner's fee simple interest in the land (the "Premises") on which these buildings are situated together with all improvements, equipment, furniture, and fixtures owned by Owner and located on the Premises (the "Collateral"). Lender will be named as a loss payee as its interests appear on policies insuring the Collateral against such risks as customary and appropriate but in any event, in an amount sufficient to prepay the Secured Notes in the event of a casualty.

Use of Proceeds: The proceeds will be used to refund a like amount of debt owing to Former Lender and to fund the expenses of this transaction.

Special Counsel:

Principal Covenants: On a consolidated basis:

    (1) The annual long-term debt service coverage ratio (sum of: (i) revenues less expenses, (expenses to include capitalized development expense); (ii) depreciation, amortization and the write-off of noncash development expenses deducted as an expense; (iii) debt service deducted as an

FIGURE 16.1 *(Continued)*

Principal Covenants:
(Continued)

expense; and (iv) cash accommodation fees received less the amount amortized divided by debt service (interest and principal)) shall not be less than 1.25:1 and Owner shall levy charges sufficient for this purpose;

(2) The current ratio (adjusted to include unbilled receivables due within thirty (30) days and to exclude from current maturities of long term debt all but three months thereof); maintained at 1.3 to 1.0;

(3) The sum of cash, marketable securities and the available unused portion of bank revolvers shall not be less than $1,500,000;

(4) The fund balance (total assets less total liabilities) shall not be less than $17,000,000 plus the sum of: (i) a cumulative amount equal to 100% of excess revenues over expenses (without regard to losses); and (ii) an amount equal to the difference, from time to time, between the current value basis as acceptable by Owner's independent auditor of properties and equipment and the book value of such property and equipment on an original depreciated cost basis;

(5) The ratio of total liabilities to fund balance shall not be greater than 1:1, accounting for properties and equipment using current value basis as acceptable by Owner's independent auditor;

(6) No liens will be incurred except: (i) those existing at 9/30/87; (ii) those incurred in the ordinary course of business other than to secure debt for money borrowed; (iii) those in connection with Lender's Collateral; (iv) purchase money liens on after acquired property including improvements that lien will secure debt limited to the cost of the property and improvements and that may extend to encumber the assets to which the improvement is an integral part, and (v) extensions and renewals of the above (except for the lien in favor of _____ _____ on the _____ retirement residence, which lien may not be extended or renewed); and

FIGURE 16.1 *(Continued)*

Principal Covenants: *(Continued)*	(7) Owner will maintain its status as a nonprofit public benefit corporation and will maintain its present line of business.
	(8) Guarantees will be treated as debt and will be further limited to 1% of the fund balance.
	(9) Restricted payments are limited to 5% of total assets.
	(10) Mergers are permitted only if the survivor is a U.S. nonprofit public benefit corporation, is exempt from taxation as an organization described in Section 501(c)(3) of the Internal Revenue Code, assumes this obligation, and, on a proforma basis, no default or event of default exists.
	(11) Sale of assets, other than in the normal course of business, are limited to 5% of total assets in any one year.

2. A cooperative consists of the residents' ownership of stock in a corporation that owns the entire development. The ownership of stock gives the resident the right to occupy a particular unit in the development. The resident does not directly own real estate but, rather, owns an interest in a corporation that owns real estate. Therefore, the resident cannot finance the purchase of the unit by means of a mortgage or deed of trust, and cooperatives are financed by means of one of two methods. The cooperative itself may borrow the money and grant a security interest in the entire development, passing through the obligation for repayment to the residents. This method potentially exposes each resident to foreclosure if other residents fail to make their payments. Alternatively, each resident may borrow the purchase price separately and pledge shares of stock in the cooperative corporation.

§ 17   RATINGS AND CREDIT ENHANCEMENT

Debt is judged by lenders on the basis of its quality, the higher quality debt being more attractive and bearing a lower interest rate than lower quality debt. Debt can be either rated by a rating agency or unrated. The quality of debt can be judged solely on the basis of strengths and weaknesses of the borrower, or it can be enhanced by such means as insurance, a letter of credit, or a guarantee.

§ 17.1   UNRATED DEBT

Most debt does not carry the credit rating of an agency but, rather, is evaluated directly by the lender or purchaser. Much of this debt consists of private placements, wherein the transaction is negotiated directly with the ultimate holder, which independently evaluates the credit of the borrower. Unrated debt may also be publicly offered, in which case the purchasers make their decisions based on information disclosed in an official statement, including financial statements and feasibility analyses by reputable consulting firms.

In private placements, the purchasers are often banks or insurance companies and have well defined underwriting criteria that they expect their borrowers to follow. Thus, the standards that the borrower is expected to meet and the business covenants that are written into the loan documents are often rigidly prescribed and not susceptible to much negotiation.[77] However, in most cases, these standards can be negotiated to fit the circumstances of individual transactions.

§ 17.2   RATED DEBT

Most publicly offered debt is rated by prominent rating agencies, which assign a rating based on standard criteria developed by the agency. These criteria include a large number of factors, such as financial performance projections, the nature of the business, strength of management, characteristics of the service area, and the terms and conditions of the debt itself. Thus, where the rating is based entirely on the borrower, the rating agency will inquire into the strength of its management, demand for services and potential for growth in demand, the prevalence and strength of competitors, and numerous other factors. The rating agency will also impose strict standards on the debt itself, requiring certain covenants, such as those relating to debt service coverage ratios, insurance, and establishment of reserves.

The most prominent rating agencies are Standard and Poors and Moody's Investors Service. Neither of these agencies currently rates life care facilities or nursing facilities, since they appear to believe that they have no standard tests for ascertaining the credit strength of such a facility. Fitch Investors Service does rate life care facilities, however, and currently imposes the conditions set forth in Figure 17.1.

§ 17.3   BOND INSURANCE

Bond insurance constitutes a contract whereby an insurance company agrees to make required payments of principal and interest in the event that the borrower should default. There are several potential sources for

---

[77] See summary of typical business covenants in Figs. 15.1 and 16.1.

insurance of debt. Once debt is insured, it will generally be evaluated by purchasers based on the strength of the insuring entity. Thus, debt that is insured by an insurance company which is rated AAA trades at AAA interest rates, even though the borrower's rating, standing alone, would not be so favorably treated.

Examples of insurers are the federal government,[78] state agencies,[79] and private insurance organizations (such as AMBAC, MBIA, etc.). The difficulty with many private insurance programs is that their ratings are based, in part, on the strength of their portfolios and, since Standard and Poors and Moody's do not rate life care facilities, they do not rate insurance companies that insure more than a small percentage of life care facility debt. Rental facilities, which do not bear actuarial risk, can more easily qualify for the various municipal bond insurance programs now in existence.

In determining whether to purchase bond insurance, a borrower should calculate the present value cost of issuing debt based on its own credit and compare it with the present value cost of issuing the debt with bond insurance. Bond insurance should be purchased only if a savings results.

§ 17.4 LETTERS OF CREDIT

An irrevocable letter of credit is a commitment on the part of a bank to advance funds to a named party upon application by that party in certain special circumstances. A letter of credit can serve as a form of credit enhancement if it is purchased by the borrower in favor of the lender or the lender's trustee, to be drawn upon in the event that the borrower defaults. Because the letter of credit is irrevocable, the bank remains committed to advance funds even if the borrower is in default and, at the time of the default, has no means of making payment. Banks enter into this type of arrangement for a fee, usually in the form of a one-time commitment or participation fee plus an additional annual fee ranging from 0.5 percent to 1.5 percent of the total amount payable under the letter of credit, payable by the purchaser of the letter of credit. Letters of credit are not available on a long-term basis, but, rather, can be obtained for a maximum term of five to seven years. For this reason, this form of credit enhancement cannot be used with respect to long-term fixed rate debt. However, a letter of credit can be used for long-term variable rate debt, since at its expiration, if it has not been extended or replaced, the letter of credit can be drawn upon for the purpose of calling the bonds.

A letter of credit is issued pursuant to the terms of a reimbursement agreement, whereby an obligor, usually the borrower or a corporation related to the borrower, agrees to reimburse the letter of credit bank for

[78]Through various FHA programs, see § 14, above.

[79]Such as the California Health Facility Construction Loan Insurance Program. Cal. Health and Safety Code § 436, et seq.

draws under the letter of credit. Usually, a drawing required to permit the Trustee to purchase demand bonds is not immediately reimbursable but, if the bonds cannot be remarketed within a reasonable amount of time (e.g., 90 days), the obligation is converted to a term loan and is repayable at a specified interest rate (usually pegged to the bank's prime rate) over a fairly short period of time. Drawings for other purposes, such as those necessary to pay principal and interest or to repay the bonds upon a default, are repayable immediately, giving the bank immediate rights, since these drawings are a good indication that the debt is deteriorating rapidly.

The reimbursement agreement is the vehicle whereby the letter of credit bank obtains security for its advances and imposes covenants on the borrower that are more stringent than those imposed under the principal transaction documents. It is advantageous that the more stringent covenants be placed in this agreement rather than in the document in which the bondholders have an interest (such as the indenture or loan agreement), since it is easier to obtain waivers and consents from the bank than from several thousand bondholders. In addition, changes in the covenants may be introduced on expiration or termination of the letter of credit by substituting a new letter of credit.

The letter of credit bank usually requires security for the reimbursement obligation over and above that of the promise of the obligor. The following are often demanded:

A pledge of the tendered bonds held by the trustee. Thus, if the drawing is for the purpose of repurchasing tendered bonds, the bank is entitled to acquire those bonds on the occurrence of a default, giving it the advantage of the security pledged for the benefit of bondholders.

A deed of trust. This deed of trust usually encumbers the facility financed by the bond issue, but it may cover other property deemed necessary. The lien is usually on a parity basis with that in favor of the bondholders.

Other security interests usually on a parity basis with bondholders. These may include liens on gross revenues.

§ 17.5 GUARANTEES

A guarantee can serve somewhat the same function as bond insurance in that it constitutes the promise by a third party to repay the debt and, therefore, if the third party is more creditworthy than the borrower, the debt should be more attractive to the lender.

One effective type of guarantee arrangement consists of a master indenture, whereby two or more corporations agree to cross-guarantee the obligations of other parties to the master indenture. These obligations are secured on a parity basis with all other such obligations and the holders have recourse against any member of the obligated group, not only the member that originally incurred the debt.

FIGURE 17.1

FITCH RATING GUIDELINES FOR CCRCs

1. *Pre-Sale:*
   A minimum number of apartment units are required to be presold, as explained below, at the time of the rating application. The presale should be evidenced by a deposit at least equal to 10% of the entrance fee. It is suggested that not more than 80% of the 10% deposit or $1000, whichever is higher, is refundable prior to the date the apartment unit is available for move-in. This requirement has been established to ensure a "valid" presale and to verify the existence of a "Market." Exceptions can be made to the above penalty refund requirements for reason of death or health or applicable state legislation.

   A. A corporation which has been in operation for 5 years or less is required to have a minimum of 60% of the entire project being financed, presold at the time of the rating application.

   B. A corporation which has been in operation for more than 5 years is required to have a minimum of 50% of the entire project being financed, presold at the time of the rating application.

   C. A multi-corporate operator or multi-facility corporation which has been in operation for 5 years or more will have a required presale established by Fitch after a review of the most recent 5 years of certified audited financial statements and related statistical information. The presale will range between 40% and 60% at the sole discretion of Fitch.

2. *Entrance Fees:*
   Entrance fees and any equity contributions should generate an amount equal to 60% of the total project costs excluding the debt service reserve fund and funded interest. This requirement can be changed upward or downward at Fitch's sole discretion depending upon the scope of the services that will be offered at the facility.

3. *Escrowed Funds:*
   A minimum percentage of the entrance fees must be escrowed and restricted for specific purposes.

   A. An organization which has been in operation for 5 years or less:

      (1) During start up and construction, a minimum of 85% of the received deposits/entrance fees are to be escrowed until the project is completed and operating. The 85% of the received deposits/entrance fees can only be used for refunds. The remaining 15% of the received deposits/entrance fees may be used for an initial working capital reserve fund.

      (2) Upon completion of the construction and commencement of operations, 80% of all the received deposits/entrance fees must be escrowed and restricted for refunds, debt service, additional

242

FIGURE 17.1 *(Continued)*

working capital (to be considered a loan and repaid within 24 months), and plant, property and equipment replacement.

   B. An organization which has been in operation for 5 years or more will be required to escrow a minimum percentage of received deposits/entrance fees. The required escrow percentage will be established by Fitch after a review of the most recent 5 years of certified audited financial statements and related statistical information is considered. The range for this requirement will be between 40% and 80%. The restriction in A.(2) above will then apply.

4. *Debt Service Reserve Fund:*

A minimum of one year's maximum annual debt service is to be funded at the time of the closing for the bond issue, or, in lieu thereof, an irrevocable Letter of Credit must be obtained from a bank or bank-holding company, acceptable to Fitch and/or rated "AA" or higher by Fitch, for the full amount or for any deficit in this Fund. The Letter of Credit must remain in effect until such time the Debt Service Reserve Fund has been fully funded from other sources (i.e., equal to the maximum annual debt service requirement).

5. *Reserve Ratio:*

Facilities which offer any type of health care guarantees of service that are not completely covered by patient/resident charges are required to produce and maintain a ratio of Total Cash Reserves (inclusive of Letters of Credit) available to Total Debt (Reserve ratio) equal to the higher of a minimum of 35% of outstanding total debt or at least 3 times the amount of the annual debt service (principal and interest). Facilities which offer any type of health care guarantees/services and completely cover such related costs through user charges or a facility which does not offer any type of health care guarantees/services could possibly have a lower minimum reserve ratio requirement determined by Fitch.

6. *Funded Interest:*

Funded Interest during construction must be equal to the anticipated interest expense during the construction period. It is favorable to have three to six months of additional interest expense also funded. Upon completion of the project, any excess Funded Interest should be transferred from the designated Funded Interest account to an appropriate debt reduction account or applied to completion of construction. The three to six additional months of funded interest requirement can be changed due to Federal, State or State agency requirements.

7. *Project Participants:*

   A. The architect, the construction company, the management company, the marketing/developer group, the feasibility consultant, and the investment banker must have prior experience in CCRC

FIGURE 17.1 *(Continued)*

projects or related types of projects. The experience and track records of the above mentioned project participants, as well as the costs associated with the project, will be heavily scrutinized.

B. The construction company must have a guaranteed maximum price type contract with a daily penalty clause equal to the minimum of the daily interest expenses if the construction is not completed on time.

C. Professional management should be obtained by contractual arrangements to operate the facility. The management fees must be subordinated to debt service.

D. Should contractual arrangements not be made with outside professional management and an individual is selected as administrator, he/she must have a successful track record of prior management responsibilities and experience at a CCRC or related types of projects. Verifying information must be made available to Fitch.

E. Only a marketing/developer group with prior successful experience in marketing and developing CCRC's will be considered. Their fees and method of compensation will be reviewed.

F. The feasibility consultant should be nationally recognized (regionally recognized consultants will be considered) and have prior experience with the preparation of feasibility studies of successful CCRC projects.

8. *Residency Contract:*
   Residency contract should provide for the following:

   A. Maintenance/monthly service fee increases to be made at management's sole discretion. The fee increases should not be limited in any way by the contract.

   B. Minimum entry age should be set at 62 years. If a husband and wife enter the facility at the same time, the older spouse should be at least 62 years of age.

   C. Apartment entrance fee refund provisions should not exceed a pro-rated 5-year period. Justified alternative prorated periods will be considered.

   D. A refund should not be paid until the resident's unit is resold.

   E. Resident's lien, if any, must be subordinated to lender's lien.

   F. It is not expected that the contract provide for acute care health services (hospitalization). However, consideration will be given to those contracts which do provide for acute care health services where adequate resident health insurance or participation in a Health Maintenance Organization (HMO) is required.

9. *Marketing of the Apartment Units:*
   We will review the marketing strategy and actual performance of the

FIGURE 17.1 *(Continued)*

marketing efforts to date. Our analysis of the marketing strategy will include, but are not limited to, the review of the following components:

A. Type of marketing techniques utilized (i.e., direct mail, television, radio, etc.).
B. Number of sales people involved with the project.
C. The direct sales approach developed and used.
D. How the sales people are compensated.
E. Number of accepted resident applications.
F. Comparison of monthly acceptance resident applications versus monthly projections from inception to date.
G. A review of the average age of accepted residents to date. (This is an important component since the actual average age of accepted residents will help support the turnover/attrition assumptions in the feasibility study.)

10. *Financial Screening Criteria:*
The criteria used to screen the prospective resident's financial ability to meet his/her future needs and obligations will be reviewed. It is favorable that the prospective resident not need to rely upon the sale of his/her home to meet the entrance fee requirement. A qualifying prospective resident's initial monthly service fee should not be in excess of 50% of that prospective resident's monthly income. The screening should be done by a Board Committee—*not by a developer.*

11. *Nursing/Health Care Facility:*
A. If the residency contract includes the provision for nursing care, then this nursing care facility must be provided either as a part of the retirement community or by contractual arrangements with an affiliate offering a similar quality life style as offered at the resident's facility. Also, if it is part of the retirement community, the organization must have an *unrestricted* "Certificate of Need" (CON) from the appropriate health planning agency. Should any other type of "Certificate of Need" be issued (i.e., conditional or restrictive), such conditions or restrictions applicable to such issued "Certificate of Need" will be reviewed by Fitch as to the reasonableness of such conditions/restrictions and the acceptance of such conditions/restrictions will be made solely by Fitch.
B. If the residency contract provides for nursing care services not covered by the monthly service fee, then the potential health care liability must be covered by an established health care fund which is adequate to cover such deficit on an on-going basis.
C. The number of nursing beds to residency units should not ordinarily exceed a 1 to 4 ratio or 20% of the total resident population,

FIGURE 17.1 *(Continued)*

whichever is less. Should the total nursing beds exceed this ratio, justification is required.

12. *Feasibility Study:*

A feasibility study prepared by a nationally recognized consulting/CPA firm with experience in CCRC's is required. It is also required to submit a copy of any and all feasibility studies which were prepared in connection with the proposed project. In addition, an actuarial study should be conducted, by an organization experienced in the preparation of such studies, to provide the residents' mortality and morbidity assumptions for the feasibility study based upon the residents' characteristics gathered from a minimum of 50% of the pre-sales. The feasibility study should present the following in addition to the usual financial, demographic, and statistical information.

A. Market area including population characteristics for the over-age-65 groups preferably in 5 year increments with income/assets statistical ranges.

B. A survey result of the existing presold prospective residents as to the number dependent upon sale of their homes before the entrance fee requirement can be made. In addition, we require the number of residents who do not need to sell their homes in order to pay the full entrance fee and will not satisfy the entrance fee requirement until their home is sold.

C. Resident turnover, segregated by reason for (i.e., death, health, etc.) and utilization of the nursing facility, both on a permanent and temporary basis.

D. A review of the screening criteria utilized and their opinion of its reasonableness.

E. Marketing of units as of the date of the study, by month.

F. Information regarding area competition—both for the residential units and the nursing facility. This would include any CON's or Permits in process.

13. *Legal Provisions:*

The following should be included in all appropriate legal documents and other provisions required as necessary:

A. *Annual Reports*—We require that the name, Fitch Investors Service, Inc., be included in the appropriate legal documents to receive the annual certified financial statements *and* other information as may be reasonably requested within 120 days of year end.

B. *Rate Covenant*—We require a rate covenant of at least 110% based upon revenues available for debt service on a cash flow basis from annual operations to commence by the third full year of operation. The rate covenant should not include the entrance fee

FIGURE 17.1 *(Continued)*

---

reserves in the calculation even though they are available. If debt service coverage falls below a 110% level, it then becomes mandatory to retain a consultant to make appropriate recommendations. Also, Fitch's name is to be included in this section to receive a copy of the management consultant's report.

C. *Security*—The Bonds should be secured by a revenue pledge and grant the bondholders a first mortgage lien.

D. *Maintenance of reserves at an adequate level*—This would include the entrance fee reserve fund, debt service reserve fund, health care liability fund, plant, property and equipment replacement fund, and maintenance fund.

E. *Additional Debt Test*—The Additional Debt Test should be reasonable but sufficiently restrictive to ensure that the bondholders are adequately protected. The tests should be based upon a debt service coverage test and others, as may be appropriate.

F. Allowances should be provided for completion bonds.

G. *Actuarial Update*—An Actuarial Analysis is required to update the mortality and morbidity study every 3 years until the facility reaches maturity, after which, the minimum requirement will be for every 5 years until the bonds are called or mature. The update studies must be conducted on only the residents then living in the financed project.

Source: Reproduced with permission from Fitch Investors Service, Inc.

A master indenture typically involves a pledge of gross revenues of the obligated group (all of the parties to the Master Indenture) and, rather than pledging a security interest in real and personal property, contains a negative pledge, whereby each party agrees not to encumber any, or at least most, of its property. This master indenture form of security offers substantial flexibility where the organizational structure of the business involves several affiliated corporations, the business of which are aggregated for purposes of borrowing.

§ 18   DEBT TERMS AND COVENANTS

§ 18.1   VARIABLE RATE VERSUS FIXED RATE DEBT

Traditionally, long-term capital debt bears a fixed interest rate that is established at the time the debt is incurred. In recent years, a substantial market has developed for variable rate debt, and numerous borrowers have found this type of debt to be advantageous. To understand this phenomenon, one must look at the economics of the capital markets as they have worked over the past several years. Except in unusual circumstances (such as a situation in which a long-term deflationary trend is perceived), short-term debt is more desirable to lenders than long-term debt because it provides lenders with greater flexibility, permitting them to avoid adverse interest rate trends. The price is, of course, that they cannot lock in advantageous trends. Therefore, lenders are willing to accept less interest in return for a shorter term. For example, when interest on bonds is readjusted to market every 30 days and sells at four percent, long-term debt with an equal rating may sell at seven percent. This differential is substantial and many borrowers find that it is worthwhile to explore variable rate debt.

(a) Publicly Offered Variable Rate Debt

Variable rate debt is usually structured by the use of variable rate demand bonds. This means that bonds are issued that bear an interest rate that is good for a short period, such as 30 days. Every 30 days, a remarketing agent, usually an investment banking firm, establishes a new interest rate that is good for the next 30 days. The rate is set at the lowest level possible that will result in the bonds being marketable. The bondholders are notified of the rate and, on short notice, they may put the bonds back to a trustee, or tender agent (if the trustee is not located in New York City), and obtain repayment of the principal. If the bonds are put back, the remarketing agent is required to resell the bonds to another investor. Thus, the establishment of the right interest rate is essential in order not to give bondholders a disincentive to hold the bonds and to assure that the remarketing agent can remarket the bonds once they are put back.

Because the borrower is unlikely to have sufficient cash on hand to repurchase the bonds on short notice, it is necessary to provide in advance for the funds to expeditiously repurchase the bonds in the event that they cannot be immediately resold. This is accomplished by providing a liquidity facility, in the form of a bank letter of credit. This letter of credit can be drawn upon by the trustee to repurchase bonds and, if the bonds are resold, the bank is repaid. If the bonds are not resold in a reasonable period of time, the bank either makes a term loan (upon very unfavorable terms) or purchases the bonds directly (also upon very unfavorable terms). Because the bondholders will look to the bank to repay the bonds in the event they desire to sell them, the liquidity facility also serves as credit enhancement on the bonds in most cases,[80] although in some cases the liquidity facility bank does not have a sufficiently high credit rating, and a guarantor bank provides a guarantee to improve the rating.

Unlike fixed rate bonds, variable rate bonds are not marketed to individuals and small investors but, rather, are marketed to large institutional

---

[80] *See* § 17.4, above.

investors—either large corporations needing short-term investments or tax exempt money market funds. For this reason, the bonds are usually issued in $100,000 denominations. Variable rate debt usually has at least one conversion feature, the ability to convert to fixed rate debt. Upon conversion, an interest rate is established that is sufficient to market the bonds, and the bonds are sold on a fixed rate basis. At that time, they are converted to the more standard $5000 denominations. There are numerous other possible conversion features, including conversion to daily, weekly, monthly, and semiannual periods. In addition, one investment banker permits conversion to short- or long-term periods of any specified length, in order to tailor the term of the bonds to the need of the investors. The flexibility resulting from these conversion features permits the remarketing agent to shop the market for the most attractive interest rates that may be available.

(b)   Institutional Variable Rate Debt

The foregoing discussion involves variable rate debt that is structured as a public offering, even though it may be placed privately. A very different type of variable rate debt involves long-term debt with a variable rate of interest that can be prepaid without premium by the borrower but cannot be put by the lender. This type of arrangement, which is most frequently in the form of taxable privately placed mortgage debt, can be a fairly simple transaction involving a note and deed of trust. Rather than being based directly on market experience, the interest rate is calculated based on an index that, itself, reflects market conditions. This type of debt is most frequently used for taxable debt, although it has occasionally been used for tax exempt debt held by a single institution.

(c)   When Variable Rate Debt Should Be Used

The use of variable rate debt has been approached cautiously by retirement home sponsors because of its potential volatility. While it may be true that variable rate tax exempt debt, even during the period of highest interest rates, did not exceed about nine percent, the possibility of extremely high rates compared with the relative inability of most retirement homes to increase fees significantly discourages this form of financing except for a minor portion of debt. However, the judicious use of variable rate debt can significantly lower interest expense.

Devices have been developed for the purpose of limiting the risk of variable rate debt while maintaining a substantial amount of its cost-saving. One such device is the purchase of an interest rate cap, whereby the borrower pays another institution, such as a bank, a given percent for assuming the payment of interest over a given cap. Prior to the 1986 Tax Reform Act, it was possible to lock in a fixed rate by means of an advance crossover defeasance, whereby a second bond issue would be issued at a fixed rate, the proceeds of which were used to purchase investment securities at maturities that would yield interest sufficient to service the debt. If the variable rate interest rose to an unacceptable level, the securities would be liquidated to pay off the variable rate debt, and the borrower would be obligated only under the fixed rate debt. However, the new law, by requiring prompt repayment of the old bonds with the proceeds of the new debt, limits the use of this device.[81]

§ 18.2   CONDITIONS PRECEDENT TO CLOSING

Certain conditions imposed on the borrowers must be met before the financing transaction will be closed. Some of these conditions relate specifically to the transaction itself, such as the receipt of legal opinions and title insurance policies. Other conditions are of broader application, assuring that the borrower and the specific project meet the underwriting standards applicable to the transaction.

(a)   Conditions Relating to the Financing Transaction

Conditions relating to the financing transaction are largely of a technical nature and need not be explained in detail here. The following is a partial list:

Various opinions of legal counsel (see § 15.6(a)).

A policy of title insurance (usually the ALTA Mortgagor's policy) insuring the lender, trustee for benefit of the bondholders, and credit enhancer, as appropriate. The lender will possibly request one or more endorsements that go beyond the basic ALTA policy terms. These endorsements, which are standard and are referred to by number, provide additional protection beyond that afforded by the basic policy. Because some lenders are prone to request endorsements whether or not they are needed, borrowers should determine which endorsements are reasonably necessary to protect the lender, given the characteristics of the project, and negotiate to exclude the others.

If the financing is to be closed following the commencement of construction, the title insurance policy will probably make an exception for mechanics liens, since mechanics liens relate back to the start of construction. The lender will not want its lien to be junior to mechanics liens, and may reject the exception. If the project is properly bonded, the title company may be willing to remove the exception in consideration of an indemnification agreement provided by the borrower.

Audited financial statements and comfort letters (see § 15.6(a)).

Financial feasibility study.

---

[81] *See* § 15.4(e).

Officer's Certificates. These certificates, executed by officers on behalf of the borrower, make certain representations of fact. They also may contain conclusions stated in absolute terms, which the borrower may not know absolutely. It may be possible to qualify the statements so that they are represented "to the best of such officer's knowledge." However, lenders usually want representations to be absolute in recognition that the borrower has ultimate responsibility to the lender with respect to the debt.

Articles of Incorporation of the borrower certified by the secretary of state of the state of incorporation.

Bylaws of the borrower, certified by its secretary.

A Good Standing Certificate from the secretary of state, to the effect that the corporation is in good standing and qualified to do business. If the project is in a state other than the state of incorporation, it will have to provide a certificate from the secretary of state of the state in which the project is located to the effect that the borrower is in good standing as a foreign corporation qualified to do business in the state.

A resolution of the borrower approving the transaction and authorizing officers of the borrower to execute appropriate documentation.

(b)   Presales

In the case of a new facility or a substantial expansion, the lender will be concerned about the ability of the borrower to market the new units at the prices indicated in the feasibility study and within the period of time during which capitalized interest is budgeted. Facilities with a substantial entry fee are perceived as more difficult to market and, therefore, lenders desire assurance that the projected occupancy will be met. For this reason, they often require that, as a condition to closing, a certain number of units be presold. Beyond selling the units, they will require that substantial nonrefundable deposits have been received in order to assure that the buyers will not be likely to back out. A typical closing condition of this type requires that 60 percent of the units be presold with nonrefundable deposits of at least $10,000 each.

(c)   Construction Contract

In a financing involving new construction or remodeling, it is crucial to know that the project can be built with the amount of money available, since an unfinished project can generate little revenue, and additional debt incurred to finish a project that has cost overruns could either be unobtainable or jeopardize the borrower's financial condition. Therefore, a common condition of closing is that the borrower will have obtained governmental approval of its plans and specifications and that it will have entered into a construction contract having a fixed cost of construction or a guaranteed maximum price.

§ 18.3 BUSINESS COVENANTS

In any financing transaction, the borrower will be required to enter into certain agreements, or covenants, designed to restrict its financial operations in order to assure the lender that the company will continue to operate in a financially responsible manner. Business covenants vary considerably between the different types of financing transactions, and will occasionally be tailored to the peculiarities of the company and project in an individual transaction. There is enough common ground between the types of transactions that a discussion of covenants in general avoids much repetition that would be involved in discussing the covenants for each type of transaction.

Covenants are usually subject to at least some negotiation. The exception is the case of standards set forth in a federal or state statute[82] or a requirement set down by a rating agency or credit enhancer or lender that is made nonnegotiable. In general, the covenants in an unrated public offering offer the borrower the most flexibility. They are established between the borrower and the investment banker, who is interested in satisfying the borrower. The constraints in this type of transaction are (1) the ability to obtain buyers for the securities on the terms offered, and (2) the investment banker's concern about its own reputation.

A rated transaction is subject to rating agency-prescribed covenants. These covenants are standard between transactions and, in addition, the rating agencies may request particular provisions related to the particularities of the transaction. The Fitch rating agency criteria are set forth at Figure 17.1.

Structuring financial covenants for rated and unrated stand-alone public offerings should be done with utmost care because if a covenant causes problems in the future, generally the only way it can be amended is to obtain consent from the holders of at least a majority of the debt, which could amount to literally thousands of people, or to defease or refinance the debt, which may be costly or even prohibited by the tax laws or by the debt instruments themselves. Therefore, covenants for such a transaction are broadly written and are designed to remain appropriate through the life of the debt, even if very substantial changes occur to the borrower.

Such covenants either contain absolute requirements or prohibitions (such as those requiring maintenance of tax exempt status or the license to operate the facility) or set forth requirements in relative terms (such as ratio tests) so that as the size of the borrower grows or inflation diminishes purchasing power, limitations are adjusted proportionately. Both types of covenants should be considered in light of potential changed circumstances. A few years ago, a requirement that certain types of insurance be carried or that a nursing facility be qualified to receive Medicaid payments was considered standard.

---

[82]For example, the California Health Facility Construction Loan Insurance Program Law mandates a community service obligation. Cal. Health and Safety Code § 436.82.

Now, many borrowers are insisting on out provisions that, for example, allow self-insurance or no insurance if a consultant certifies that the premium for such insurance is not reasonable, or permit the facility to decide not to be qualified for Medicaid if the terms of reimbursement are inadequate.

It may be desirable to convert an absolute requirement into a ratio covenant so that changes over time do not distort its original intent. A prohibition against incurring more than $100,000 of short-term debt could be recast with the limit expressed in terms of a given percentage of net revenue. Even ratio tests should be looked at carefully. A requirement that a debt service coverage test be met may seem innocuous if the required ratio is well below the actual existing ratio. However, if in 20 years market or regulatory pressures preclude the maintenance of the ratio, an out provision should be included.[83]

When negotiating with a credit enhancer or with a lender or bond purchaser in a private placement, more flexibility is possible in structuring the financial covenants, since the party at risk is literally at the negotiating table. However, such parties usually have definite underwriting standards, and will often insist on very restrictive covenants, reasoning that because there is only one or a small number of parties to deal with, it is possible to come back for approval in the event there is a good business reason to obtain waiver of a covenant. Sometimes the documents contain, besides a general waiver provision, a provision relating to waiver of specific financial covenants, requiring the approval of the lender or credit enhancer to the waiver to "not be unreasonably withheld." The risk to the borrower of a general waiver provision is that, in the event interest rates have risen since the transaction was entered into, the lender will have an interest in not approving a waiver, either to force the borrower to get out of the covenant by paying off the debt or to require the borrower to adjust the interest rate as the price of obtaining the waiver. The borrower will want to avoid the possibility of this happening by first avoiding covenants that may, at some future point, not be capable of being complied with and, secondly, by including in the loan documents requirements that the lender act reasonably, possibly in accordance with certain standards, in acting on requests for waiver.

Covenants may take the form of straight mandates or prohibitions, such as the requirement that the borrower maintain prescribed insurance or that it refrain from incurring certain encumbrances. They may also take the form of ratios or prescribed limits, such as the covenants that require the maintenance of a prescribed debt service coverage ratio or the requirement that a specified level of net worth be maintained. The covenants may also take the form of an absolute mandate or prohibition coupled with a ratio or prescribed level exception, for example, a prohibition against incurring additional indebtedness, with the exception that such indebtedness may be incurred if, after its incurrence, a prescribed debt service coverage ratio is maintained. The following is a discussion of covenants that are often contained in financing documents.

---

[83] See § 18.2(d).

(a) Limitation on Consolidations, Mergers, Sales, or Transfers

The corporation is prohibited from merging or consolidating with another corporation and from dissolving, selling, or otherwise disposing of all or substantially all of its assets unless certain conditions are met. Typically, at least the following conditions will be imposed:

1. The surviving corporation (if other than the borrower) must agree to assume the borrower's debt obligations.

2. The transaction must not result in a violation of the other covenants. The effect of this depends on the content of the other covenants. For example, if there is a net worth covenant, the resulting corporation must comply with it. Some merger covenants require that the new corporation be capable of incurring at least one dollar of additional indebtedness without violating a covenant. The purpose of this requirement is to impose on the merger the additional indebtedness tests.

3. The most common financial restriction in publicly offered tax exempt debt is that the debt service coverage ratio after the merger may not be less than a specified level. Often, this level is the same as that required by the rate covenant, in which case the requirement is merely a statement of the requirement that there be no covenant breach after the merger. However, on occasion, the ratio is placed at a higher level.

4. If the borrower is a nonprofit corporation, the successor corporation will be required to be a nonprofit corporation with appropriate tax exempt status. This covenant is particularly important with respect to tax exempt bonds, because the tax exempt status of the borrower is usually the factor that results in tax exempt status for bond interest. Even if the debt is not tax exempt, it is usually required that the successor be a tax exempt corporation, because (1) any change in tax status would significantly change the nature of the transaction, and (2) tax exempt status may result in exemption from property tax and other benefits that would be advantageous from the standpoint of the project.

5. If the debt is tax exempt, an opinion of bond counsel confirming that the debt will remain tax exempt and that the borrower's obligations under the bond issue have been properly assumed may be required.

6. If the debt is insured or guaranteed, or if it is privately placed, additional tests may be required. For example, the projected long-term debt service coverage ratio (as calculated by an independent consultant) for the next three years will be at least equal to the ratio of the borrower prior to the proposed transaction and the resulting corporation's net worth will be at least that of the borrower.

7. In some cases, a lender or credit enhancer may be so concerned about the possible effects of mergers and transfers that it will prohibit them or require that approval be obtained on a case-by-case basis.

(b) Limitation on Encumbrances

Whether security for the debt is a mortgage or deed of trust or a pledge of gross revenues, the borrower typically is prohibited from creating or permitting any liens or encumbrances on the project (usually defined to include the complete facility financed by the proceeds of the indebtedness) and, in some cases, certain or all of its other properties. Usually, there is an exception for certain liens and encumbrances defined as permitted encumbrances, which may include:

Various liens, easements, and other encumbrances that typically exist (e.g., mechanics liens, liens for nondelinquent taxes, easements for utilities) and that do not in the aggregate materially affect the operation of the project.

Occasionally, any encumbrance of record disclosed in the title policy issued in connection with the transaction. This is favorable to the borrower, in that it grandfathers any matters already on record that the parties have not otherwise arranged to remove. It forces the parties to deal with those items that may be objectionable to the lender, and removes the possibility of open questions of interpretation with respect to preexisting matters.

Liens resulting from the indebtedness itself.

Liens for permitted indebtedness. Often any lien in connection with other indebtedness, which is junior to the primary indebtedness, is automatically permitted if the other indebtedness itself is permitted under the indebtedness covenant.

Purchase money deeds of trust and security interests. The borrower can acquire real or personal property for which it grants a security interest for all or a portion of the purchase price. In some instances, the amount of the lien is limited to a percentage of purchase price less than 100 percent. Also, a limit may be imposed as to the amount of the borrower's property that may be so encumbered (e.g., 10 percent).

Nonrecourse indebtedness; that is, the lender's remedies are limited to its lien, and the lender cannot go against the borrower.

Leases and contracts related to the operation of the facilities. These are usually limited to obligations entered into in the ordinary course of business. For example, resident contracts may constitute a form of an encumbrance and would be covered by this exception.

The rights of the state under any regulatory scheme. While the residents of a life care facility usually subordinate their rights to the rights of the bondholders,[84] such a subordination may be limited or supplanted by state legislation designed to protect the interests of the residents.

---

[84] *See* § 21.9.

Additional liens and encumbrances that may be approved by the lender or credit enhancer.

(c) Limitation on Indebtedness

The ability of a borrower to incur additional indebtedness, whether junior to or on a parity with the principal indebtedness, is usually restricted in order to protect the security of the debt holders. In multifacility borrowers, the lender occasionally imposes restrictions on indebtedness incurred with respect to facilities other than the one financed because of potential adverse impacts on the financed project. The following are typical covenants:

1. The borrower may incur parity debt only if it meets a certain debt service coverage ratio (that is, maximum annual debt service compared with net revenue available for debt service). This ratio test is often structured in the form of two alternative tests: (1) a comparison of historical net income available for debt service with the maximum annual debt service for both existing debt and the proposed parity debt; or (2) a comparison of projected net income available for debt service following completion of the new project, as developed by a consultant, with maximum annual debt service for both existing debt and proposed parity debt. The ratio for the former is usually less than for the latter, since the former does not depend on yet-to-be-realized revenues. The former test assumes no additional revenues from the new project but may be impossible to meet if the object of the borrowing is the development of additional revenue-producing capacity. The latter test has a higher ratio, but permits the borrower to count revenues from the project. It requires the hiring of a management consultant to prepare projections and calculate the ratio.

2. In calculating maximum annual debt service, one point of negotiation is often the extent to which it is necessary to take into account debt of other corporations that is guaranteed by the borrower. A conservative lender will require that 100 percent of such debt be counted, on the theory that the borrower could be liable for its payment. A more generous perspective is that since there is only a possibility that the borrower will be called upon to pay the debt, only a fraction of the guaranteed debt should be taken into account. Thus, some covenants require debt service on 25 percent of guaranteed debt to be counted. Another often used approach is to vary the percentage counted by the quality of the prime obligor under the guaranteed debt. Thus, if the prime obligor has a high debt service coverage ratio, the percentage that must be claimed by the guarantor would be small, in recognition of the reduced risk, and vice versa. Finally, some lenders prohibit guarantees altogether on the theory that the borrower should not guarantee the debt of other companies but should devote its assets only to its own business.

3. In a privately placed transaction, a limit may be placed on the amount of the debt as well as on debt service. Such a limit may be expressed, for example, in terms of a percentage of the original cost of assets, a percentage of appraised value, or other terms.

4. There are usually separate tests for short-term debt. Short-term debt, which is defined as debt that is not outstanding for one year, with a requirement that all (or all but a specified minor percentage) must be cleaned up for a specified period of time each year, is generally limited by some percentage of total annual revenues.

(d) Rate Covenant

The borrower often has to promise to establish rates and charges sufficient to provide a debt service coverage ratio of at least a specified amount (often 1.10). Two important exceptions should be included in this covenant: (1) an exception for free or reduced-rate services provided in order to maintain the borrower's tax exempt status, and (2) a provision that if the required ratio is not met, a management consultant will be retained, and that if the consultant's report (assuming the board of the borrower finds it to be reasonable) is adopted, the ratio requirement is waived. In some documents, it cannot be waived below 1.0.

(e) Limitation on Disposition of Properties

The borrower is usually limited as to its disposition of properties. The covenant is stated as a general prohibition, subject to certain exceptions, which may include:

Disposition in the ordinary course of business. This includes such things as selling goods to customers.

Disposition of property that has become inadequate, obsolete, or unnecessary. This is often accompanied by a requirement that such disposition be at fair market value.

A further exception is often stated as a percentage of total property plant and equipment (e.g., 5 percent during any one year with an aggregate total of 15 percent).

In recent years, it has been a common practice to restructure health care corporations in such a way as to provide for a parent corporation or sister corporations that may not be subject to the indebtedness of the borrower, and to require that the borrower pay over surplus cash to such other corporations. In response, lenders have required that dispositions of cash be subject to the foregoing covenants or be subject to separate covenants. A stringent covenant applied to nonprofit corporations requires that net worth be increased each year by an amount equal to net earnings. A more liberal form of this covenant restricts dispositions to a given percentage of net worth or specified dollar amount each year.

(f)   Other Ratio Covenants

While the debt service coverage ratio is most frequently encountered in both property backed and gross income backed debt, additional ratio covenants are often required, especially by credit enhancers and private lenders. The function of these ratios is to test other indicators of financial stability, security, and ability to service the debt. Two of the most common ratios are:

1. *Debt Equity Ratio.* This ratio, usually applied in the case of debt backed by a security interest in property, assures that total debt will not exceed a certain percentage (e.g., 75 percent) of the value of the property. Usually value is book value—acquisition price less depreciation. Some borrowers, especially those that have owned property that has appreciated considerably since acquisition, have successfully argued for substitution of appraised value for book value.

2. *Current Assets to Current Liabilities Ratio.* This ratio assures that, apart from long-term financial condition, the borrower has the ability to pay its obligations when due.

(g)   Insurance and Condemnation

The borrower is required to carry certain specified insurance coverage and to apply insurance benefits and condemnation awards so as to provide adequate security.

Required Insurance. The borrower usually is subject to a general obligation to carry insurance of a type and amount customarily carried by like businesses. This standard has the advantage of being flexible. Thus, if a particular type of insurance is no longer available or is no longer generally carried because it is no longer available, the borrower need not carry it. However, it is also a vague standard and if challenged, a borrower may be hard-pressed to demonstrate what insurance is customarily carried.

Often as an adjunct to the above requirement, the borrower will be required to carry certain types of insurance with certain minimum limits. These include:

Comprehensive property insurance in an amount equal to the lesser of replacement cost or the remaining principal amount of indebtedness.

Public liability insurance (including, with respect to health care facilities, professional liability insurance), with specified limits.

Various other types of insurance, including business interruption insurance, boiler insurance, and fidelity bonds for officers and employees who handle money.

In California, earthquake insurance. Because of the high cost of this coverage and the high co-insurance provisions, borrowers often try to have this requirement waived.

The insurance requirement may be subject to a provision requiring review of the borrower's insurance coverage by a recognized insurance consultant on an annual (sometimes biannual) basis. Because insurance availability and cost can change over time, a desirable feature is to permit the borrower to reduce its coverage if the insurance consultant reports that the insurance is not available at a cost that is reasonable given the risks insured against. Finally, the borrower can be given the ability to substitute self-insurance for required insurance coverage with a favorable report of the insurance consultant.

(h)   Disposition of Insurance and Condemnation Proceeds

Debt instruments treat the disposition of insurance and condemnation proceeds in detail, because such money is substitute value for property that otherwise would have secured the debt or provided the means of generating revenue to service the debt. The lender or credit enhancer wants to assure that the money is used in such a manner as to maximize the borrower's chances of servicing the debt. The borrower wants to preserve maximum flexibility in the use of the money. The following are types of covenants typically encountered dealing with disposition of insurance and condemnation proceeds.

1. The most restrictive covenant encountered provides for the proceeds paid over to the lender to be applied as the lender sees fit. In less arbitrary terms, it could provide that the lender may, at its discretion, apply the proceeds either to repayment of debt or restoration of the premises. Borrowers usually reject this covenant, because it gives all power to the lender. They contend that it can be used by the lender to unfairly change the terms of the debt in exchange for releasing the funds for needed construction. Lenders argue that after destruction or taking of the premises, conditions are changed to such an extent that the lender needs to reassess its status and decide whether repayment of debt or reconstruction makes sense.

2. The covenant may give the borrower the right to choose between repayment of principal or reconstruction of the building in substantially its original value, condition, and character. While this formulation gives the lender essentially what it bargained for, it may be inefficient or even absurd from the borrower's point of view. It may be that a building of the same value but very different use or character would be more appropriate.

3. The covenant may provide for restoration of a facility of equivalent value. This permits the borrower to determine what is built. This covenant is certainly necessary where the debt is publicly sold and there is no lender with which to negotiate in the event that a pure replacement project is not appropriate.

4. Most covenants permit a certain amount of insurance or condemnation proceeds to be paid to the borrower with no further requirements. This de minimus amount depends on the total size of the facility involved.

5. To the extent that proceeds are not otherwise utilized, they are required to be used to pay principal on the debt.

§ 18:4   TIMING, FUNDING, AND DISBURSEMENTS

When obtaining capital for a project, it is necessary to reconcile the needs of the project with the demands of the capital markets. This often results in a structure of the transaction that appears unnecessarily complex but that is essential if the disparate interests are to be served in one transaction.

(a)   Timing

In the development of a project, it is never too early to investigate financing options and include the results of the investigation in the planning of the project. Feasibility determinations necessarily include ascertaining the cost and availability of financing and its terms and restrictions.

When the general availability of financing on acceptable terms is ascertained, planning for the project can proceed. Once a schematic design is developed, it should be possible to determine with a fair amount of precision the economics of the project, including the cost of construction, the cost of operating the project, and the expected revenues. At this point, it is desirable to obtain a commitment for the financing, because the next step, producing working drawings, is an expensive proposition. It may even be desirable to obtain some form of bridge financing in order to accomplish this step. But closing on the financing itself usually must await completion of the working drawings and the execution of a firm construction contract, in order to obtain assurances that the project can be completed with the amount of money available.

(b)   Construction Financing and Permanent Financing

In many cases (including publicly offered and tax exempt debt), only one loan is obtained, which is used to construct the project and remains in place thereafter. However, the most common practice for conventional financing is for one loan to remain in place during construction and, on completion, to be replaced by a permanent loan. The permanent loan is either in place with the proceeds being deposited in escrow, or committed prior to the commencement of construction, the proceeds being used to pay off the construction loan on completion. The reason for having two loans is that each represents a distinct lending risk for which there are two different capital markets, having different objectives. Construction loans are made by lenders that have a desire to keep money out for a short term and at fairly high risk. In return, they get a high interest rate. To control their risk, they exercise a supervisorial role over the project, inspecting the work and disbursing only when they are satisfied that progress has been made as represented and liens have been removed. If the project is not completed as planned, the construction loan is not paid off with proceeds of the permanent loan. The permanent lender desires a low-risk, long-term investment. Its interest rate is lower, but the lender does not bear the risk of construction. However, it does have to bear the risk of the successful operation of the project.

(c) Lender Control of Construction

As noted above, the construction lender assumes significant risk with respect to completion of the project. Therefore, in lending documents, it will assert various elements of control. Prior to loan closing, it will want to be comfortable that the contractor is competent, that a valid and binding construction contract has been entered into, that performance and payment bonds are in place, and that provision has been made for reasonable contingencies. During construction, the lender will want to inspect the site periodically, be informed of and have the right to approve changes in the plans or construction contract (or at least to be assured that funds are sufficient to pay for such changes), and approve disbursement of loan proceeds. Usually, loan proceeds, plus such equity as may be necessary to yield the total construction cost, are placed into a trust fund, to be disbursed by the trustee upon receipt of a certificate for payment. This certificate is presented by the borrower and is certified by the architect (see Figure 18.1).

Occasionally, the lender requires additional documentation at the time of each disbursement, including an endorsement from a title company assuring that no unpermitted liens have been filed against the property and certificates submitted by the contractor and subcontractors releasing or partially releasing their mechanics liens.

§ 18.5 CALL PROTECTION AND PREPAYMENT PREMIUM

One crucial term of any indebtedness relates to the issue of whether the borrower is permitted to call the debt, that is, to repay the principal of the debt prior to its maturity and, if so, whether a premium is charged for the privilege of doing so. Restrictions on these rights are often included in the terms of long-term fixed rate debt in order to provide equity to the borrower. In the event that market interest increases above that of the debt, the borrower

FIGURE 18.1

BORROWER'S AFFIDAVIT
(TO BE FURNISHED WITH EACH ADVANCE)

STATE OF _____,)

                                : ss.:

COUNTY OF _____)

_____, being duly sworn, deposes and says:

That affiant is the _____ of _____ (the "Borrower"), and has made due investigation as to matters hereinafter set forth and does hereby certify the following to induce _____ (the "Lender") to make and advance the sum of _____ ($_____) Dollars to the Borrower pursuant to the terms of a Building Loan Agreement, dated April _____, 19_____, between the Lender and the Borrower, and Request for Advance number _____, dated _____, 19_____, between the Lender and the Borrower, and Request for Advance number _____, dated _____, 19_____, the day on which this Affidavit is sworn to be affiant, being submitted to the Lender herewith:

1. All representations and warranties contained in the Building Loan Agreement are true and accurate in all material respects as of the date hereof.

2. No event of Default exists under the Building Loan Agreement, the Note, the Mortgage, the Guaranty, or under any other security document, and no event or condition has occurred and is continuing or existing or would result from the advance about to be made which, with the lapse of time or the giving of notice, or both, would constitute such an Event of Default.

3. Construction of the Improvements has been carried on with reasonable dispatch and has not been discontinued at any time for a period of Unavoidable Delay for reasons within the control of the Borrower, the Improvements have not been damaged by fire or other casualty, and no part of the Premises has been taken by eminent domain and no proceedings or negotiations therefor are pending or threatened.

4. Construction of the Improvements is progressing in such manner so as to insure completion thereof in substantial accordance with the Plans on or before the Completion Date.

5. All funds received from the Lender previously as advances under the Building Loan Agreement have been expended or are being held in trust for the sole purpose of paying costs of construction ("Costs") previously certified to the Lender in Requests for Advances; and no part of said funds has been used, and the funds to be received pursuant to the Request for

FIGURE 18.1 *(Continued)*

Advance submitted herewith shall not be used, for any other purpose. No item of Costs previously certified to the Lender in a Request for Advance remains unpaid as of the date of this Affidavit.

6. All of the statements and information set forth in the Request for Advance being submitted to the Lender herewith are true and correct in every material respect at the date hereof, and all Costs certified to the Lender in said Request for Advance accurately reflect the precise amounts due, or where such Costs have not yet been billed to the Borrower, the same accurately reflect the Borrower's best estimates of the amounts that will become due and owing during the period covered by said Request for Advance. All the funds to be received pursuant to said Request for Advance shall be used solely for the purposes of paying the items of cost specified therein or for reimbursing the Borrower for such items previously paid by the Borrower.

7. Nothing has occurred subsequent to the date of the Building Loan Agreement which has or may result in the creation of any lien, charge or encumbrance upon the Premises or the Improvements or any part thereof, or anything affixed to or used in connection therewith or which has or may substantially and adversely impair the ability of the Borrower to make all payments of principal and interest on the Note, the ability of the Borrower to meet its obligations under the Building Loan Agreement or to the best of its knowledge, the ability of the Guarantor to meet its obligations under the Guaranty.

8. None of the labor, materials, overhead, or other items of expense specified in the Request for Advance submitted herewith have previously been made the basis of any Request for Advance by the Borrower or of any payment by the Lender.

9. The status of construction of the Improvements is as follows:

10. The estimated aggregate cost of completing the Improvements including but not limited to labor, materials, architectural and engineering fees, management, financial and other overhead costs and expenses, does not exceed _____ dollars ($_____).

11. All conditions to the advance referred to above and to be made in accordance with the Request for Advance submitted herewith in addition to those to which reference is made in this Affidavit have been met in accordance with the terms of the Building Loan Agreement.

The capitalized terms used herein have the meaning given thereto in the Building Loan Agreement.

BORROWER

By _____

enjoys a savings and will likely not prepay the debt. However, if market interest drops below that of the debt, the borrower has an economic incentive to prepay the debt with the proceeds of cheaper debt. This is perceived as unfair to the lender, locking in an interest rate favorable to the borrower but not favorable to the lender. From the perspective of the borrower, restrictions on the right to prepay are important because, even if it intends to leave indebtedness outstanding for the entire 30 year term, unforeseen events, such as lower prevailing interest rates, the need for expansion or renewal, the need to revise business covenants, or the sale of the facility, may make refinancing desirable or necessary.

Call protection consists of a prohibition against prepayment of debt for a given period of time. In publicly offered, tax exempt 30 year debt, typically call protection is for a period of 10 years. The last 20 years is left unrestricted because a call protection during that period does not currently buy a borrower a lower interest rate. In a privately placed transaction in which the lender has more bargaining power, the prepayment prohibition may extend for the entire term of the debt. Rather than a prohibition against prepayment, the borrower may be permitted to prepay with a prepayment penalty, which is an amount of money in excess of the principal that must be paid in consideration of the right to prepay. It is often calculated on the basis of a percentage of the principal paid. Thus, the premium will be, for example, 10 percent of the principal. It is also expressed in terms of a combined sum, for example, principal may be repaid at 110 percent. The premium usually declines over a period of time to the point that, in the final years, it becomes 0 percent. An example of a combined call protection and prepayment premium is as follows: No prepayment permitted for the first 10 years; prepayment premium of 10 percent in the eleventh year, declining by one percent a year for 10 years; no prepayment premium for the twenty-first through thirtieth years.

In the case of publicly offered tax exempt debt, the typical prepayment premium is negligible. Typically, these transactions contain a 10 year call protection and thereafter a two percent prepayment premium, declining by one percent a year. In essence, the modest prepayment premium is in place for only two years. More complex forms of prepayment premiums are sometimes encountered that attempt to measure the loss of interest and compensate the lender accordingly.

In some transactions, especially privately placed issues, exceptions are made to the absolute prohibition. The following are examples of exceptions which are typically permitted:

A borrower might be permitted to make prepayments on any principal payment date equal to twice the amount of principal owing on that date.

In the case of taxable debt, the borrower might be permitted to prepay the principal from the proceeds of tax exempt debt.

If all or a portion of the facility is destroyed by fire or taken by eminent domain, and it is not reconstructed, principal may be prepaid. This provision, even in a liberal form, is accepted in the tax exempt market but is resisted in the taxable market.

In some cases, prepayment of principal is permitted so long as it is not for the purpose of obtaining a lower interest rate. This sort of covenant usually involves either a straight comparison of interest rates or a formula test that the new transaction must meet, whereby the premium is adjusted depending on the differential in rates.

§ 19 EQUITY FINANCING

Capital may be obtained for a project by means of either debt or equity. Debt financing involves a loan of money by a lender to the owner. Equity financing involves raising capital through the sale of ownership interests in the project. The demarcation between debt and equity is blurred in some of the more innovative capital structuring techniques, such as:

Convertible debentures, whereby a corporation issues debt that is accompanied by an option, exercisable at the will of the creditor, to convert the debt into a specified number of shares of stock;

Preferred stock, which is an equity interest, but with limited voting rights and a guaranteed rate of return;

Debt for which a portion of interest consists of a share of net earnings and capital appreciation.

The decision as to how much equity and how much debt financing to include in a given project depends upon a number of factors and is often dictated by the availability of capital, financial markets, requirements of lending programs, and the economics of the project. The following are some of the considerations that may apply to particular types of projects:

1. Nonprofit projects, especially those that pursue social goals (such as housing for lower income persons) and that are not prone to generating excess revenues, may not be able to generate sufficient amounts of revenue to service debt at levels that would attract debt capital. However, in some cases, federal tax incentives may make equity investment attractive notwithstanding little or no economic return from the project. Moreover, such projects may be able to attract governmental or private grants and gifts that could be invested in the project without expectation of return. Thus, many such projects have very high proportions of equity, if not 100 percent equity financing.

2. Many debt financing programs contain a requirement that there be a certain minimum percentage of equity investment.[85] Even where the

---

[85]*E.g.*, the California Health Facility Construction Loan Insurance Program requires 10 percent equity investment for nonprofits.

program has no formal requirement, lenders usually require the borrower to have some stake in the project in order to assure that the borrower will have an incentive to properly manage it, and to give the lender some cushion in the event of a foreclosure. An exception to the foregoing is the case of certain federal loan guarantees, which permit 100 percent financing (see § 14).

§ 19.1   OWNER CONTRIBUTION

The simplest form of equity financing is by the infusion of capital by the owner of the project. Whether the owner is an individual or an existing corporation, the owner may contribute capital by paying for that portion of the project that is not otherwise financed. This capital may come from surplus earnings from other ventures or be in the form of property already held. Examples of such equity financing are:

A church determines that a portion of the site on which the church is located is not needed for church purposes and decides to build a retirement home on the property. That property is an equity contribution by the church.

A' hospital utilizes revenues from its operations to pay architect, engineering, feasibility, and legal costs to start a retirement home project. The payment of those expenses is an equity contribution.

A corporation that owns an existing retirement home pays a portion of the cost of expansion of the facility out of its surplus revenues.

In determining how much of one's own money to invest in a project, two factors are important: (1) the amount of equity required to be invested, and (2) the opportunity cost of the invested equity as compared with the cost of outside financing. Thus, if the project owner can use its capital in a manner that will give it a higher rate of return than it would have to pay for debt or equity capital in the financial markets, it would be wise to finance a larger portion of the project. But if it cannot earn a higher rate, it may be wise to use a higher proportion of its capital to finance the project.

Because different parties are differently situated, the rate of return will vary notwithstanding the equilibrium otherwise created by the market. For example, a nonprofit sponsor might receive a six percent return on its investment in the project, but could receive an eight percent return · by investing its capital elsewhere. However, a for profit investor may be willing to contribute debt or equity capital to the project and be happy with the six percent return because it can take advantage of tax treatment that results in a higher effective yield. The nonprofit corporation and perhaps other for profit investors may not be able to take advantage of such tax treatment because of their individual situations.

§ 19.2 CORPORATE STOCK

The issuance of stock by a corporation is the typical method whereby it raises capital in the market. The issuance of stock is a very heavily regulated activity subject to very particular requirements imposed by both state and federal governments, which will not be dealt with in detail here. There are several good treatises on this subject that should be consulted for further information. However, the following is a general discussion of some of the elements of corporate equity finance.

A corporation that is considering the raising of equity capital, either on a private or public basis, must engage in careful preparation, including the preparation of a business plan with projections of growth of the enterprise and financial results. A private offering usually involves approaching a limited number of prospective investors and negotiating the terms of the investment, which may include issues of control, buy-out, and the nature of future offerings. Public offerings are usually structured in conjunction with an investment banking firm, which assists the corporation in developing the terms of securities that the market will accept. The investment bankers, often through a syndicate, will market the stock utilizing their retail capabilities.

The issuance of stock is governed by the registration and disclosure scheme set out under the Securities Act of 1933[86] and under the Blue Sky laws of the states in which the stock is offered for sale, unless exempt under the provisions of those laws. A for profit corporation issuing stock may not rely on the exemption for securities of a public agency, typically relied upon in tax exempt debt offerings. However, several other exemptions from registration may be available principally those for private offerings. In general, private offerings are those made to a limited number of persons deemed capable of both evaluating the nature of the investment risk they are taking and of bearing that risk. Such offerings must be made without general advertisement or public solicitation. Because some issuers find it difficult to determine whether or not they have in fact complied with the vaguely worded standards of the generic private offering exemption, the SEC has also certain detailed "safe harbor" exemptions from registration for offerings made to institutional investors such as banks, insurance companies, investment companies, employee benefit plans and wealthy individuals (accredited investors), or others determined to have sufficient knowledge and experience, so long as it is reasonably believed that there will be no more than 35 of such other purchasers.[87] If the entire offering is less than $5,000,000, it is not necessary that the 35 purchasers who are not accredited meet any particular requirements. The exemptions for private offering available in the federal securities laws

---

[86] 15 U.S.C. § 77a *et seq.*
[87] 17 C.F.R. § 230.506.

usually have parallel provisions in the laws of the various states. There is also a federal exemption for a stock offering that "comes to rest" in a single state. However, state law may then be a concern.

If the issue is not exempt and therefore is subject to registration with the Securities and Exchange Commission pursuant to the Securities Act of 1933, it is necessary, as a condition to the offering, for the securities to be registered with the SEC and for a prospectus that has been approved by the SEC to be disseminated to prospective investors. In addition to these conditions to the offering of stock, companies with registered stock must file with the SEC annual, quarterly, and periodic reports, some of which must be disseminated to stockholders and all of which will be available for public inspection. These companies also become subject to the proxy rules promulgated by the SEC.

§ 19.3   GENERAL PARTNERSHIPS

A partnership is a venture carried on between two or more persons (who may be corporations). In a partnership, two persons may contribute capital to and share the management and control of a project. Characteristic attributes of a general partnership (in contrast to a corporation) include:

1. *Limited scope.* The partnership will usually be established to own and operate a particular project rather than having the authority to engage in unlimited business enterprises.

2. *Limited duration.* The partnership may have a limited term of existence, for example, for the duration of a 65 year ground lease of the property from one of the partners. It may be capable of being dissolved by either party on certain terms. Limited duration is a partnership characteristic taken into account in the taxation of partnerships (see discussion of tax treatment of partnerships, below).

3. *Liability of partners.* General partners, unlike corporate stockholders, members of nonprofit corporations, and limited partners, are jointly and severally liable for the debts and obligations of the partnership.

4. *Management of the partnership.* Unless otherwise set forth in the partnership agreement, general partners have equal rights to manage the business of the partnership. Because of the general liability feature, all of the partners will probably want to exercise at least some ability to manage.

The advantage of a general partnership is that the parties can pool their equity, share the risk, and each contribute their expertise and management capability. For example, a housing developer may have some capital and a knowledge of how to develop and operate a housing project but know nothing of the development and operation of health facilities. Likewise, a hospital may have some capital and a knowledge of how to develop and operate health facilities but know nothing of housing. If the two form a partnership to construct a retirement home, they can pool their capital, share the risk of the project, and each contribute its unique expertise in the operation of the completed facility. The risk of this type of enterprise is that in a general partnership, both partners have control over the partnership, unless one of them is given managerial rights. Such a partnership could be unstable and, in the event of a conflict between the parties, could be ungovernable.

§ 19.4 LIMITED PARTNERSHIPS

A limited partnership is a partnership containing at least one general partner (that is, a partner that is generally liable for the debts and obligations of the partnership and that has the right to control the partnership) and at least one limited partner (that is, a partner whose liability is limited to the amount of his investment and who does not generally have the right to control the partnership). Limited partnerships have been extensively used, especially in real estate development, because they offer some of the benefits of both a general partnership and a corporation.

Like a general partnership, a limited partnership is not taxed directly, but its partners are taxed on their share of its earnings. This avoids the so-called double taxation, whereby corporations are taxed and their earnings are again taxed when distributed to shareholders as dividends. Like a corporation, investors are shielded from liability except to the extent of their investment. Because of the tax benefits of this form and its similarity to a corporation, a limited partnership must be careful not to be considered an association by the Internal Revenue Service and thereby be taxed at corporate rates. A limited partnership will not be treated as an association taxable as a corporation unless the organization has more major corporate characteristics than noncorporate characteristics.[88] The four major relevant corporate characteristics are: (1) continuity of life; (2) centralization of management; (3) limited liability; and (4) free transferability of interests. The Tax Court has held[89] that where only two of the four above listed characteristics are found to exist, the organization will not be deemed an association taxable as a corporation, but instead will be classified as a partnership.

With respect to continuity of life, the regulations[90] provide that "if the death, insanity, bankruptcy, retirement, resignation or expulsion of any member will cause a dissolution of the organization, continuity of life does not exist." In order to come within this provision, the partnership agreement often provides that the partnership will dissolve upon the dissolution of a general partner, if a corporation, or the death or incompetency of an individual general partner, or the general partner's retirement, resignation,

[88]Treas. Reg. § 301.7701-2(a)(1).
[89]*Larson v. Comm'r*, 66 T.C. 159 (1976).
[90]Reg. § 301.7701-2(b)(1).

removal or bankruptcy, unless the limited partners elect unanimously to continue the partnership. Treasury regulations further provide that a limited partnership organized pursuant to a state law corresponding to the Revised Uniform Limited Partnership Act is deemed to lack the corporate characteristic of continuity of life.[91]

In order to avoid a finding of "free transferability of interests," partnership agreements often contain a provision requiring the consent of the general partner prior to any limited partner transferring a partnership interest.

Centralization of management and limited liability are two corporate features that are usually present in a limited partnership. However, if the other two characteristics are missing, a partnership should be able to avoid corporate taxation.

Unlike a general partnership interest, which is considered to be the ownership of the business itself, limited partnership interests are considered to be securities under the Securities Act of 1933 and the Securities Exchange Act of 1934.[92]

As a consequence, public offerings limited partnerships interests must be accompanied by disclosure documents and may be required to be registered with the SEC if no exemption is available, State Blue Sky laws will also be applicable.

With the enactment of the Tax Reform Act of 1986, restrictions on limited partnerships that had as their predominant economic rationale the avoidance of federal income tax are of less importance than in the past. However, to the extent that such transactions continue to be developed, projects that anticipate inordinately great tax benefits must be registered and the at risk rules, requiring investors to be at risk with respect to the capital on which they are claiming tax benefits, will be applied. The overriding consideration is that tax benefits are not available for those "activities not engaged in for profit."[93] It has been suggested that the partnership must be engaged in the activity with the *predominant* purpose and intention of making a profit (excluding tax benefits).[94] However, the IRS has ruled that the construction and operation of an apartment project for low and moderate income housing under Section 236 of the National Housing Act is not an activity to which Section 183 of the Code applies. Congress, in limiting the amount of rental that could be charged in Section 236 projects assumed that deductions of tax losses would be allowed to encourage investment in such projects.[95] This same reasoning would

---

[91]Treas. Reg. § 301.7701-2.

[92]*Mayer v. Oil Field Systems Corp.*, 721 F.2d 59 (2d Cir. 1983); *Goodman v. Epstein*, 582 F.2d 388 (7th Cir. 1978); *McGreghar Land Co. v. Meguiar*, 521 F.2d 822 (9th Cir. 1975).

[93]I.R.C. § 183.

[94]*Sanderson v. Comm'r*, 50 T.C.M. 1033 (1985).

[95]Rev. Rul. 79-300; 1979-2 C.B. 112.

probably also apply to Section 42, relating to low income housing tax credits, since congress, by limiting rental rates to very low levels, must have intended that credits rather than profit would provide the necessary incentive for an investment in low income housing projects.

§ 19.5 REAL ESTATE INVESTMENT TRUSTS

While most real estate syndication utilizes the limited partnership mode (see § 19.4) a significant amount of syndication is accomplished by means of real estate investment trusts (REITs). A REIT is a trust, rather than a partnership, and can be used both for equity and debt investment in real estate.

As distinguished from a limited partnership, a REIT is generally subject to federal income tax. However, it is not subject to tax on earnings distributed to its shareholders so long as 95 percent or more of its ordinary taxable income and foreclosure property income is distributed. Furthermore, at least 75 percent of the REIT's annual gross income must be derived from passive real estate or real estate mortgage investments. An additional 20 percent must be from either the foregoing or dividends or interest from any source or gain from the sale or other disposition of stocks and securities.[96]

The recent growth of REITs has been directed towards pension funds and IRA investments. REITs have evolved that pursue specialized objectives, appropriate to the aims of their investors. Therefore, there are, for example, REITs that make leveraged equity investments, in the manner of limited partnerships, REITs that focus on all equity (unleveraged) investments, and REITs that make loans secured by mortgages or deeds of trust. The latter are often characterized by provisions that result in a current return plus a share in excess cash flow and sale proceeds of the financed project.

§ 19.6 FOR PROFIT-NONPROFIT JOINT VENTURES

In an effort to raise a greater amount of equity capital than they can raise on their own, many nonprofit organizations have entered into joint ventures with for profit investors. This device enables the nonprofit organization to develop its project, usually under its management and control, using equity capital that would otherwise be unavailable.

The structure of such an enterprise is that of a limited partnership in which the nonprofit, with little equity contribution, is the general partner and the investors are limited partners, contributing the capital but not

---

[96]For a more detailed description of REITs and the applicable tax restrictions, see Jarchow, *Real Estate Syndication*, § 2.4. (New York: John Wiley & Sons, 1985).

sharing in the management of the project. In this type of partnership, there is often a for profit cogeneral partner that has a fiduciary responsibility to the limited partners, especially regarding tax matters.

In a limited partnership involving a nonprofit general partner, there is a potential conflict of interest in that, as a general partner, the nonprofit organization has a fiduciary duty to the limited partners but, as a nonprofit organization, to the objects of its charitable purposes. In fact, questions have been raised in the past as to whether a nonprofit could function as a general partner in that it could be said to impermissibly benefit private investors. The Internal Revenue Service has recently found, however, that such an arrangement is permissible if it follows the guidelines described in § 12.1.

§ 19.7 LOW INCOME HOUSING TAX CREDITS

Federal tax laws have traditionally contained provisions giving favorable treatment to real estate investments generally and, in particular, to low income housing.[97] These provisions have included accelerated depreciation, producing paper losses that could be used to shelter ordinary income from tax. As a result, it was possible to structure transactions in which most, if not all, of the return to an investor consisted of favorable tax treatment. While generally a transaction must have economic substance—that is, it must produce economic return notwithstanding tax treatment—the Internal Revenue Service has ruled that favorable treatment of low income housing is intended as a subsidy to produce an investment that would not otherwise be made and, therefore, no economic substance need be shown.[98] Thus, it was possible to raise capital for such a facility by, in essence, selling the tax writeoff to private investors. Such a sale occurs by selling limited partnership interests in a partnership that owns the facility.

The 1986 Tax Reform Act eliminated special depreciation benefits for low income housing, and lengthened to 27.5 years the period over which residential real estate improvements generally must be depreciated. The Act also severely restricted the extent to which depreciation and other tax benefits could be used to shelter ordinary income. As a consequence, a major source of equity capital has dried up.

Congress did, however, provide for a low income housing tax credit,[99] which provides a substantial new potential source of capital. This credit is discussed in detail in § 8.3. The credit can be used to raise capital by structuring a limited partnership and selling the limited partner shares to investors who can use the credit. To be able to use the credit, a corporate investor must have sufficient tax so that, after the credit is taken, its

[97]I.R.C. § 42.
[98]Rev. Rul. 79-300; 1979-2 C.B. 112.
[99]I.R.C. § 42(c)(1)(D).

resulting tax is not less than the alternative minimum tax. Individual investors are restricted to the amount of credit that can be taken on tax levied with respect to income other than passive income.

At the time of this writing, it is uncertain as to how effective the tax credit program will be in stimulating the development of low income housing. Except in cases of smaller rehabilitation projects, it is usually not possible to structure an economically feasible project without additional subsidy. However, in those cases in which private or local government subsidy is available (federal subsidy reduces the amount of credit available), the tax credits can make the difference between a feasible and an infeasible project.

Seven

Regulation of Retirement Facility Development and Operation

Retirement facilities may be regulated in some degree by federal, state, or local governments. Federal laws are usually tied to a funding source such as a HUD loan or loan guarantee, or Medicare or Medicaid payments, but may also include commerce-related concerns such as securities registration or antitrust laws[1] (see, e.g., §§ 20.4, 20.5, 22, 24). Most regulation occurs at the state level and is concentrated in the areas of licensure for the provision of personal care or health care, regulation of continuing care agreements, and control of health planning.[2] To the extent there is local government regulation, it is usually limited to zoning and land use planning, construction standards, rent controls, and similar real property development issues.

§ 20 LICENSING OF CARE PROGRAMS

Facilities and organizations that offer health care or personal care are heavily regulated by the states. Often, the source of state regulations is federal

[1] Antitrust laws are discussed in Part V in the context of joint venture issues.

[2] Although states frequently regulate housing subdivisions, these generally do not have distinctive features affecting elderly housing and are therefore not discussed.

law imposing requirements on the states as a condition of receiving funding pursuant to the Medicare or Medicaid programs. Regulation may encompass such subjects as construction of facilities, addition of licensed beds, purchase of substantial equipment, construction standards, staffing requirements, resident rights, reimbursement for services, transfer of residents, and other issues touching on almost every aspect of the operation of such facilities.

§ 20.1   CERTIFICATE OF NEED

CAUTION: In the final days of the 99th Congress, the entire federal health planning law, contained at 42 U.S. Code Section 300k-1 through Section 300n-6, was repealed by Public Law 99-660, effective January 1, 1987. Nevertheless, many states still have programs in effect that were patterned after the federal program. The effect on state programs of the loss of federal funding remains to be seen. The following discussion of the former federal program requirements is offered as a general guide to those still subject to state laws.

Public Law 93-641, effective beginning in 1975, established a system of national health planning and development designed to encourage states to control the distribution, efficiency, and costs of health care services, and thereby reduce spiraling increases in federal health expenditures.[3] States that did not comply with federal health planning parameters were subject to loss of federal funding for various health programs and, as a result, all states but Louisiana had enacted health planning programs by 1981.[4]

A chief product of federal health planning, as implemented by the states, is Certificate of Need programs.[5] Certificate of Need programs are administered by the state's health planning and development agencies, and review and determine the need for certain capital expenditures for health care projects, major medical equipment purchases, and additions of institutional health services.[6] States developed a state plan that inventoried existing resources and evaluated each state's needs and long-term goals for health care. The state plan is composed of health systems plans (HSPs) created by local health systems agencies (HSAs). Those who planned to add new institutional health services or make certain capital expenditures or purchases for health care equipment or facilities were reviewed and required to secure a certificate of need before undertaking the project or committing to the expenditure.

For retirement facilities in development, the principal issue has been whether a new institutional health service is being proposed or whether a capital expenditure is being made in excess of the statutory threshold.

---

[3] *See* former 42 U.S.C. §§ 300k, *et seq.*

[4] *See, generally, Hospital Law Manual,* "Health Planning," Vol. IIA, ¶ ¶ 1-5, *et seq.*, Aspen Systems (1983).

[5] *See* former 42 U.S.C. § 300m-6.

[6] Former 42 U.S.C. § 300m-6(a)(1).

Institutional health services were defined to include health services offered by nursing homes, rehabilitation facilities, and other health facilities, as defined by the Secretary of Health, Education and Welfare, and that meet a minimum annual operating expenditure threshold of $306,750.[7] Any obligation of a capital expenditure, by or on behalf of a health facility, of $600,000 or more during a specified 12 month period was also subject to review under federal law.[8] Health facilities are defined in federal regulation to include skilled nursing and intermediate care facilities.[9] However, a certificate of need could not be required with respect to a health service offered by certain qualifying health maintenance organizations (HMOs).[10]

A project requiring a certificate of need is reviewed with regard to numerous criteria, such as its relation to the applicable health systems plan, the needs of the population to be served, the availability of less costly alternatives, the project's financial feasibility, and the needs of underserved groups such as low income persons, the handicapped, or ethnic minorities (elderly are not specified).[11]

Generally, the process of determining need has involved a detailed application, public hearings with the right to have legal counsel and to present evidence, written findings, and the opportunity for full judicial review of any decision.[12]

Although their impact has been felt less acutely among retirement facilities than in the hospital industry, certificate of need laws generally have required any retirement facility developer contemplating construction of a skilled nursing or intermediate care facility to show that such a facility is needed in the particular health planning area in which the project is to be located. Usually, the determination of need includes an assessment of the number of existing facilities of the same type in the area, their census or occupancy figures, as well as a demographic prediction of future health care needs in the locale. Facilities offering care at a level below that of skilled nursing or intermediate care—for example, personal care facilities—generally are not included within the certificate of need requirements, except in a few states. Home health agencies are, however, subject to certificate of need review under the laws of approximately 27 states.[13]

A determination of the need for a particular facility can involve contested, trial-like hearings in which other providers opposed to the project

---

[7]See former 42 U.S.C. § 300n(5), and 50 Fed. Reg. 14,027 (1985) raising the statutory expenditure minimum from $250,000.

[8]42 C.F.R. § 123.401.

[9]Id.

[10]Former 42 U.S.C. § 300m-6(b)(1).

[11]42 C.F.R. § 122.412. ·

[12]42 C.F.R. § 123.410.

[13]"How to Establish a Home Health Agency: Some Preliminary Considerations," National Association of Home Care (1984).

present evidence and opinion showing why the project is not economically feasible, why it would lead to underutilization of resources already in the community, or why, for other reasons, it would waste the health resources of the particular area. However, retirement facilities tend to be less subject to these kinds of arguments from competitors than freestanding health facilities, because retirement facility health services are usually offered as part of an overall residential and services program that does not offer services to the general public and thus does not directly compete with typical nursing facilities.

In some states, statutory provisions have been adopted giving special preferences in the application of certificate of need laws to retirement facilities, and particularly to continuing care facilities. Because retirement facilities with health centers tend to have a captive market for their health facilities, the population to be served may be considered to be the retirement community residents themselves, rather than the general public. Health planning agencies therefore may look to the needs only of the retirement community, rather than those of the entire planning area. As a consequence, a health planning agency may determine that new health beds are needed for a retirement facility despite the absence of a need in the community at large, and it may ignore retirement facility health care beds in calculating the inventory of health resources for the planning area.

Another reason for granting certificate of need preference to a retirement facility can arise when some form of financial security device for health care costs is provided. This may be in the form of a prepaid, self-insured continuing care program, or use of an HMO or long-term care insurance policy. Because of the favored treatment once given in federal regulation to prepaid health plans and cost-efficient payment mechanisms, states may give special treatment to retirement facilities, either by rule or regulation, or on the basis of a case-by-case review.

Many commentators feel that the certificate of need program has failed in controlling the costs of health care and, in fact, simply adds additional administrative burdens to the already climbing costs of providing health facilities.[14] With the repeal[15] of the federal program, and the funding that goes with it, it is likely that most states will eventually repeal their own certificate of need laws. And in some instances, states abolished their certificate of need programs in anticipation of the possibility of federal action.[16]

For the retirement facility developer contemplating a program that includes health care services in a state where certificate of need is still a prerequisite to construction, determination of the state's published calculation of the need for skilled nursing or other facilities in the area where

[14]See, generally, Sfekas, "Can Health Planning Survive the 1980's?" Aging Network News, June 1986.

[15]P.L. 99-660.

[16]See, e.g., Cal. Stat. of 1986, ch. 1084, eff. Jan. 1, 1987.

construction is contemplated is a necessary first step. It should be determined whether any exemptions are available for retirement facilities of the type contemplated, and steps must be taken immediately to put the appropriate state agency on notice of the intention to build, so that, in the event any need for beds is shown in the state or local area plan, a competitor does not preempt the project by submitting an earlier application to fill the same need.

§ 20.2   NURSING FACILITY LICENSURE

Most nursing facility licensure standards adopted by the states have their genesis in federal Medicare and Medicaid laws, which are imposed as a condition of receiving funding from the federal government.[17] States normally have adopted licensing statutes that incorporate federal requirements and make them applicable to all nursing facilities seeking to do business within the state, irrespective of their status as a provider certified under one or both of the federal programs. In addition to skilled nursing facilities, intermediate care facilities are also heavily regulated.[18] Intermediate care facilities are essentially skilled nursing facilities with a less intensive level of nursing services.

Most states require nursing facilities to obtain licenses from a regulatory agency in order to do business. Although regulation varies from state to state, virtually all have numerous elements in common due to the federal standards.

Under federal law, eligible skilled nursing facilities must provide 24 hour nursing service, with at least one registered nurse employed full time, have policies and procedures developed and carried out by one or more physicians and nurses, require patients to be under physician supervision, have a physician on call for emergencies, maintain clinical records, have a utilization review program in effect, maintain accounts of patient funds, meet fire safety standards, and have a budget, among other requirements.[19] The extensive regulatory conditions of participation in the Medicare or Medicaid programs for nursing facilities expand dramatically upon the statutory fundamentals to include such diverse topics as minimum standards for facility administrators, and for various categories of nurses, dietary service supervisors, medical record practitioners, and assorted therapists and practitioners, governing body and management criteria, personnel policies and staffing patterns, patient rights standards, required basic services and amenities, protocols for handling pharmaceuticals, transfer agreements with hospitals, numerous physical plant requirements, linens and infection control,

---

[17] See, generally, 42 U.S.C. § 1396a(a)(28) (Medicaid) and 42 U.S.C. § 1395x(j) (Medicare).
[18] See, e.g., 42 C.F.R. Pt. 442, Subpt. F.
[19] 42 U.S.C. § 1395x(j).

disaster planning, and a host of other subjects covering every aspect of facility and program design and operations.[20]

A typical state statute expands even further on the federal regulatory framework. Staffing standards are usually set at a minimum ratio of daily nursing hours per patient in the facility. Basic services standards may elaborate on the performance of such functions as dining, housekeeping, laundry, dietitian services, and physical therapy. Physical plant criteria may relate to the basic requirements for sterilization facilities, water temperatures, fireproofing requirements, emergency power systems, and other similar health and safety minimums. State regulations also routinely require implementation of facility policies and standards relating to admissions and discharges, records of storage and use of medications, keeping patient care plans and nursing notes, logging physician orders and visits, documenting patient falls and other incidents, reporting grievances to an ombudsperson, and other recordkeeping requirements.

(a) Admitting the General Public

Of particular interest to retirement facilities is the patients' rights standard set forth in 42 Code of Federal Regulations Section 405.1121(k)(4), which requires that a patient be "transferred or discharged only for medical reasons, or for his welfare or that of other patients, or for nonpayment of his stay (except as prohibited by titles XVIII and XIX of the Social Security Act)."

Often, new retirement projects with a health care unit cannot fill the health care beds with retirement home residents. Because the facility is new, all the residents are likely to be healthy, independent, and comfortable in their residential units. Only after the facility population matures over many years is there likely to be a stream of residents in need of care sufficient to keep the health center reasonably full. Therefore, it is common for facility operators, especially in the early years of operation, to make health center beds available to members of the general public, with the idea that general public patients will, with time, increasingly need to make way for facility residents in need of nursing services.

The problem, of course, is that a general public patient apparently cannot be discharged, under the federal patients' rights rules, simply to make room for another patient unless, for example, (1) there is a change in the level or type of care needed by the person in the nursing facility that warrants the patient's transfer, (2) he or she fails to pay the charges for care and the care is not covered by the Medicaid program,[21] or (3) the patient's continued stay in the facility endangers another patient.

---

[20] See, generally, 42 C.F.R. Pt. 405, Subpt. K.

[21] A Medicaid provider is required to accept the government payment as payment in full for covered services, even though the usual charges may be higher, see § 9.2(b)(4).

Facilities cannot be arbitrary or cavalier in discharging patients for medical reasons, especially discharges to a lower level of care that could result in ineligibility for government benefits. Although the Supreme Court has held that a nursing home patient threatened with transfer does not have a constitutional right to due process notice and hearing procedures prior to transfer,[22] the provider must allow the patient's physician to participate in the utilization review committee's determination of the appropriateness of a transfer, and must report any transfer to the appropriate state agency.[23]

Probably the only practical and lawful solution to the dilemma of transferring patients to make room for residents in need is to admit as patients from the general public a sufficient ratio of persons whose need for nursing care is not likely to be long term, but rather convalescent in character. For example, an experienced nursing administrator can screen entering patients and admit only those recovering from surgery, but not those suffering from degenerative diseases from which a hope of speedy recovery appears dim. In this way, it should become possible to control with reasonable accuracy the rate with which beds will become available for use by occupants of the residential facilities, or for temporary refilling by another outsider.

(b) Construction Standards

Any retirement facility developer contemplating construction of any type of health care facility as a part of the project should carefully review state and local construction standards applicable to the particular facility. Depending upon the jurisdiction, health facilities may be required to be built to much higher construction standards than those that would be imposed upon purely residential structures. For example, in California, where earthquake safety is a concern, a very elaborate set of construction standards has been established for hospitals, so that in the event of a serious earthquake, the hospitals will remain standing and be able to treat the injured. In California, these seismic standards apply to skilled nursing facilities that are more than one story in height. The kind of steel and concrete construction required to conform a skilled nursing facility to hospital seismic safety standards can be so much more expensive than, for example, conventional wood frame construction as to be prohibitive.

Statutes or regulations such as this can also pose particular problems in multiple story buildings where a health care facility is to be incorporated into the structure as one or two floors of an otherwise residential building. Depending upon the location of the health care unit within such a highrise structure, it may become necessary to build the entire structure to the heightened standard required for the health facility component.

---

[22] *Blum v. Yaretsky*, 457 U.S. 991, 73 L. Ed. 2d 534, 102 S. Ct. 2777 (1982).
[23] *See* 42 C.F.R. §§ 456.336(f), 456.337.

Another consideration for health facility construction is the ability to convert structures to different uses over time. For example, facilities initially used for personal care may be designed so that they are convertible to skilled nursing standards for use later on when the retirement facility population has matured and a higher level of care is generally needed.

The intricacies of these types of regulations, which vary from state to state, and deal with such matters as corridor widths, door size, structural strengths, fireproofing, and the like, are beyond the scope of this book. Suffice it to say that the prudent developer will inquire into these issues early in the planning process, and should consult with an architect or structural engineer with experience in constructing health facilities in the region where project development is contemplated.

§ 20.3   BOARD AND CARE FACILITY LICENSURE

Personal care facilities offer a level of care substantially below that required to be available in skilled nursing facilities. They have been called by numerous names, such as board and care, or assisted living.[24] Whereas skilled nursing facilities offer 24 hour skilled nursing care, occupants of personal care facilities may need only occasional or part-time assistance with such activities as bathing, dressing, or grooming, which can be provided by an assistant who does not have nursing training.

(a)   A Patchwork of Laws

The only significant federal legislation dealing with personal care facilities is the Keys Amendment,[25] which requires that states adopt standards for those facilities dealing with such matters as admission policies, safety, sanitation, and protection of civil rights, where they house, or are likely to house, a significant number of recipients of supplemental security income benefits (SSI). Unfortunately, the only sanction available for failure to conform to the Keys Amendment has been to deny SSI payments to needy facility residents. There is no federal enforcement mechanism against states or operators of board and care facilities, as there has been for standards imposed on health facilities as a condition of Medicare and Medicaid enrollment.[26]

A 1983 survey conducted by the American Bar Association (ABA) and the Department of Health and Human Services (HHS) revealed a crazyquilt of

---

[24]Other names used in various state statutes include sheltered care, group home, boarding home for the aged, residential care, congregate living, supervised living, rest home, domiciliary care, supportive living, community residential facility, adult family home. *See Mental Disability Law Reporter*, 7, No. 2 (March–April 1983), 158–209.

[25]P.L. 94-566, 42 U.S.C. § 1382e(e).

[26]*See, Mental Disability Law Reporter*, note 24, above, at 159.

state laws regulating board and care types of facilities.[27] Not only does the nomenclature vary widely from state to state,[28] but statutes cover facilities for the elderly, children, mentally and developmentally disabled, and drug dependents or delinquents, and includes residential and day-care formats, and operations ranging from massive institutions to mom and pop programs operated in the owners' personal residences. Some states have statutes affording only piecemeal coverage of the various possible permutations, while others prescribe as many as six separate categories of licensure tailored to the size, purpose, and clientele of each class of facility.

Licensure provisions generally include an application and screening process. Physical plants are inspected for conformity with construction standards, including fire safety, sanitation, and accessibility. Basic staff qualifications and levels, criminal record clearance, and bonding may be prescribed. Basic services may be required, such as meals, supervision and observation, planned recreational activities, assistance with personal activities, housekeeping, and so on. Patient rights may be established, including the rights to have visitors, privacy, and personal possessions, to be free from restraint or involuntary work, and to certain procedures prior to eviction. Recordkeeping requirements can involve patient care plans, incident reports, medications records, and accounting of patient funds. Finally, enforcement mechanisms are usually present, including such things as grievance systems, ombudsmen, injunctions, license suspension or revocation, and criminal sanctions.

For retirement facility operators, the major problem with this patchwork of laws is that, depending on the state, applicable regulations may not be well suited to the particular realities of a residential community that may contain healthy, independent senior citizens on the same premises with those in need of substantial care.

(b) The Subtle Boundaries of Licensure

A significant step toward uniformity of licensing approaches came in 1984 with the completion of the ABA-HHS Model Act for state licensure of board and care homes. The Model Act defines a board and care home as: "a publicly or privately operated residence that provides personal assistance, lodging, and meals to two (2) or more adults who are unrelated to the licensee or administrator."[29]

Personal assistance is defined to include (1) helping with the resident's "activities of daily living," (2) assisting with daily activities necessary to access "supportive services"[30] required in the board and care plan, (3) being

---

[27] *Id.*

[28] *See* note 24, above.

[29] *See Mental and Physical Disability Law Reporter*, 8, No. 2 (March-April, 1984), 157.

[30] For example, medical, social, financial, legal, or transportation services. *Id.*, at 160.

aware of the resident's general whereabouts, but allowing for independent travel, and (4) monitoring resident activities while on the premises.[31]

Daily activities under the Model Act include such bodily functions as bathing, dressing, eating, and grooming, but also room cleaning, laundering, making appointments, and managing money. A potential problem with the Model Act, and with some state statutes, when applied to many retirement facilities is that they do not distinguish between bodily care and other services, nor between services that are provided due to the recipient's frailty or dependence, versus those furnished to independent persons as a convenience.

Laws should recognize that the receipt of personal services from a valet, concierge, housekeeper, hairdresser, or manicurist does not necessarily warrant licensure even when offered as part of the standard program in a group residence for the elderly. Some states deal with this problem by limiting the activities described in licensure-triggering definitions to hands-on bodily assistance, such as bathing and dressing, rather than extending definitions to such things as housekeeping, laundry, or transportation, which are more likely to be mere conveniences for some residents. Another possible approach is to retain the broader definition, but to require licensure only for facilities that contain·residents in *need* of such services due to physical or mental frailty.

Retirement facility developers should become familiar with the particular approaches taken by their states in determining what activity is ground for board and care licensure. Homes with units designed for a mix of independent and dependent residents should be particularly aware of licensure parameters. States may require that all facilities in a mixed use project be licensed, even though some units are designed strictly for independent living. This particularly may be true if the contractual arrangement with the resident contains a promise that initially independent residents eventually will be furnished care when needed.

While licensure of independent living facilities may seem anathema from the viewpoint of the facility operator, many with a mix of independent and personal care units have actively sought personal care licensure for the entire project on the ground that it distinguishes the facility from conventional housing and thus may constitute a basis for exemption from rent controls, property taxes, certain discrimination laws, landlord-tenant obligations, or other strictures that may not apply to licensed care facilities. From a public policy perspective, licensure of independent as well as care units can be beneficial by helping to avoid circumstances where, due to a provider's fear of licensure, residents are kept in inadequate independent facilities after having declined gradually to a state of dependence and need.

Often, the process of aging in place can pose problems for independent living facilities that do not have licensed units equipped to provide care. Facility owners can face the difficult problem of being forced to transfer, or even evict, people for whom they cannot care, and who may be reluctant to

<hr>

[31]*Id.*, at 159.

accept their advancing dependence. Although home health services may be utilized to provide care in an unlicensed residential unit, this is a temporary measure at best. All retirement facilities in development should seriously address the problems of transition from independence to the need for care, and should develop a specific plan for identifying and dealing with the social, legal, and operational consequences.

Because of the growing elderly cohort, the current lack of uniformity among state laws, and the continuing need for an alternative to nursing facility placement for those in need of assistance but not ready for 24 hour care, one can expect to see increased efforts to regulate personal care.[32]

§ 20.4 HOME HEALTH REGULATION

Home health is a well defined concept nationally due to its eligibility for reimbursement through the Medicare program. The Medicare conditions of participation set forth the salient features of an approved home health care program as follows:

1. It must provide part-time or intermittent skilled nursing care, plus one or more of the following:
   a. Physical, speech, or occupational therapy,
   b. Medical social services, or
   c. Home health aid services, which may include such services as personal care, household services essential to health, exercise, and assistance with medications.
2. It must be provided on a visiting basis, to people in their homes (homebound or confined to home).
3. Services must be rendered pursuant to a plan and periodically reviewed by a physician, at least every two months.[33]

If qualified, home health services are reimbursed retroactively, based on the lesser of the provider's costs or reasonable charges. There is no limit on the number of days the benefit may last, no prior hospitalization requirement, and no deductible to the patient. Meals on Wheels, nonmedical domestic care, drugs, and transportation are not covered.

The Medicare homebound requirement limits reimbursable services to persons unable to leave home without the assistance of medical devices or another person.[34] A retirement facility unit can be considered the person's home. However, if a resident of a retirement facility needs, for example, personal assistance to be bathed, groomed, and dressed, but then is able to

---

[32] See, e.g., Cal. S.B. 185, 1985 Stats. ch. 3.3.

[33] List compiled primarily from 42 C.F.R. §§ 405.1201, et seq. and Home Health Agency Survey Report, HCFA Form 1572.

[34] HIM-11 § 208.4.

leave the facility, the personal assistance may not be reimbursable as a Medicare home health service.

The intermittent requirement can also pose problems in the retirement facility context. In an unlicensed congregate living community, as the population ages in place, the facility can employ home health services to provide intermittent care. However, if the residents' need for care becomes ongoing, the facility could face the dual prospect of loss of Medicare reimbursement and the necessity for licensure as a personal care facility (see § 20.3(b)). While interpretations may vary locally, a rule of thumb is that home health services of up to three days per week for up to three weeks should be considered part time. Daily care for an indefinite period is beyond the limit of coverage.[35]

Home health is a growing segment of the continuum of care available to seniors in retirement facilities. There are now over 6000 Medicare-certified providers, generating an estimated $2.3 billion in Medicare expenditures for 1985, rising to $4 billion by 1990.[36] In response, the federal Health Care Financing Administration (HCFA) is reportedly considering a prospective payment system to replace the current retrospective payment of cost method. Prospective payment could take a form such as a fee schedule, diagnosis related groupings (DRGs), or a daily rate.

While home health was not specified in federal certificate of need laws (now repealed: see § 20.1, above), 27 states require new home health services to obtain a certificate of need review.[37] In addition, some 28 states have home health license laws. The Joint Commission on Accreditation of Hospitals (JCAH) is in the process of developing accreditation standards for home health agencies, which may be utilized by states as a uniform standard for licensure.

Home health can be utilized by retirement facilities as an interim measure for residents in need of short-term care. While it may forestall a move to continuous or long-term care for residents as they grow more dependent, home health cannot take the place of a plan for transition to ongoing licensed care for those who need it.

§ 20.5   REGULATION OF HEALTH MAINTENANCE ORGANIZATIONS

Health maintenance organizations, or prepaid health plans, are entities that provide health care services to enrollees who, for a fixed periodic membership fee, are entitled to receive various health care services, with no adjustment in fee based on the frequency, extent, or type of an individual's utilization of the

[35]See HIM-11 §§ 204.1 and 206.6 and Regan, J., *Tax, Estate and Financial Planning for The Elderly* (New York: Bender, 1985).

[36]*"Home Care Fact Sheet,"* National Association for Home Care, April 1986. However, Medicare denials for home care services have increased 133 percent from 1984 to 1986. *See* "Hospitals Travel Some Rough Ground in LTC," *Hospitals*, December 20, 1986, 70.

[37]*"How To Establish a Home Health Agency: Some Preliminary Considerations,"* National Association for Home Care, Jan. 1984.

services. The classic and familiar model of an HMO is the Kaiser health plan. Various forms of HMOs have evolved over the years (see § 27.2(c)(2), regarding "SHMOs"), but a basic trait is that they combine the risk pooling and set premium characteristics of insurance with the control over service delivery enjoyed by a health care provider.

HMOs should be distinguished from conventional insurance carriers in that insurers generally do not control the delivery of health services, but simply indemnify the insured for health care expenses in the marketplace. Recently, however, many insurers are offering favored benefits, such as waiver of deductibles, when insureds use the services of preferred providers of health care, with whom the carrier contracts to provide cost-efficient or discount services. The theoretical distinctions between HMOs and insurance companies fade as insurance carriers obtain more control contractually over the delivery of health care services.

Legally, HMOs are defined by the federal Health Maintenance Organization Act of 1973,[38] which established federal financial assistance for HMOs in the form of grants and loans. Importantly, the Act also exempted federally assisted programs from any state laws that required, among other things, that HMOs conform to minimum capitalization and reserve requirements for insurance companies, or that prohibited solicitation of members through advertising.[39] Instead, the federal Act established many of its own criteria for HMOs, including that they provide a range of basic health services such as physician, hospital, diagnostic, home health, and preventive services.[40] In addition, the law requires eligible HMOs to enroll persons broadly representative of age, social, and income groups, not to expel or refuse to reenroll a member due to his or her health status or need for services, and to insure or make other arrangements for funding its health care contingent liabilities.[41] State laws governing HMOs that are not applying for federal assistance generally mimic basic federal requirements.

Retirement facilities may utilize HMOs as a means of providing health services to residents on a group basis at a predictable cost. However, existing HMOs are likely to be designed, or even legally required, to offer broad-based services to the community at large, including maternity and pediatric services, for which elderly members must pay. On the other hand, a broadly based membership pool may economically favor older enrollees, who tend to use health services more frequently than their younger counterparts. States may also permit specialized service plans that do not offer the full panoply of health services but concentrate in a single area such as dental or ophthalmological services. Service packages could be custom tailored for the elderly, and recently senior care health plans have begun to emerge.

[38] 42 U.S.C. §§ 300e *et seq.*
[39] 42 U.S.C. § 300e-10(a).
[40] 42 U.S.C. §§ 300e-1(1), 300e(b).
[41] 42 U.S.C. § 300e(c).

One further distinguishing feature of health plans is that they are based almost universally on an annualized financial model. That is, premiums and eligibility may often be determined on an annual rather than a lifetime actuarial basis. Elderly enrollees seeking a lifetime hedge against the costs of health care may find HMOs more susceptible than continuing care arrangements, or some of the newer noncancelable long-term care insurance products, to substantial increases in premiums or to cancelation.

§ 21 REGULATION OF CONTINUING CARE AGREEMENTS

§ 21.1 JURISDICTION

At least 22 states have some form of regulation covering continuing care or life care arrangements.[42] Generally speaking, the type of activity regulated is the promise to furnish health care or personal care for the life of a resident, or for an extended period of time, in exchange for a prepaid entrance fee, a fixed periodic fee, or both. Some states may look to whether the promise for care is actually for life, and others to whether it is for more than a year, or for more than a month. Some cover all entrance fee arrangements, regardless of duration. (See Table 21.1 for a comparison of statutes.) Usually, fee-for-service arrangements are not subject to this form of regulation, unless there is a promise or implication that fee-for-service care will be available, on a priority basis not extended to the general public, in the future or for an extended period of time beyond a year.

With the many different varieties of arrangements recently being introduced in the marketplace, jurisdictional definitions are taking on added importance. Whereas traditional continuing care facilities usually involved a single organization that furnished housing, comprehensive health care, and services in a single facility for an entrance fee and a regular monthly fee, many providers are now experimenting with different organizational structures, service packages, and fee mechanisms, all of which pose a challenge to regulatory agencies.

Among the issues to be considered by government is whether regulations should cover only transactions where there is some entrance fee or other

---

[42]Eighteen state laws are reviewed in Table 21.1. In addition, Arkansas, Louisiana, North Carolina, and Texas all passed CCRC legislation shortly before this book was published. In addition, several states regulate limited portions of life care arrangements. Oregon requires a refund of entry fees for six months on withdrawal from a facility (Or. Rev. Stat. § 91.690 (1984)). New York's nursing home regulations currently prevent the offering of life care contracts by prohibiting any provider from contracting for prepaid life care for longer than three months (N.Y. Comp. Codes R. & Regs. tit. 10 §§ 415.1(f), 730.2(f), 730.3(b), 414.16(b) (1987)).

States that are in various stages of movement toward some form of regulation include Iowa, Massachusetts, Nebraska, New York, Ohio, Oklahoma, Oregon, and Washington. *See, generally,* "Current Status of State Regulation of Continuing Care Retirement Communities," American Association of Homes for the Aging (Jan. 1987).

prepayment in return for a promise of future health care, or whether a statute or regulation should also cover the promise merely that fee-for-service care will be available on a priority basis in the future. Another concern is whether the regulatory mechanism can be avoided by having entrance fees allocated to housing, rather than health care. Some argue that if a large entrance fee or purchase price is paid in addition to a monthly fee for housing, but there are nursing facilities on the premises, the consumer will expect health care to be available on some priority basis or at a reduced rate irrespective of the express terms of the contract, and that licensure is therefore appropriate.

In legislation effective January 1, 1987, California addressed some of these concerns in its adoption of S.B. 1620.[43] The legislation was needed in large part to address gaps in the already comprehensive statute to account for new facility formats and structures that looked like continuing care, but did not mesh with the statute that had been designed around traditional facility models. The new statutory mechanism is designed to cover, in addition to express promises of care for life or more than one year, those transactions, or series of transactions, in which residents prepay a sum greater than the value of one year's services.

The statute also makes clear that not only promises of the licensee to provide care, but promises to make care available (for example, via another entity), are regulated. Transactions are subject to licensure whether or not there is an entrance fee. Licensable providers may include homeowner's associations and similar types of cooperative formats.

Similarly, the American Association of Homes for the Aging (AAHA) has adopted stricter guidelines for state continuing care regulations in apparent recognition of the many new forays into the field.[44] These recommendations are reflected in Table 21.1 and the following text. As diversity continues, one can expect more states to enact new laws or adjust or reinterpret old ones to meet the changing marketplace.[45]

§ 21.2   APPLICATION SUBMISSIONS

Virtually all state statutes require some form of disclosure as part of a license application or registration procedure. Usually, this involves at a minimum basic information about the business entity and owners, and submission of audited financial statements. In states that more thoroughly regulate

---

[43]Stats. 1986 c. 1093, amending Cal. Health and Safety Code §§ 1770 *et seq.* (West 1979 & Supp. 1987).

[44]*See* American Association of Homes for the Aging, "Guidelines for Regulation of Continuing Care Retirement Communities" (May 1987).

[45]*See, e.g.,* Fox & Ritchie, "Watch Your Language: Regulators Scrutinize Resident Contracts and Advertising Materials," *Retirement Housing Report,* (Oct. 1986), 8, regarding expansive interpretation of activities subject to life care licensure in Pennsylvania. *See also Moravian Manors, Inc. v. Commonwealth of Pennsylvania,* 521 A.2d 524 (1987).

these facilities, projected budgets, feasibility studies, marketing projections, forms of resident agreements, and advertising copy also may have to be submitted. States may require license applicants to adhere strictly to their own projections of marketing progress, construction schedules, and income and expenditures, and may tie conformance to projections to the ability to release escrowed funds, admit residents, or obtain final state approval. Regulations may also require that evidence of application for appropriate facility licenses (e.g., skilled nursing and personal care) accompany the continuing care license application.

Although state regulation limited to a process of registration and disclosure was recommended by AAHA in its Model Act published in 1980, the Association has more recently recommended in guidelines for state regulation of continuing care retirement communities a more extensive form of regulation, including filing of audited financial statements, pro forma budgets with actuarial analysis, a market review and marketing schedule, and state approval prior to the taking of deposits.[46]

§ 21.3 ESCROWS OF RESIDENT DEPOSITS

Resident deposits on entrance fees prior to completion of project construction have traditionally served at least two purposes: (1) They are an indication of the prospective buyer's interest in the development and are used to secure a place on the waiting list, or to reserve a particular unit, pending completion of development, and (2) the funds are often used to help retire construction debt or to actually fund some of the construction or start up operational costs of the facility. Often, developers require progress payments on entrance fees as construction proceeds, with the final increment due upon move-in. State license procedures may track a two-step process in which a provisional license or permit is required to collect deposits, and a final certificate of authority is required before residents are permitted to move in or to sign long-term care agreements.

Many influential people in the continuing care facilities field believe that some of the more restrictive provisions contained in state law reflect sound business practices necessary to the successful development of any continuing care facility. Accordingly, to help prevent facility failures, and to protect the consumer and the reputation of such facilities, business practices such as escrow of entrance fee deposits, and minimum levels of presales (see next section) have been adopted as law with the concurrence and assistance of facility owners and operators.

When continuing care facility developers collect preconstruction deposits from prospective residents, most states with license statutes require that such deposits be placed in approved escrow accounts. Various conditions are then placed upon the release of the deposits out of escrow for use

[46]AAHA Guidelines at 25–27.

by the developer to pay down construction debt or for other expenses of development or operations. Some states may allow the developer to post a surety bond or letter of credit in lieu of escrowed deposits.

In Florida, for example, at least 75 percent of entrance fee deposits must remain in escrow until payment in full has been received for no less than 70 percent of the total units, and a certificate of occupancy has been received.[47] California, on the other hand, permits monies to be released from escrow when the developer has received a deposit of at least 20 percent of the total entrance fee from at least 50 percent of the total units planned to be constructed, with 50 percent of facility construction completed.[48] As an alternative, the developer may collect as little as 10 percent of the entrance fees for 75 percent of the units, but must wait until completion of construction before releasing escrowed funds.[49]

It is generally acknowledged that linking release of escrow monies to presales and construction progress is prudent because they are a measure of the eventual success of the project. In addition, progress in the construction of the facility may give prospective residents a tangible asset that can be tapped in the event of a marketing failure, and construction has a tendency to encourage further sales. In addition to presales and construction progress, some states may require financing commitments or funding for the full cost of construction before escrowed funds can be released.

Occasionally, despite having made initial deposits toward entrance fees early in the development process, some prospective residents may later decide against making additional deposits and moving into the facility. Most states require that entrance fee deposits be refundable, although some, such as Florida,[50] may permit the developer to charge a penalty for the prospective resident's withdrawal. Other states may permit the developer to withhold refunds from escrow until the particular unit is resold. Even after occupancy is commenced, most state laws require an initial trial period during which a resident may withdraw from the facility, with or without cause, and receive a refund of entrance fees on a pro rata basis, or less the actual cost of services actually delivered (see §§ 21.6(b) and 21.6(c)).

Provisions for refund of escrowed deposits should permit some penalty, such as withholding of interest or refund deferral, until the unit is resold, so that prospective residents are motivated not to make deposits at several projects with the intention of dropping out of all but one. Most project failures occur during development due to lack of enrollment, and presales should be firm so that developers and applicants for residence may proceed with confidence.

[47]Fla. Stat. Ann. § 651.023(2) (West 1984 & Supp. 1986).
[48]Cal. Health & Safety Code § 1773.6.
[49]Id.
[50]Fla. Stat. Ann. § 651.055(g) (West Supp. 1986).

AAHA's guidelines recommend escrow of resident deposits, with release only upon receipt of at least 10 percent of the entrance fee for 50 percent of the units, arrangement for 100 percent of construction financing, and when construction costs have been fixed by contract. AAHA also recommends that a penalty be assessed against prospective residents who withdraw.[51]

§ 21.4   PRESALES IN GENERAL

Because one of the most vulnerable periods for any retirement facility, and especially continuing care facilities, is in the initial marketing, many states have extensive regulation of this process to help protect consumers' monies and to help assure that facilities will be financially sound.

Presales requirements are often used as a condition of release of escrowed entrance fees (see § 21.3). Some observers feel that presales are so important to the success of a new continuing care facility that substantial presales are necessary prior to commencement of any construction, or even before obtaining any commitment of financing for the project development. For example, in Florida, 10 percent of the fee for 50 percent of the units must be collected to apply for a certificate of authority.[52] Similarly, when resident deposits are to be used for construction in California, construction may not commence until 60 percent of the units projected to be occupied upon the facility's opening are reserved with a 20 percent deposit on the entrance fee.[53]

Although many facilities traditionally have been constructed using the proceeds of presales deposits, states will be facing with increasing frequency circumstances where continuing care facilities are financed by other means. It will become more common, for example, for such facilities to be financed from the holdings of a major corporate developer. In addition, conversions of filled condominium projects or other existing structures into continuing care facilities will become more commonplace. In these situations, resident presales deposits will not serve construction financing purposes so much as they will be intended as an indication of the seriousness of a prospective buyer's interest in the project. While it makes sense to preserve resident funds in escrow if deposits are collected prior to admission, it may not be necessary to mandate that a developer collect resident deposits prior to construction or opening when the developer is risking only its own funds on the venture.

Presales requirements may also be a condition for obtaining final state approval for the project, or for executing contracts with residents. Pennsylvania

---

[51]AAHA Guidelines at 56.
[52]Fla. Stat. Ann. § 651.023(c).
[53]Cal. Health & Safety Code § 1773.7.

law requires a minimum 35 percent payment for at least 50 percent of the units to obtain a certificate of authority.[54] California requires full payment for 80 percent of the units, or lesser amounts with a business plan or collateral satisfactory to the state, in order to obtain a final certificate, although a provisional certificate is available sooner to permit a gradual move-in of residents.[55] The apparent concern underlying such statutes is that facilities that do not reach certain optimum levels of occupancy that are sufficient to sustain operations may fail or convert to another use. The state may be able to extend escrows, impose resident liens, or possibly even take over management in an effort to preserve resident deposits or facility assets for resident refunds or claims.

§ 21.5   RESERVES

The unique characteristic of most continuing care facilities is that they offer future health care or personal care in exchange for some form of prepayment or predictable periodic payment. To the extent that such facilities act as self-insurers of the health care risks and needs of their resident populations, it is prudent for facilities to set aside reserves, usually out of entrance fees, for such future contingencies. Many states have mandated reserve requirements by law.

Most statutes relate reserve requirements directly to such expenditures as debt service. For example, Missouri requires that the reserve amount never fall below 150 percent of the annual principal and interest payments of the provider on long-term debt.[56] Similarly, Minnesota requires that at least an amount equal to the total of all principal and interest payments due for the upcoming year on any first mortgage be reserved.[57] Florida requires a reserve equal to one-half the principal and interest payments due during the upcoming year plus taxes, insurance, and any leasehold payments.[58]

Another approach is to base reserves on the facility's operating costs. Florida, for example, requires a reserve of 30 percent of annual operating costs in addition to debt service.[59] California requires that facility operators set aside reserves sufficient to cover all life care contract obligations.[60] In practice, however, to the extent a facility operator can show that future

[54]Pa. Cons. Stat. Ann. § 3212(2)(c) (Purdon 1986).
[55]Cal. Health & Safety Code § 1780.5.
[56]Mo. Ann. Stat. § 376.945 (Vernon. Supp. 1987).
[57]Minn. Stat. Ann. § 80D.06 (West 1986); *see also* Ariz. Rev. Stat. Ann. § 20-1806 (1985).
[58]Fla. Stat. Ann. § 651.035.
[59]Fla. Stat. Ann. § 651.035(2)(a).
[60]Cal. Health & Safety Code § 1775.

health care needs will be paid out of monthly fees, or out of fee-for-service payments, reserves need not be set aside. Colorado and Missouri require that specified percentages of resident entrance fees be set aside as reserves.[61]

One state court has ruled that a life care contract implied that the provider could not use fees paid by members of one facility to fund other operations, but that fees must be based on services rendered to the residents.[62]

Reserve requirements in state statutes should take into account the extent to which different structures may lessen the risk inherent in a pure self-insurance type of format. For example, one facility may provide all needed health care, including hospitalizations, in return for the entrance fee, and at no charge in addition to the regular monthly fee required for residents. Another facility may offer only a limited number of days of nursing care per year for the regular monthly fee, and may charge an additional per-use fee for all services beyond that threshold. A third facility may guarantee access to nursing care as a benefit of residence, but charge on a fee-for-service basis for all care, and provide residents with group health insurance, purchased from a third party, as part of the regular monthly fee. These three examples all have different degrees of risk, and whereas significant reserves may be appropriate in the first case, no reserves may be necessary in the third case, where the facility has not assumed the risk respecting future health care costs.

California has also recognized that refundable entrance fees represent a distinct additional future liability for which reserves may have to be set aside.[63] Although entrance fee refunds for residents leaving the facility normally could be payable from new entrance fees received from resale of the unit being vacated, the California statute assumes that the limited useful life of retirement facility building will prevent the provider from selling contracts after 40 years and that, at that time, the facility operator will be required to comply with refund obligations. Therefore, the reserve mechanism is designed to yield a fund sufficient to refund all entrance fees at the end of 40 years. Arguably, a reserve for plant replacement would also solve this problem, but in most cases, total facility replacement costs are likely to equal or exceed entrance fee refund obligations. This statutory reserve for refundable entrance fees is valid only for two years while state government and industry representatives determine whether such a fund, or a variation of it, is effective or needed on a permanent basis.

AAHA's guidelines state that reserves should include, in addition to the debt service reserve, two to six months of normal operating expenses,

[61]Colo. Rev. Stat. § 12-13-110(1)(1978); Mo. Ann. Stat. § 376.945.

[62]*Onderdonk v. Presbyterian Homes of NJ*, 85 N.J. 171, 425 A.2d 1057 (1981).

[63]Cal. Health & Safety Code § 1775.5.

major equipment refurbishment or replacement costs, health reserves where future costs are to be prepaid or substantially discounted.[64]

§ 21.6   CONTRACT REQUIREMENTS AND DISCLOSURES

Many states define the parameters of certain provisions that must appear in the contract between the resident and the facility operator. These are designed primarily to require certain minimum disclosures by the provider and to protect the resident from loss of substantial funds in the event the transaction was ill-considered or entered into hastily. Virtually all states regulating continuing care require that contract forms be submitted to the state agency for review. Many states also have enacted laws prescribing in detail required contract provisions or subjects that must be addressed in every agreement.

(a)   Financial Statements

Most states with continuing care regulation either require that the provider furnish financial statements directly to prospective residents prior to contract execution, or allow public inspection of financial statements and other provider information filed with the state. Those requiring that copies be furnished include Arizona, California, Florida, Illinois, Indiana, Maryland, Minnesota, Missouri, and Pennsylvania. Florida, Indiana, Michigan, and Wisconsin permit public inspection.

Some states, such as Minnesota, Missouri, and Virginia, require that financial statements be updated annually and furnished to residents.

One state supreme court has found that life care contracts by their nature impose on the provider an obligation to furnish residents with meaningful financial information sufficient for them to determine if fee increases are reasonable.[65]

(b)   Contract Termination

Many states have specific provisions dealing with termination of the contract by the resident, by the facility, or by reason of death of the resident. These statutes often further provide for certain specified refunds of any entrance fees, and possibly of monthly fees paid to the facility operator.

Several states require that care agreements be terminable at will (with or without cause) during a specified number of days of initial residence, with a full refund to the resident of entrance fees and possibly monthly fees, except that the operator may be able to retain a pro rata portion of the fees, or the actual cost of care for the period. These cooling off, or

---

[64] AAHA Guidelines at 59–60.

[65] See note 62, above.

probationary, periods are intended to give the resident, and in some cases the facility, the opportunity to rescind the transaction in the event that it appears to either party that it was a serious mistake for the individual to take up residence at the facility. Rescission periods mandated by statute may range from seven to 90 days.

Some states require that, once the probationary or cooling off period has expired, the provider may dismiss the resident, after notice, only upon a showing of good cause (e.g., California, Florida, Maryland).[66] Others state only that the termination provisions must be set forth in the contract (e.g., Colorado, Missouri).[67]

(c) Refunds

Refunds present special problems and issues depending upon when they occur. As discussed in the previous section, some states require refund of all entrance fees, less perhaps some retention for the cost of care in the event of a termination during an initial probationary period. A few states also regulate in detail the amount of refunds and the manner in which they are given in the event of a termination by the facility after such a probationary period. For example, in the event of the dismissal of a resident for cause by a provider in California, the provider must refund all entrance fees except for the cost of care.[68] On the other hand, if the resident decides to leave after the initial probationary period, the provider is free to enforce whatever refund provisions are set forth by contract.

One of the most difficult refund situations encountered by continuing care facilities and residents has been that of entrance fee refunds upon the death of the resident early in the life of the continuing care agreement. Traditional continuing care agreements have been based upon a pure self-insurance model, which relies upon an actuarial assumption that each person of a given age has a predictable life expectancy. The economic viability of the facility and the entrance fee structure are based on the assumption that for every person who dies sooner than expected, there will be another facility resident who outlives her or his life expectancy. Therefore, when a resident dies shortly after moving into a facility, it is important, in theory at least, to retain that person's entire entrance fee in order to pay the expenses for that other person who is likely to greatly outlive the actuarial average.

While this basic philosophy of insurance has traditionally been accepted by many courts,[69] there has been growing reluctance to permit a continuing care community to retain an entire accommodation fee of a person who has died shortly after moving into the facility, when that entrance fee may be

---

[66]Cal. Health & Safety Code § 1779(d), 1779.6; Fla. Stat. Ann. § 651.061; Md. Ann. Code art. 70B, § 14(c) (1986).

[67]Colo. Rev. Stat. § 12-13-106(b); Mo. Ann. Stat. § 376.920(13).

[68]Cal. Health & Safety Code § 1779.8.

[69]*See, generally,* 44 ALR 3d 1174.

several times the value of services actually received by the resident. These cases give essentially no value to the provider's promise to care for the resident for life and the risk, inherent in each transaction, that the resident may live far beyond anyone's expectations. Instead, once the resident has died and disgruntled heirs, who were not a party to the transaction, surface with charges that the retirement facility took advantage of the elderly decedent, courts are increasingly finding retention of accommodation fees after an early death to constitute forfeitures, which the law abhors. Courts may also find such provisions to be unconscionable, or may look for some ambiguity in the contract in an effort to find a way to interpret the agreement against the retirement facility draftor.[70] Although the issue arises relatively infrequently, due in part to the health screenings of applicants performed by most facilities, it has received a good deal of critical attention from courts and other observers.[71]

Florida, Maryland, Michigan, Minnesota, Pennsylvania, and Wisconsin have responded by requiring that when a resident dies after signing the care agreement but before taking occupancy, the facility must refund the entire entrance fee.[72] However, legislatures generally have not dealt with the concerns about the absence of refunds in the event of death after a short period of residence. Facilities offering fees that are refundable no matter when the resident dies or leaves the facility are one solution to the issue, but there are tradeoffs, such as the necessity of charging higher entrance fees, and securing the ability to pay the refunds when due. AAHA recommends in its guidelines that states establish minimum refund criteria, but allow a broad variety of provisions, provided they are clearly spelled out in the contract.[73]

§ 21.7   ADVERTISING

All states probably have some form of statute generally prohibiting false or misleading advertising. Many states, however, have specific provisions relating to the advertising of continuing care retirement facilities. In some cases, these may require prior review and approval of advertising materials by the state. Many states also specifically deal with the issue of the liability of facility sponsors.

One of the most publicized failures of a continuing care community was that of Pacific Homes, Inc., a nonprofit organization that had several facilities in California, Arizona, and Hawaii and that filed in bankruptcy court

---

[70]See Howe v. American Baptist Homes of the West, 112 Cal. App. 3d 622, 169 Cal. Rptr. 418 (1980).

[71]See, generally, 44 ALR 3d 1174, and Schact, "Protection for the Elderly Person and His Estate: Regulating and Enforcing Life-Care Contracts," 5 Prob. L. J. 105 (1983).

[72]Fla. Ann. Stat. § 651.055(5); Md. Ann. Code art. 70B, § 14(b); Mich. Comp. Laws. Ann. § 554.810(1)(a) (1986); Minn. Stat. Ann. 80D.04(3)(b); Pa. Cons. Stat. Ann. § 3214(c); Wis. Stat. Ann. § 647.05(6)&(7) (West Supp. 1986).

[73]AAHA Guidelines at 47–48.

for a Chapter XI reorganization in 1977. One of the principal issues in the ensuing class action lawsuit for damages was whether the United Methodist Church was in fact an alter ego of Pacific Homes and had any financial responsibility for performance of the contracts.[74] Pacific Homes, Inc. was originally established by members of what came to be known as the Pacific and Southwest Conference of the Methodist Church, and advertising materials referred to Pacific Homes' affiliation with the organization, but the Conference denied any legal liability for resident agreements. The United Methodist Church argued that it was not a suable entity, because it is not a hierarchical church but a confederation of regional conferences and national or global entities, all separately incorporated. The Supreme Court refused to prevent prosecution of the case against the Church entities and eventually Church sources contributed $21 million to settle the case. (See § 5.1 for further discussion of this case.)

As a result of the Pacific Homes situation, California enacted a statute in 1978 prohibiting any developer of a facility from mentioning the name of any other organization or person in its contracts or advertising materials unless that other person or organization had first filed a written statement of financial responsibility for continuing care agreements with the state.[75] An exemption was made for church sponsored facilities already in existence, but these are required to state expressly in their agreements the precise scope and extent of financial responsibility of any sponsor or other organization referred to in advertising or contract materials. Colorado, Florida, Indiana, and Missouri have adopted similar requirements.[76] It is wise to avoid references to entities other than the contracting parties without setting forth the extent of their responsibility for contract obligations.

In general, developers of facilities should review advertising materials carefully to make sure that representations comport with the service program that is actually going to be provided under the terms of the resident agreement. Abbreviated descriptions of contract features appearing in brochures can be characterized as misleading or viewed to modify contract language. In addition, developers should be careful not to use phrases or terminology in advertising materials that imply a certain kind of service that is not in the contract, or licensure that the provider does not intend to obtain. For example, developers occasionally use words such as "continuing care" or "care for life" in advertising materials when they have no intention of providing a program that would meet definitions and requirements of the particular state's continuing care or life care regulations. While the developer's use of such jargon may not intentionally be misleading, the state, a dissatisfied

---

[74]See *United Methodist Council v. Superior Court*, 439 U.S. 1369, 99 S. Ct. 36, 58 L. Ed. 2d 77 (1978).

[75]Cal. Health & Safety Code §§ 1789, 1789.2.

[76]Colo. Rev. Stat. § 12-13-113; Fla. Stat. Ann. § 651.095(3); Ind. Code Ann. § 23-2-4-4(8) (West Supp. 1986); Mo. Ann. Stat. § 376.920(8).

resident, or the operator of a competing facility may find that the use of such terms in advertising materials is misleading and bring an action to enjoin the advertising, change the program to comply with license standards, or seek damages.

AAHA's recommendation is that state legislation require licensees to explain their legal relationship with other organizations mentioned in advertising, but suggests that advertising should not be subject to prior state review.[77]

§ 21.8 RESIDENT RIGHTS

Some states require that residents be given certain rights of organization or participation in facility management. These provisions may be contained in statute or regulation.

Several states give residents the right to form a residents' association. Florida, Pennsylvania, and Virginia further require that management meet quarterly with the organized residents.[78] Michigan and Missouri, on the other hand, require that one resident be a member of the board of directors of the retirement facility.[79] In Michigan, it is specified that that member has an advisory status only.[80]

There is some objection in the industry to placing residents on boards of directors, and with good reason. As directors, residents inherently face a continuous problem of conflict of interest and self-dealing that most state corporations laws recognize as a handicapping, if not prohibited, status for any corporate director. Residents certainly should be able to organize and refer suggestions and grievances to facility management. This may include attendance at board meetings as invited guests. However, voting membership on the board of directors may hamper the effective functioning of the board when dealing with matters of resident policy or the application of policies to individuals in the community. AAHA's guidelines agree that while residents should have the right to organize and to meet with the facility management, it may be inappropriate to require that residents be appointed to the governing board or have formal representation at owners' meetings.[81]

§ 21.9 PROTECTIVE FINANCIAL PROVISIONS

Some states have provisions dealing with the circumstances of a possible facility bankruptcy or other failure. An example is the type of provision that

[77] AAHA Guidelines at 70.
[78] Fla. Stat. Ann. § 651.081, .085; Pa. Cons. Stat. Ann. § 3215(b); Va. Code § 38.1-965.
[79] Mich. Comp. Laws Ann. § 554.812; Mo. Ann. Stat. § 376.950.
[80] Mich. Comp. Laws Ann. § 554.812.
[81] AAHA Guidelines at 71–72.

specifies that the rights of residents under continuing care agreements constitute liens or preferred claims against the assets of the failed community. A preferred claim gives residents priority over general creditors, but is usually subordinate to any creditor with a lien, such as a mortgage lender. Some states, such as Arizona, Colorado, and Minnesota, give the residents an automatic statutory lien against facility assets.[84] In other states, such as Pennsylvania and California, such liens are imposed only in the event that the state determines that a particular facility's financial condition warrants it.[85] In all states but Minnesota, such statutory liens may be subordinated to other prior liens, such as those of construction lenders.[86] California even has a provision that permits the state to take over management of a facility that, in its opinion, appears to be on the verge of financial collapse.[87]

As a practical matter, liens are of questionable use in protecting residents from retirement facility failures. Many failures occur during facility development, due to poor financial management or overly optimistic assumptions about the ability to sell the product. In these situations, there may not be assets of sufficient significance to insure that residents do not lose their entrance fees or some portion of them. In fact, in many such facility failures, it has been the assets of a sponsoring organization, a lender, or the residents themselves that have made it possible for facilities to rebound and return to a financially sound status.

Even if there are facility assets of any substance, they are likely to be contained predominantly in the physical plant of the facility itself. If resident entrance fees have been used to pay off construction loans, there may be equity in the building that can be reached by residents, but there is no guarantee that entrance fees will be used for such purposes, and residents may find themselves in a second position behind a secured lender. Moreover, buildings that have been designed specifically for use as life care communities are not readily salable for other purposes, and it may make little sense to attempt to liquidate such an asset in an effort to pay off construction lenders, residents, and other creditors in the event of a dissolution. It makes more sense for all concerned, and is more common, for a retirement community with any substantial assets to be reorganized and operated as a going business under new management and possibly after renegotiation of care agreements.

§ 21.10 ACCREDITATION

The American Association of Homes for the Aging has established an independent commission to develop and implement a comprehensive accreditation program for use by nonprofit and for profit continuing care facilities.

---

[84]Ariz. Rev. Stat. Ann. § 20-1805; Colo. Rev. Stat. § 12-12-112(a); Minn. Stat. Ann. § 80D.08.

[85]Cal. Health & Safety Code §§ 1772, 1775; 40 Pa. Cons. Stat. Ann. § 3211.

[86]Minn. Stat. Ann. § 80D.08, as amended by Laws 1981, c. 135, § 80D.08.

[87]Cal. Health & Safety Code §§ 1790–1790.6.

The program, modeled in part after the Joint Commission on Accreditation of Hospitals program, includes an extensive self-evaluation process in the areas of governance and administration, finance, health care, and resident protections. The survey includes review by a visiting team and evaluation by an accreditation committee.

Eligibility for the process, which is estimated to take approximately eight months, is limited initially to common entrance fee models with an ongoing monthly service fee. Other financial structures will be included as the program develops. Applicants must have had one year of 90 percent occupancy and must have completed an audited fiscal year, or, if less than 90 percent occupancy, must demonstrate financial viability. Facilities are also reviewed for compliance with applicable state regulation.

Accredited facilities are required to file annual reports, including financial audits, and pay a fee to maintain their status. Facilities denied accreditation may appeal the denial to a committee of the commission. The accreditation process has been considered by at least one state licensing agency as a substitute for or supplement to certain state regulatory functions that might duplicate accreditation.

§ 21.11   JURISDICTIONAL OVERLAP WITH HMOS, INSURANCE CARRIERS

Where a retirement facility developer intends to provide some form of guaranteed access to health care, or coverage of health care costs, there may be problems of jurisdictional overlap, or gaps in coverage between two or more state agencies. Even in states where there is extensive regulation of continuing care facilities, a given product may raise questions as to whether the financial transaction with the resident constitutes a prepaid health plan, a continuing care arrangement, a contract of insurance, or all or none of the foregoing. State laws should be carefully reviewed by the developer's legal counsel to determine which state statutes may be applicable.

In states where there are multiple layers of regulation covering continuing care facilities, prepaid health plans, and insurance companies, it is sometimes a difficult task, both for the regulatory agencies and for the developer, to determine which agency, if any, has jurisdiction over the arrangement. This situation is complicated by the current variety of new approaches being explored by facility developers. Facility developers who have structured their programs to avoid a particular kind of licensure, such as continuing care, have sometimes found themselves subject to more burdensome regulation under a more general statute, such as the state's insurance code. Generally, licensure as an insurance carrier can be the most onerous form of regulation from the facility's perspective due to the stringent reserve requirements that are usually applicable.

Another problem encountered in forum shopping among multiple state authorities is that certain agencies are unfamiliar with and perplexed by

Table 21.1 Continuing Care Statute Provisions

Statute	AAHA Guidelines (May 1987)	Arizona Ariz. Rev. Stat. Ann. § 20-1801	California Cal. Health & Safety Code § 1770
1. Definition			
a. For life	—	—	—
b. 1 year	X	X	X
c. Entrance fee required	X	X	—
d. Priority admission	Optional	—	X
e. Health or health related services	X	X	X
f. Personal care	X	—	X
2. Application			
a. Disclosure statement	X	X	X
b. Financials	X	X	X
c. Financial feasibility study	X	X	—
d. Actuarial study	X	X	—
e. Market study	X	—	—
f. Accreditation in lieu of regulation	X	—	—
3. Escrow of Fees			
a. Required	X	X	X
b. Basis for release	Presales, financing, construction price	Varies	Presales, construction
c. Construction	Fixed price	Completed	Percentages vary
d. Financing	Commitment	Commitment	—
4. Presales			
a. To close escrow	At least 10 from 50%	—	20% from 50% or 10% from 75%
b. For final certification	Yes	—	100% from 80%; alternatives
c. To begin development	—	—	20% from 60% of initial occupants to start construction; alternatives
5. Reserves			
a. P & I	1 year	1 year	1 year
b. Percent of deposits	—	—	—
c. Operating costs	2–6 months, plant replacement, health liabilities	—	All unfunded contract liabilities
d. For refunds	—	—	Present value of all refunds in 40 years
6. Bonds			
Surety	—	—	If necessary
7. Disclosure to Residents			
a. Financial report	X	Before signing	Before signing
b. Public inspection of filings	—	—	—
8. Contract Terms			
a. Submit form	X	X	X
b. Detailed contents	X	X	X
c. Probation period	X	7 days	90 days
d. Refunds in general	X	—	X
e. Required amortization of refund	—	—	All but cost
f. Full refund if resident dies before occupancy	Option	—	—
9. Advertising			
a. Prior approval	No	—	Filing only
b. Sponsor liability	X	—	X
10. Residents' Right to Organize			
a. Association	X	X	X
b. Meetings with management	Annual	—	—
11. Liens			
a. For residents	—	X	If necessary
b. Subordinated to priors	—	X	X
12. Agency	One with financial review capability	Insurance	Social services

Colorado	Connecticut	Florida	Illinois Ill. Ann. Stat.	Indiana	Kansas
Colo. Rev. Stat. § 12-13-101	1986 Conn. Acts 252	Fla. Stat. Ann. § 651.011	Ch. 111-1/2, § 4160-1	Ind. Code Ann. § 24-2-4-1	Kan. Stat. Ann. § 16-1101
X	—	Any duration	—	—	—
—	X	Any duration	X	1 month	X
—	X	X	X	X	—
—	—	—	—	—	—
X	X	X	X	X	X
—	—	X	X	—	X
X	X	X	—	X	X
X	X	X	—	X	X
—	—	X	—	—	—
—	—	—	—	—	—
—	—	X	—	—	—
—	—	—	—	—	—
X	X	X	X	Or letter of credit	—
Financing, construction	Formula	Final certif., construction, presales	Presales, construction, financing	Formula	—
Completed	—	Completed	Schedule	—	—
Commitment	—	Commitment	Commitment	—	—
—	75% reserved	100% from 70%	50% reserved	—	—
—	—	100% from 70%	—	—	—
—	5% from 50% to begin construction	10% from 50% to apply for license	—	—	—
—	1 year	1 year	6 months	—	—
65%	—	—	—	—	—
—	1 month	30% of annual	—	—	—
—	—	—	—	—	—
—	—	—	—	—	—
On request	Before signing	Posting and before signing	Before signing	Before signing	Annually on request
—	—	X	—	X	—
X	—	X	X	X	—
X	X	X	—	—	—
60 days	30 days	7 days	14 days	—	—
X	—	X	—	—	—
X	—	Pro rata basis	—	—	—
—	Less costs	X	—	—	—
—	—	X	—	—	—
X	—	X	—	X	—
—	—	X	—	—	—
—	—	Quarterly	—	—	—
X	—	Preferred claim	—	—	—
X	—	X	—	—	—
Insurance	Aging	Insurance	Public health	Securities	Insurance

Table 21.1   Continuing Care Statute Provisions (Continued)

Statute	Maryland Md. Ann. Code art. 70B, § 7	Massachusetts Mass. Gen. Laws Ann. ch. 93 § 76	Michigan Mich. Comp. Laws Ann. § 544.801	Minnesota Minn. Stat. Ann. § 80D.01
1. *Definition*				
a. For life	—	—	—	—
b. 1 year	X	X	X	X
c. Entrance fee required	X	—	—	$100
d. Priority admission	X	—	—	—
e. Health or health related services	X	X	X	X
f. Personal care	X	—	X	—
2. *Application*				
a. Disclosure statement	X	X	X	—
b. Financials	X	—	X	X
c. Financial feasibility study	X	—	X	—
d. Actuarial study	—	—	—	—
e. Market study	—	—	—	—
f. Accreditation in lieu of regulation	—	—	—	—
3. *Escrow of Fees*				
a. Required	X	Disclosure to resident of voluntary reserve & escrows	Or surety bond	X
b. Basis for release	Construction, final certification	—	—	Formula
c. Construction	Complete	—	—	—
d. Financing	Complete	—	—	—
4. *Presales*				
a. To close escrow	10% from 65%	—	—	—
b. For final certification	10% from 65%	—	—	—
c. To begin development	—	—	—	—
5. *Reserves*				
a. P & I	—	—	—	1 year
b. Percent of deposits	—	—	—	—
c. Operating costs	—	—	—	—
d. For refunds	—	—	—	—
6. *Bonds*				
Surety	—	—	If necessary	—
7. *Disclosure to Residents*				
a. Financial report	Two weeks before signing	Before signing	—	Before signing and annual
b. Public inspection of filings	—	—	X	—
8. *Contract Terms*				
a. Submit form	X	—	—	X
b. Detailed contents	X	X	—	—
c. Probation period	30 days	—	—	—
d. Refunds in general	X	X	—	—
e. Required amortization of refund	—	X	—	—
f. Full refund if resident dies before occupancy	X	Less costs	X	X

	Missouri	New Jersey	New Mexico	Pennsylvania	Virginia	Wisconsin
	Mo. Ann. Stat. § 376.900	N.J. Stat. Ann. § 52-27D-33	N.M. Stat. Ann. § 24-17-1	40 Pa. Cons. Stat. Ann. § 3201	Va. Code § 38.1–955	Wis. Stat. Ann. § 647.01
	X	X	X	X	X	X
	—	X	X	X	—	$10,000 or 50% of estate
	—	—	—	—	—	—
	X	X	X	X	X	X
	—	—	X	—	—	X
	—	X	X	X	X	—
	X	X	X	X	X	X
	—	—	—	—	—	—
	—	—	—	—	—	—
	—	—	—	—	—	—
	—	X	—	X	—	—
	X	Letter of credit, securities, or bond	X	Letter of credit, securities, or bond	—	—
	Formula	—	Occupancy of unit by resident	—	—	—
	—	—	—	—	—	—
	—	—	—	Secured	—	—
	—	35% deposits equalling 50% of total fees	—	35% deposits equalling 50% of total fees	—	—
	—	—	—	—	—	—
	—	—	—	—	—	—
	1.5 × annual	Greater of 1 year P&I or 15% of operating expenses	—	Greater of 1 year P&I or 10% of operating expenses	—	—
	50%	—	—	—	—	—
	—	Greater of 1 year P&I or 15% of operating expenses	—	Greater of 1 year P&I or 10% of operatingexpenses	—	—
	5% of move-outs/year	—	—	—	—	—
	—	—	—	—	—	—
	Before signing and annual	Before signing	7 days before signing and annual	Before signing	Annual	On request
	—	—	—	—	—	X
	X	—	—	X	X	X
	—	X	X	—	—	X
	—	30 days	7 days	7 days	—	10 days
	—	—	—	—	—	—
	—	—	—	—	—	X
	—	Less costs	—	—	X	Less costs

305

Table 21.1   Continuing Care Statute Provisions (Continued)

Statute	Maryland Md. Ann. Code art. 70B, § 7	Massachusetts Mass. Gen. Laws Ann. ch. 93 § 76	Michigan Mich. Comp. Laws Ann. § 544.801	Minnesota Minn. Stat. Ann. § 80D.01
9. *Advertising*				
a. Prior approval	X	—	Filing only	—
b. Sponsor liability	—	—	—	—
10. *Residents' Right to Organize*				
a. Association	Permissive	—	X	—
b. Meetings with management	—	—	Board seat	—
11. *Liens*	.			
a. For residents	—	—	—	X
b. Subordinated to priors	—	—	—	No
12. *Agency*	Aging	—	Corporations and Securities	None, file with County recorder

Notes to Table 21.1

In General: This chart was derived principally from information compiled by AAHA. It summarizes statutory language and may not reflect regulatory or other interpretation. Rules are generally much more complex than chart indicates. "X" indicates there is a provision on point; "—" indicates there is no provision on point.

1. *Definition*

    a & b. Shows what duration of contract is required to be subject to licensure. If a statute covers contracts for life *or* greater than one year, chart shows only "1 year" checked.

    c. Statute applies only where there is some form of entrance fee.

    d. Priority admission to services, even if not prepaid, triggers licensure.

    e & f. Chart refers to the kind of activity that is considered to trigger licensure. Health related services and personal care may be similar activities in some states.

2. *Application*

    a. Disclosure to residents of various information about the provider and/or project plans.

    b. Financial statements or budgets required to be submitted to the state.

    c, d, e. These studies required to be submitted to the state may contain overlapping information depending on state definitions.

    f. Accreditation accepted in lieu of state review.

3. *Escrows*

    a. Some escrowing of entrance fees required, at least for initial facility sell-out.

    b. Factors considered in releasing money from escrow can be very complex and not susceptible to simple summary, but see below for more detail..

    c. Construction standard required for escrow release.

    d. Financing standard required for escrow release.

4. *Presales*

    a. Shows whether certain levels of presales are required to close escrows. First figure indicates percentage of total entrance fee that must be on deposit. Second figure is percentage of total units required to have the specified deposit.

    b. Presales required to obtain final certification.

    c. Presales required to begin development or license application.

5. *Reserves*

    a. Required reserve of principal and interest payments or other real property expenses for facility; required amount of reserve in months of payments.

    b. Reserve calculated as percentage of deposits received from residents.

    c. Reserves measured by costs of operation.

    d. Reserves measured by entrance fee refund obligation.

Missouri	New Jersey	New Mexico	Pennsylvania	Virginia	Wisconsin
Mo. Ann. Stat. § 376.900	N.J. Stat. Ann. § 52-27D-33	N.M. Stat. Ann. § 24-17-1	40 Pa. Cons. Stat. Ann. § 3201	Va. Code § 38.1–955	Wis. Stat. Ann. § 647.01
—	—	—	—	—	—
X	—	—	—	—	—
—	X	—	X	X	—
Board seat	Quarterly	—	Quarterly	Quarterly	—
—	If necessary	—	If necessary	—	—
—	—	—	X	—	—
Insurance	Community affairs	Aging	Insurance	Insurance	Insurance

6. *Bonds*

   Surety bond for contract obligations required when deemed necessary by state.

7. *Disclosure to Residents*

   a. When operator's financial report must be given to residents.

   b. License statute provides specifically for public inspection of licensee's filings with state; other states may permit this by reason of other general statutes.

8. *Contract Terms*

   a. Contract form must be submitted to state.

   b. Statute sets forth detailed requirements for the contents of contracts, for example, services offered, fees, cancelation, terminations for cause, consequences of death, and so on.

   c. Statute provides for period in which resident can rescind contract without penalty, usually measured after contract execution or commencement of occupancy.

   d. General statutory treatment of refunds to residents in the event of voluntary cancelation, termination for cause, or death, often with differing amounts due depending on circumstances.

   e. Statute sets forth a refund schedule based on resident length of stay.

   f. Full refund required if resident dies before taking occupancy, sometimes less actual cost of care.

9. *Advertising*

   a. Advertising must be submitted to state and approved, or filed only. Some states have express prohibitions against false advertising; these are not noted in the chart.

   b. State requires that if a sponsoring organization, or other organization in addition to the licensee, is mentioned in the contract or in advertising, the other organization must file a statement of financial responsibility for contract obligations.

10. *Resident Right to Organize*

    a. Provision for resident right to organize in an association.

    b. Statute sets forth minimum meet and confer requirements between management and residents or establishes resident seat on home's board of directors.

11. *Liens*

    a. A statutory lien is established against facility assets, giving priority over general creditors; may be in state's discretion.

    b. The statutory lien is recognized to be subordinate to prior recorded liens or to secured lenders (e.g., holders of mortgages).

12. *Agency*

    State agency in charge of continuing care licensure process.

the hybrid of insurance, annuity, residential, and health care concepts represented by a single facility's operational plan. Trying to fashion a continuing care facility, which may be heavily regulated, as a prepaid health plan, which may be subject to less regulation, can lead to costly delays, as bureaucrats unfamiliar with lifetime actuarial risks ponder the implications of a project that is strange to them. Sometimes, therefore, it may be economically and legally prudent to accept, rather than avoid, the jurisdiction of an agency that is best equipped to regulate the project. One of the motivations for real estate developers to seek a joint venture with an insurance company, prepaid health plan, or hospital or other health care provider, is that these partners are usually already familiar with many of the regulatory requirements, and may already be licensed to provide the kind of services, or coverage of services, that the developer intends to offer to facility residents.

States should clarify, either administratively or by amendment of their statutes, the jurisdictional parameters of insurance, continuing care, and health plan regulations.

In analyzing a given retirement facility structure, regulators should find the statutory structure that most closely fits the circumstances. Providers should not be subject to multiple regulation for a single transaction between resident and retirement facility. For example, if a retirement facility is offering to purchase group health insurance for its resident population through a carrier that is already licensed by the state's insurance department, and that retirement facility operator is not directly engaged in the provision of health care, and is not promising to provide the health care covered by the insurance carrier, the program should not be subject to licensure as a continuing care facility or health plan.

§ 22   HUD REGULATION

Despite the overall cutback in federal funding for elderly housing, there has been some recent acknowledgment by the federal government of the desirability of combining housing and services, including care, in a single retirement facility product (see §§ 22.1, 22.2).

In addition to the financial requirements imposed by the federal government as a condition of receiving loans or loan guarantees for construction of such retirement facilities (see § 14), the Department of Housing and Urban Development (HUD) imposes numerous conditions on eligibility that affect the structure and operations of the project. Some of the programs listed in Table 22.1 and discussed in the following sections are not available for new facility development, but they are described because they have been used by many facilities already in the marketplace.

Table 22.1 HUD Elderly Housing Finance Programs

Program	Statute	Regulations	HUD Handbook	Other
Mortgage Insurance				
Section 221(d)(4) ReSC new construction and substantial rehabilitation	12 U.S.C. § 1715(l)	24 C.F.R. § 251	4561.1; 4560.2	Notices H-85-33, 84-41, 83-58 (HUD)
Section 223(f) ReSC moderate rehabilitation and conversion of existing facilities	12 U.S.C. § 1715z-9	24 C.F.R. § 255	4565.1	HUD Fact Sheet
Section 232 Board and care homes	12 U.S.C. § 1715(w)	24 C.F.R. § 232	4600.1	Notice H86-20 (HUD); P.L. 98-181
Cooperatives				
Section 221(d)(3)	12 U.S.C. § 1715(l)	24 C.F.R. § 251	4560.1	
Section 213	12 U.S.C. § 1715(e)	24 C.F.R. § 213	4550.1	
Section 231 New construction or rehabilitation of elderly rental housing (inactive)	12 U.S.C. § 1715(v)	24 C.F.R. § 231	4570.1	
Section 236 Interest reduction payments (inactive)	12 U.S.C. § 1715z-1	24 C.F.R. § 236	N/A	
Subsidy Programs				
Section 202 Direct loans	12 U.S.C. § 1701(q)	24 C.F.R. § 885	4571.1 REV-2	Annual HUD Appropriations legislation
Section 8 Housing assistance payments	42 U.S.C. § 1437(f)	24 C.F.R. § 880	7420.1 REV-1	
Congregate housing services program	42 U.S.C.§§ 8001–8010	N/A	N/A	HUD Fact Sheet; P.L. 95-537; HUD Appropriations

§ 22.1   RETIREMENT SERVICE CENTERS

(a)   Section 221(d)(4)

(1)   Generally

The U.S. Department of Housing and Urban Development has in recent years developed regulations to provide for a new housing insurance program within the current Section 221(d)(4) program to cover the gap between the totally independent living arrangements of noncongregate housing for the elderly and the health care-oriented nursing home. The Section 221(d)(4) program is designed to assist in financing the construction or substantial rehabilitation of rental housing for low and moderate income families.[86] Under this program, HUD and the FHA insure mortgages made by approved lenders, which is intended to increase the mortgage credit available from private lenders.[87] The Retirement Service Center (ReSC) program builds on the existing Section 221(d)(4) mortgage insurance to provide meals, services, and an amenities package that exceeds that normally submitted under this program.[88]

ReSC facilities are developed for the frail elderly of 70 years and up who no longer desire to prepare their own meals and are willing to pay a substantial part of their income—in excess of 30 percent—for shelter, amenities, and services. There are four major differences between ReSCs and basic Section 221(d)(4) elderly housing projects:

1. Prospective mortgagors must prove experience and ability to manage retirement housing.
2. ReSCs involve modified market and rental analysis techniques.
3. ReSCs can provide a broader range of amenities and services.
4. ReSCs require special reserve funds.

HUD has indicated that ReSC project applicants must be familiar with this type of retirement housing and the special needs and expectations of the target occupancy group. HUD is also concerned that the mortgagor group be able to effectively promote rentals and handle the long rent up periods and complex services and expenses of retirement housing.[89] All mortgagors eligible under the Section 221(d)(4) program, which include both for profit and nonprofit developers, may develop ReSCs. All mortgagors must meet the requirements of and be processed under both the Section 221(d)(4) and the special ReSC procedures.

[86]For a full discussion of the financing aspects of the Section 221 program, *see* text at § 14.1(d), above.

[87]*See, generally*, 24 C.F.R. § 251; HUD Handbook 4560.1.

[88]*See* HUD Handbook 4561.1, ch. 17; Notices H85-33, 84-41, 83-58 (HUD); and May 15, 1984 HUD Memorandum of Assistant Secretary Maurice L. Barksdale.

[89]HUD Handbook 4561.1, ch. 17-5.

ReSC projects must consist of five or more dwelling units, which may be detached, semidetached, row houses, or multifamily structures. Projects must be on real estate held either: (1) in fee simple, (2) under a renewal lease for not less than 99 years, (3) under a lease running at least 75 years from the date the mortgage is executed, or (4) under a lease executed by a government agency or HUD-approved lessor for a term of not less than 50 years.[90] The property must be free and clear of all liens other than the insured HUD mortgage. New construction projects must comply with local requirements and HUD minimum property standards. Rehabilitation projects must comply with local requirements. All projects must comply with applicable local zoning or deed restrictions.

(2) Services and Amenities

Each ReSC unit must contain kitchen and bathroom facilities. Kitchens must contain at least a small sink, refrigerator, and a two-burner stove; no oven is required. Bathrooms in five to 10 percent of the project units must generally be designed for handicapped eligibility. Weekly linen and housekeeping services are permitted as part of the services package. It is also expected that amenities such as arts and crafts spaces, lounges, recreation rooms, and similar facilities will be included to a greater extent than in noncongregate housing for the elderly. Reasonable charges to ReSC tenants and facilities may be made only after obtaining any lender approval required by HUD's administrative procedures.[91] No part of the project may be rented for transient or hotel purposes, and single-room occupancies (SROs) are prohibited. Commercial rentable area in any project may exceed five percent of the total rentable area only with HUD's approval, and in no event may exceed 20 percent.[92]

No medical services are permitted as part of the ReSC project itself or as part of the service package without prior approval by HUD. With approval, a small number of infirmary beds may be included. Access to a nursing home, hospital, or other medical facility may be part of a ReSC; however, any charges to ensure access are prohibited.

ReSCs offer meals to their tenants by operating a congregate dining facility. Where there is an identity of interest between the owner of the ReSC and the operator of the congregate dining facility, the purchase of meals by each tenant may be made a mandatory condition of occupancy in order to assure stability of demand for meals. The charges to the tenants must be sufficient to exceed the expense shown by a small safety factor or margin of proprietary return for managing the provision of meal services. Even if the meal service is run by a commercial food service vendor independent of

---

[90]HUD Handbook 4561.1, ch. 3-1.

[91]24 C.F.R. § 251.703(c).

[92]24 C.F.R. § 203(a)(5).

the ReSC sponsor, the sponsor may determine that a mandatory meal requirement will contribute to the success of the facility. However, in exchange for making meals mandatory, the commercial lease must provide the ReSC sponsor with a right to concur with changes in service and charges for meals. Certain additional requirements apply to a commercial lease of restaurant space in a ReSC.[93] A Meals on Wheels type approach to providing meal service can also be used in conjunction with a ReSC.

(3) Rents and Fees

Projects may not charge a founder's fee, initial admission fee, or similar charge beyond normal security deposits associated with standard rental projects. Security deposits must be maintained in a trust account separate from all other funds in the project. The owner must comply with any state or local laws regarding investment of security deposits and the distribution of interest or other income earned thereon.[94]

The mortgagor of the property sets the charges for ReSC project accommodations, which are expected to be market rate. No HUD subsidy of rents is provided in the form of Section 8 payments or direct loans, nor are there any income limitations for tenants. However, as noted above, the mortgagor must obtain HUD approval for any charges for services or facilities. Mortgagors may also be subject to state and local rent control regulation of project rents (see discussion in § 22.5(a)). Mortgagors and their agents must also comply with federal law and HUD-FHA regulations prohibiting discrimination on the basis of race, color, creed, or national origin. The mortgagor must also comply with state and local laws and ordinances prohibiting discrimination[95] (see also discussion at § 23).

All rents and other receipts of the project must be deposited in the project's name in accounts that are fully insured by an agency of the federal government. Project funds may only be used for payment of mortgage obligations, payment of reasonable expenses necessary to the proper operation and maintenance of the project, and certain distributions of surplus cash under HUD procedures.[96]

Because of what HUD perceives as the extremely narrow market band for ReSCs (which results in slow initial rent up), limited market comparables, and industry experience, substantial reserves are required in the program. ReSC projects require one of the following: (1) an operating deficit escrow funded at 200 percent of HUD's determination of the initial operating deficit, (2) a six-month debt service reserve, or (3) an operating deficit escrow and a six-month debt service reserve.

---

[93] See May 15, 1984 HUD Memorandum, note 88, above.

[94] 24 C.F.R. § 704(d).

[95] See HUD Handbook 4560.2, ch. 1-5.

[96] 24 C.F.R. § 251.704, 705.

The reserve requirements for ReSC projects are determined by calculating the initial operating deficit and a six-month debt service reserve. If the operating deficit is less than the six-month debt service reserve, the amount of reserve funds required will be the greater of two times the operating deficit calculation or the six-month debt service reserve. If the anticipated operating deficit equals or exceeds the debt service reserve amount, both an operating deficit escrow and debt service reserve are required.[97] Funds remaining in the operating deficit escrow and/or debt service reserve can be released after sustaining occupancy has been maintained for 90 days.

(b) Section 223(f)

HUD also permits the financing of existing structures as ReSCs under the Section 223(f) program. Section 223(f) authorizes HUD to insure mortgages in connection with the purchase or refinancing of existing multifamily projects without requiring a program of substantial rehabilitation.[98] Substantial rehabilitation projects for ReSCs must be coinsured under the Section 221(d)(4) program, outlined above.

Section 223(f) coinsurance applies to any existing rental housing of more than five units that is more than three years old. The property must consist of at least eight living units, and have a remaining economic life long enough to permit at least a 10 year mortgage. The cost of repairs cannot exceed the greater of:

15 percent of the property's value after repairs; or

$6500 per dwelling unit (adjusted by applicable high cost area factor), plus equipment; and

No more than one major building component may be replaced.

Applications have to meet the financial reserve, marketing, and sponsor criteria currently required for ReSC financing under Section 221(d)(4).

Because the extension of the ReSC program to Section 223(f) is a relatively recent development, HUD is still in the process of formulating explicit processing instructions for this program. HUD expanded the ReSC program to include Section 223(f) because of the growing interest in converting existing elderly projects and residential structures that do not need substantial rehabilitation into retirement centers.

§ 22.2 SECTION 232 BOARD AND CARE HOMES

The Housing and Urban-Rural Recovery Act of 1983[99] amended the Section 232 program to permit federal mortgage insurance to help finance the

[97] Notice H85-33 (HUD).
[98] See 24 C.F.R. § 255.233.
[99] P.L. 98-181.

construction or improvement of board and care homes. Section 232 had previously been limited to nursing homes and intermediate care facilities (ICFs). Board and care homes are known by many different names in different states, such as domiciary care, shelter care, adult congregate living care, personal care, and residential care. This type of facility provides living arrangements for individuals who cannot live independently but who do not require the more extensive care offered by ICFs or nursing homes.[100] For a full discussion of the financing aspects of Section 232 board and care facilities, see Section 14, above.

Board and care homes may be privately owned and operated for profit, or owned by a private nonprofit corporation or association, to qualify for FHA financing. Board and care facilities may either be freestanding structures or can be attached to—but form an identifiable and separate portion of—an ICF or nursing home. Nursing home or ICF services may not be carried out in a board and care home, or in the board and care portion(s) of an ICF or nursing home. In addition, a separate entrance must be provided for a board and care facility where it is part of a nursing home or ICF.[101] Boarding houses providing only food and shelter, and single room occupancy hotels are not eligible. HUD emphasizes that good accessibility to residential areas is important when evaluating the suitability of board and care home sites, as well as where family, friends, social support groups, health services, and recreation facilities are located.

Eligible facilities must certify that the state in which the home will be located is in compliance with Section 1616(e) of the Social Security Act (Keys Amendment) (see discussion in § 20.3(a)).

Facilities must contain a minimum of five bedrooms. Accommodations may be bedrooms with shared living, kitchen, and dining areas, and shared bathroom facilities, or efficiency and one-bedroom dwelling units. Each bedroom must be for not more than four persons. Congregate dining facilities must be provided for all board and care facilities, including those with dwelling units with kitchen and dining space. Kitchen and dining space must be provided in efficiency and one-bedroom dwelling units. These units must also have a full separate bathroom. In congregate facilities, a full bathroom must be provided for at least every four residents. Dormitory or communal-type bathroom facilities are not permitted.

Interior space must also be provided for passive activities such as sitting, reading, and conversing; active pursuits, such as parlor games and crafts; and communal activities, including meetings and group entertainment. A lounge for board and care residents must be separate from any nursing home or ICF use.

Board and care homes must offer three meals per day to each resident. Residents in accommodations without kitchens must take the three meals a

---

[100] See 12 U.S.C. § 1715w; 24 C.F.R. § 232.
[101] Notice H86-20 (HUD).

day provided by the homes. Residents whose accommodations have kitchens must take at least one meal a day provided by the home.

Board and care homes must also offer continuous protective oversight for the residents, which involves a range of activities. Services for relatively independent occupants may include such things as awareness on the part of management staff of an occupant's condition and whereabouts, and the ability to intervene in the event of a crisis. Charges may be assessed for other services that are in addition to those services included in the basic residential fee. Such services may include housekeeping, laundry, supervision of nutrition or medication, assistance with daily living—such as bathing, dressing, shopping, or eating—or 24 hour responsibility for the welfare of the resident.

No founder's fees, lifecare fees, or any other similar charge can be allowed in any insured proposal. Any proposal that requires the client/tenant to give or deposit money or other property, other than the normal security deposit and the first month's charges, is ineligible.

When a board and care proposal consists of independent living units (efficiency or one-bedroom units), HUD requires a six-month debt service reserve. Any independent living board and care proposal is, according to HUD, attempting to reach the same narrow market band as retirement service centers and, therefore, should have the same reserve requirement.[102] If independent living units are combined with an ICF/nursing home, only a three-month debt service reserve is required.

§ 22.3   SECTION 202/8 DIRECT LOANS

The HUD Section 202/8 program provides loans at reduced interest rates to nonprofit sponsors for the development cost of new or substantially rehabilitated housing for the elderly or handicapped. Section 202 provides 40 year loans at below-market interest rates for up to 100 percent of the total development costs of the project. Rental subsidies are offered through the Section 8 program to qualifying low income families and individuals living in approved residential facilities. With the consolidation of the application requirements of both the Section 202 and the Section 8 programs, projects that meet the requirements of the Section 202 program are deemed by HUD to have met the requirements for housing assistance payments under Section 8. Accordingly, a separate application for Section 8 assistance is not necessary.[103]

(a)   Section 202

The Housing and Community Development Act of 1974[104] amended the Section 202 program to permit construction loans and direct 40 year permanent

---

[102]*Id.*

[103]24 C.F.R. § 885.1(b); HUD Handbook 4571.1 REV-2, ch. 1-4.

[104]P.L. 93-383.

financing to nonprofit sponsors for the construction or substantial rehabilitation of housing projects for the elderly, handicapped, or disabled.[105] The loans are made at a rate based on the average interest of all interest-bearing obligations of the United States that form a part of the public debt, plus an amount to cover administrative costs. As of fiscal year (FY) 1987 the interest rate was frozen by statute at 9.25 percent.[106]

As the Section 202 program is one of direct loans, availability of federal funding is dependent on annual appropriations by Congress. The actual level of recent HUD funding for the Section 202 has been relatively low, making it difficult to get money even for projects deemed worthy by HUD. In FY1987, for example, approximately $593 million was appropriated for Section 202 loans, to provide some 12,000 housing units. The Administration has repeatedly requested that no further funding be provided for the Section 202 program, but this recommendation has been rejected by Congress.[107] Funds are also allocated on a geographical basis among the ten HUD regions, and further between metropolitan and non-metropolitan areas based on a needs formula, thus further restricting their availability to interested borrowers.

(1) Eligible Applicants

Only private nonprofit corporations are eligible to apply for Section 202 loans. The law creating the Section 202 program does allow public agencies and private, profit-motivated entities to be project developers, as well as nonprofit corporations. However, HUD regulations and annual appropriations bills have restricted the program to nonprofits.[108] The program handbook makes it clear that indirect participation by public agencies or profit-motivated groups is prohibited. A profit-motivated group may not sponsor a nonprofit borrower, and a public agency may not set up an agency or instrumentality to participate in the 202 program. The handbook says HUD will reject "applications proposing loans to groups acting as 'fronts' for profit-motivated developers or builders, and proposals based on syndications to profit-motivated investors."[109]

In addition to the private, nonprofit corporation borrower, Section 202 projects must have a sponsor that is expected to provide the funds required by the borrower to carry out the project. The sponsor is expected to pledge its financial and other support to the borrower over the full 40 year term of

---

[105] See, generally, 12 U.S.C. § 1701q; 24 C.F.R. § 885.

[106] Department of HUD-Independent Agencies Appropriations Bill, 1987, H.R. REP. No. 731, 99th Cong., 2nd Sess., at 9 (1986).

[107] Id.

[108] Id.; 24 C.F.R. § 885.5.

[109] HUD Handbook 4571.1 REV-2, ch. 2-7.

the Section 202 loan. It is largely on the basis of the sponsor's experience and its arrangements with and pledge of support to the borrower that HUD selects a borrower for a Section 202 loan.[110]

Among the groups that typically qualify as Section 202 sponsors are religious organizations, minority organizations, fraternal orders, labor unions, senior citizens' groups, and consumer cooperatives. In contrast to the borrower, HUD expects the sponsor to have a history of interest and successful activity in housing generally or housing for the elderly or the handicapped, or to have been involved in one or more other social or community activities or services that provide the background and skills that may be transferable to housing for the elderly or handicapped. A sponsor is evaluated primarily on the strength of its activities as an organization. While religious bodies may serve as sponsors, the borrower must be a separate legal entity. Moreover, no religious purposes may be included in the Articles of Incorporation or bylaws of the borrower corporation.[111]

As noted earlier, projects may be new construction or substantial rehabilitation. They must be designed in accordance with appropriate HUD minimum property standards, and should include only units that are designed for elderly or handicapped persons. Special consideration must be given to such factors as location and site, architectural and design features, and the inclusion of a wide range of services and programs. Sites must be selected to avoid steep inclines. Convenience to transportation, shopping, personal and other services critical to the residents of the projects is also to be considered.[112] Projects for the elderly generally are not approved for more than 200 units, to avoid undue concentration of senior housing and to expand the number of areas in the community in which elderly can choose to live in housing specially designed to meet their needs.[113] Moreover, in approving sites, HUD will take into account the impact of the development on fair housing and equal opportunity concerns, particularly if the project is to be located in an area of minority concentration.[114]

Finally, occupancy of housing financed under the Section 202 program is open only to elderly or handicapped families and to handicapped persons, as defined by HUD.[115] Projects are not required to be designed to serve all four groups intended to be benefited by the Section 202 program (i.e., the elderly, physically disabled/mobility impaired, developmentally disabled, and chronically mentally ill) (see discussion at § 23.2).

---

[110]*Id.* at ch. 2-2.

[111]*Id.*

[112]*Id.* at ch. 5-15, 17.

[113]*Id.* at ch. 1-5.

[114]*Id.* at ch. 4-23, 24.

[115]*See id.* at ch. 1-4.

(2)   Required Amenities

Proposals for projects may contain a mix of efficiency and one-bedroom units, with at least 25 percent of the units efficiencies. Two-bedroom units are not permitted. Architectural barriers, such as steps and narrow doorways, must be eliminated to assure ingress and egress, livability of units, and access to all areas by all residents. Buildings must be designed to meet special safety requirements, including wider corridors, nonslip flooring, grab-bars, and shelves and specially placed electrical outlets. Each unit includes a kitchenette, or a kitchen, even if central dining is provided. A complete bathroom must also be provided.

Projects financed under the Section 202 program must not be elaborate or extravagant in design or materials. Unacceptable amenities include dishwashers, individual unit trash compactors, and balconies.[116] Commercial spaces, such as beauty and barber shops, may not be provided unless they are self-sustaining, provide needed services for residents, and do not exceed five percent of total project space.[117]

Projects must be designed to include an assured range of necessary services for the occupants, such as, among others, health, continuing education, welfare, information, recreation, homemaker, counseling, and referral services, as well as transportation necessary to facilitate convenient access to such services and to employment opportunities and participation in religious activities. Projects should include special spaces such as multipurpose rooms, game rooms, libraries and reading rooms, lounges and snack bars, and central kitchen and dining facilities. These common areas should not normally exceed 10 percent of the total project space.[118] Facilities may not be set aside solely for religious purposes; however, a multipurpose room may be used for religious services and other purposes from time to time and on an equitable basis for all religious groups comprising the tenancy.[119]

Provisions for health and medical care are expected to be based primarily on the services offered in the community rather than by the project. The project may incorporate an emergency room for temporary treatment, but not to provide care overnight or for extended periods. No staff provisions for doctors, nurses, or other medical personnel are permitted under the program, although consideration may be given to renting space for medical professionals.[120]

---

[116]*Id.* at ch. 5-17.
[117]*Id.* at ch. 1-5(6).
[118]*Id.* at ch. 5-17.
[119]*Id.* at ch. 1-4(8).
[120]*Id.* at ch. 1-4(7).

(b)   Section 8 Housing Assistance Payments

Because the relatively small reduction of interest to Section 202 borrowers does not permit much reduction of rents, HUD couples this loan assistance with a reservation of Section 8 subsidies for all Section 202 units. All projects receiving Section 202 long-term loans must meet the requirements for, and receive the benefits of, leased housing assistance payments under the Section 8 program. Reservations for Section 8 funds are set aside at the time a Section 202 reservation is made, so that, as noted earlier, a separate application for Section 8 assistance is not necessary. Except for Section 202 housing for the elderly and handicapped, Section 8 is now used solely with existing housing stock, rather than for new construction.[121]

Participation in the Section 8 Housing Assistance Payments Program is required for a minimum of 20 percent of the units in any Section 202 project. However, if the borrower proposes Section 8 assistance for fewer than 100 percent of the units, HUD must review and approve the request prior to selection of the application.[122] It is important to remember that in any facility with Section 8 subsidized residents, none of the units in the building can command a rent higher than the HUD ceilings, regardless of whether the resident of a particular unit is a recipient of Section 8 assistance.[123]

Under the Section 8 program, a family pays 30 percent of its gross income for rent directly to the landlord. The federal government pays the rest pursuant to a Housing Assistance Payments (HAP) contract between HUD and the landlord. Eligible households are those with incomes under 80 percent of the median in their area, adjusted for family size. The HUD funds pay for adequate and reasonable use of all utilities, except telephone. One problem with this type of funding for elderly housing projects is that the costs of any programs provided to tenants, including meals, are not covered by the Section 8 subsidy.[124]

HUD acts to set the ceilings for the maximum rents that can be charged in facilities with Section 8 subsidized residents. As discussed, these also become the limits for facilities with Section 202 financing. For projects built with Section 202 funds, the maximum rent is 115.5 percent of the fair market rent, including utilities, and taking into consideration accessibility to the elderly and handicapped, structure type, and market area.[125] Rent increases, as well as eviction procedures, are governed by HUD regulations.[126]

---

[121] *See* Housing and Urban-Rural Recovery Act of 1983, P.L. 98-181.

[122] HUD Handbook 4571.1 REV-2, ch. 1-7(b).

[123] Ward, note 134, below, at 40.

[124] *Id.*

[125] *Id.* at 39.

[126] *See, generally,* 24 C.F.R. § 880 and discussion at §§ 22.5(a)–(b), below.

(c) Congregate Housing Services Program

The Congregate Housing Services Program (CHSP) was authorized as a demonstration project under Title IV of the Housing and Community Development Amendments of 1978.[127] Under CHSP, HUD provides for a core program of meals and minimum support services to selected public housing and Section 202 housing projects for elderly, nonelderly handicapped, or temporarily disabled persons who are frail and at risk. Actual services are provided directly by nonprofit corporation grantees or by local service providers under contract to the grantees. Each contract is for a term of not less than three years or more than five years, and is renewable at the end of such term. The nonprofit corporations applying for assistance to provide congregate services to elderly residents are required to consult with the local area agency on aging to determine the most appropriate means of providing services under the program.[128]

The CHSP was designed to test four premises: (1) that the use of appropriate community-based supportive services can help frail and handicapped people avoid premature institutionalization; (2) that the multiyear funding offered by CHSP would alleviate the need of sponsors to spend inordinate amounts of time looking for funds to keep services going; (3) that the required coordination with other agencies would prevent duplication of services and secure appropriate technical resources; and (4) that a continuing reassessment of clients and their needs would result in successful targeting of services to those in need.[129]

The key aspects of the program are that housing projects that apply for CHSP have to demonstrate that congregate services are needed because services existing in the community are insufficient or inadequate to meet project residents' needs. Participants in the program must receive two onsite meals seven days a week. Additional nonmedical services such as housekeeping, personal assistance, escort, and social services may also be provided to fill gaps in the project's service delivery system.

CHSP services are not to substitute for services already provided, but to be in addition to these services. Clients must pay at least some fee for all the services received. CHSP is generally not to cover more than 20 percent of the residents in a building in order to maintain an atmosphere of independent living. A volunteer professional assessment committee must be created at each project to screen all applicants to determine both if they are in need of services and which CHSP services are appropriate.[130]

---

[127] P.L. 95-557.

[128] See, generally, 42 U.S.C. §§ 8001-8010.

[129] "Maximizing Support Services for the Elderly in Assisted Housing: Experiences from the Congregate Housing Services Program." Hearings Before the Subcomm. on Housing and Consumer Interests of the House Select Comm. on Aging, 99th Cong., 1st Sess. at 4 (1985) (statement of Kenneth J. Beirne, General Deputy Assistant Secretary for Policy Development and Research, HUD.)

[130] Id.

In 1986, there were only about 2100 elderly and nonelderly handicapped residents enrolled in CHSP programs in some 62 projects nationwide. Both groups exhibit multiple frailties. The average age among elderly participants is about 78 years old; most are female. The nonelderly handicapped population is mostly male, with an average age of 34 years. Because the population served is not static, that is, when people are no longer at risk they are no longer eligible to receive CHSP services, only approximately 3000 people have been served by the demonstration since its inception in 1980.[131]

The Administration has proposed eliminating funding for the CHSP program in its recent budgets. Congress, however, has continued to fund the program at current levels, to continue those projects already in existence. For FY1987, some $3.4 million has been appropriated.[132] Given current budget constraints, however, it is unlikely that the present demonstration program will either be expanded or develop into a full-fledged assistance program for elderly and handicapped individuals in need of congregate services.

§ 22.4 OTHER FEDERAL HOUSING PROGRAMS FOR THE ELDERLY

(a) Section 231 Mortgage Insurance for Elderly Housing

Section 231 is a program of federal mortgage insurance to facilitate financing of construction or rehabilitation of rental housing for the elderly or handicapped.[133] To assure an adequate supply of this type of housing, HUD insures mortgages made by private lending institutions to build or rehabilitate multifamily projects consisting of eight or more units. HUD may insure up to 100 percent of project cost for nonprofit and public mortgagors, but only up to 90 percent for private mortgagors. All elderly (62 or older) or handicapped persons are eligible to occupy units in a project whose mortgage is insured under this program. The Section 231 program was intended to be used in conjunction with the Section 8 leased housing assistance payments program (see § 22.3(b)).

In terms of the availability of Section 231 insurance, statistics reveal that the program has become almost dormant. From $75 million in insured loans in FY1979, appropriations have fallen in FY1983 to $2 million, calling for insuring one project, nationwide, containing 85 units. Reasons for the program's demise include:

Lender preference for Section 221 insurance, because of cash payment in a default situation versus difficult-to-market debentures under Section 231; and

---

[131] *Id.*

[132] HUD Appropriations Bill, above, at 9–10.

[133] *See, generally,* 12 U.S.C. § 1701; 24 C.F.R. § 231; HUD Handbook 4570.1.

Existence of the Section 202 direct loan program as a 9.25 percent interest lender under Section 231.[134]

(b) Section 236 Mortgage Insurance and Interest Reduction Payments

The Section 236 program combined federal mortgage insurance with subsidized interest payments to mortgagees (lenders) in order to reduce the mortgagor's (owner) monthly mortgage payment. The interest payment subsidy lowered the effective interest rate of the mortgage to one percent. The benefits of the reduced interest payments were realized by the tenants in the form of lower rents. Eligible tenants were low income families, including the elderly and the handicapped.[135]

As originally enacted, the Section 236 program was meant to stimulate housing production by making private industry the primary vehicle for providing shelter for low and moderate income families. The Section 236 subsidy program was suspended during the 1973 subsidized housing moratorium and has never been revived as an active production program. Altogether, approximately 600,000 units were produced, which will continue to receive the mortgage subsidy until termination of their HUD contract, which usually extends 30 to 40 years. A number of Section 236 units have been shifted to the Section 8 program with owner approval.

§ 22.5 REGULATIONS GENERALLY APPLICABLE TO HUD PROGRAMS FOR THE ELDERLY

(a) Rent Control

HUD regulations regarding the applicability of state and local rent control laws to elderly housing projects depend on whether the program is classified as subsidized or unsubsidized. The principal active subsidy program is the Section 202/8 Direct Loan Program. Unsubsidized programs include:

Section 221(d)(4) ReSC New Construction and Substantial Rehabilitation (Mortgage Insurance)

Section 223(f) ReSC Moderate Rehabilitation and Conversion of Existing Facilities (Mortgage Insurance)

Section 232 Board and Care Facilities (Mortgage Insurance)[136]

With regard to subsidized programs, HUD regulations declare that "it is in the national interest to preempt . . . the entire field of rent regulation

---

[134]Ward, "Congregate Living Arrangements: The Financing Option," *Topics In Health Care Financing* (Spring 1984), 34, 42.

[135]*See, generally,* 12 U.S.C. § 1705; 24 C.F.R. § 236.1.

[136]*See, generally,* 24 C.F.R. § 246.

by local rent control boards . . . or other authority."[137] Rent increases for Section 202/8 programs, must, therefore, be submitted to the appropriate local office of HUD for approval.

For unsubsidized projects, HUD generally does not interfere in the regulation of rents by a rental control board or agency constituted under state or local laws. However, HUD preempts the regulation of rents under certain conditions. This preemption may occur for an unsubsidized project when HUD determines that the action of a rent board prevents the mortgagor from achieving a level of residential income necessary to maintain and adequately operate the project, which includes sufficient funds to meet the financial obligations under the mortgage.[138]

When a mortgagor determines that the permitted increase in rents as prescribed by the local board will not provide a rent level necessary to maintain and adequately operate the project, the mortgagor may file an application for preemption with HUD and must notify the tenants of the application for preemption. The mortgagor must also seek whatever relief or redetermination is permitted under state and local law. The HUD regulations outline in detail the type of notice that must be given to tenants and the materials that must be submitted to HUD in support of the application for preemption.[139]

(b) Eviction Procedures

HUD regulations govern evictions only from subsidized housing projects, which for the elderly is principally the Section 202/8 Direct Loan Program. Unsubsidized projects are governed by state and local law. The landlord may not terminate any tenancy in a subsidized project except for:

Material noncompliance with the rental agreement;
Material failure to carry out obligations under any state landlord and tenant act; or
Other good cause.[140]

The conduct of a tenant cannot be deemed "other good cause" unless the landlord has given the tenant prior notice that the conduct constitutes a basis for termination of occupancy. Prior notice must be served on the tenant in the same manner as that provided for termination notices.

The term "material noncompliance with the rental agreement" includes: (1) one or more substantial violations of the rental agreement, or (2) repeated minor violations of the rental agreement that disrupt the livability of

---

[137]24 C.F.R. § 246.21.
[138]24 C.F.R. § 246.5. *See also* rental rehabilitation grants, § 14.3(d), above.
[139]*See* 24 C.F.R. §§ 246.6–§ 246.12. § 14.3(d), above.
[140]24 C.F.R. § 247.3.

the project, adversely affect the health or safety of any person or the right of any tenant to the quiet enjoyment of the leased premises and related project facilities, interfere with the management of the project, or have an adverse financial effect on the project. Failure of the tenant to timely supply all required information on income and composition of the tenant household (including required evidence of citizenship or eligible alien status) constitutes a substantial violation of the rental agreement. Nonpayment of rent or any other financial obligation due under the rental agreement (including any portion thereof) beyond any grace period permitted under state law also constitutes a substantial violation of the rental agreement. The payment of rent or any other financial obligation due under the rental agreement after the due date but within the grace period permitted under state law constitutes only a minor violation.

The regulations further specify the required contents of the termination notice to the tenant and the manner in which such notice must be served.[141] Actual eviction of the tenant pursuant to these HUD regulations must be made by judicial action pursuant to state or local law. A tenant may also rely on state or local law governing procedures that provide the tenant procedural rights in addition to those provided by HUD, except where local rent law has been preempted under 24 C.F.R. § 246 (see discussion at § 22.5(a)).

(c) Pet Regulations

The question of pet ownership in elderly housing has been one of the most hotly debated topics of HUD regulation. Section 227 of the Housing and Urban-Rural Recovery Act of 1983[142] provides that no owner or manager of federally assisted rental housing for the elderly or handicapped may prohibit or prevent a tenant from owning or having common household pets, or restrict or discriminate against any person regarding admission to or occupancy of such housing because of the person's ownership of pets.[143]

In 1986, HUD issued detailed and voluminous final regulations, as directed by the statute, to establish guidelines under which owners or managers of covered housing (1) may prescribe reasonable rules governing the keeping of common household pets, and (2) must consult with tenants when prescribing the rules.[144] House pet rules must be reasonably related to a legitimate interest of the project owner, such as an interest in providing a decent, safe, and sanitary living environment for existing and prospective tenants and in protecting and preserving the physical condition of the project

---

[141] 24 C.F.R. § 247.4.

[142] P.L. 98-181.

[143] 12 U.S.C. § 1701r-1.

[144] 51 Fed. Reg. 43,270 (1986) (to be codified at 24 C.F.R. pts. 243, 511, 942) (issued Dec. 1, 1986).

and the owner's financial interest in it. In addition, the house pet rules must be narrowly drawn to achieve the owner's legitimate interests without imposing unnecessary burdens and restrictions on pet owners. Within these regulations, project owners retain a significant amount of flexibility in formulating house pet rules.

In the final regulations, HUD interprets the statutory language and Congressional intent to extend the prohibitions on discrimination on the basis of pet ownership to *all* projects that are designated for occupancy by elderly or handicapped tenants, including those projects that are only federally insured, but unsubsidized. This interpretation may be open to challenge, however, as the statutory language on its face applies only to "federally assisted rental housing."[145]

In the interim, HUD's regulations apply to HUD-insured mortgages under Sections 221(d)(3), 221(d)(4), and 231, even though these projects may be unsubsidized. The regulations exclude mortgages insured under Section 232 for board and care facilities, since HUD does not consider them to be rental housing within the meaning of the statute. Section 202/8 direct loan projects are clearly covered by the regulations. The regulations also define under what conditions a particular project is considered to be "designated for occupancy by elderly or handicapped families."

The regulations require that project owners must, at a minimum, establish rules on several important matters:

1. Pet owners must have their pets inoculated and licensed in accordance with state and local law.
2. Project owners must prescribe sanitary standards to govern the disposal of pet waste. Where the pet is duly determined to constitute, under state or local law, a nuisance or threat to the health and safety of the occupants of the rental housing project or other members of the community, removal of that pet may be required.
3. Pets must be appropriately and effectively restrained and under the control of a responsible individual while in the common areas of the project.
4. Pet owners must register their pets with project owners. Project owners may refuse to register pets if the owner reasonably determines, based on the pet owner's habits and practices, that the pet owner will be unable to keep the pet in compliance with the house rules and other lease obligations.
5. Project owners may require an additional pet security deposit, which may be used only to pay reasonable expenses directly attributable to the presence of the pet in the project. The deposit may only be required for cats and dogs. For tenants whose rents are subsidized by

[145] 12 U.S.C. § 1701r-1(a).

HUD, the Department from time to time sets a maximum deposit (currently fixed at $300[146]); the initial deposit may be paid in installments. For unsubsidized tenants, the deposit may not exceed one month's rent, and may be paid in installments at the discretion of the project owner.

The regulations are clear that project owners cannot ban all pets from a project, even if the ban were consistent with the wishes of the owner and a majority of the residents. Nor may the project owner designate "pet" and "no pet" residential areas of the project, as HUD has determined that the health threat from allergic reactions to pets in residential areas is insufficient. However, an applicant for tenancy in a project may reject a unit offered by the project owner if the presence of a pet in a nearby unit would constitute a serious health threat to the applicant. Reasonable limitations may also be placed on the presence of pets in specified common areas of the facility.

Project owners may establish reasonable limitations on the number of common household pets allowed in each dwelling unit, as well as on pet size, weight, and type. The regulations further define "common household pet," and state that the owner may limit the number of "four-legged, warm-blooded" pets to one per dwelling unit. However, the project owner may not place any quotas on overall pet occupancy. The regulations do not apply to animals that assist the handicapped. The regulations also provide detailed procedures for tenant input into the formulation of house rules, notice to tenants of the rules and rule making procedures, and for the enforcement of house pet rules.

Finally, the regulations do not preempt state and local laws designed to protect the public health and safety by establishing reasonable limits on pet ownership within their jurisdiction. The pet rules prescribed by project owners may not conflict with state or local authority and, where they do, state and local law or regulation applies. Numerous sections of the regulations further explicitly preserve state and local law. The exceptions, where state and local are not to apply, pertain principally to HUD's management and procedural responsibilities under the statute.

(d) Mandatory Meals

Subsidized elderly housing facilities sometimes offer congregate meal programs in an effort to ensure adequate nutrition and encourage socialization among residents. In order to spread overhead costs and minimize the charges necessary to the provision of central dining, many facilities require enrollment in the meal program as a condition of admission for every resident. According to federal guidelines in effect since 1963, mandatory meals were to be operated only at cost, could require purchase

[146]51 Fed. Reg. 43,306 (issued Dec. 1, 1986).

of only one meal per day (with some exceptions), and had to have prior approval by HUD.

In recent years, several court cases have been brought on behalf of residents challenging mandatory meal programs. Although plaintiffs generally had agreed to participate in meal programs to gain initial admission to their residences, they wanted to opt out for reasons of convenience, affordability, special medical needs, conflict with work schedules, dissatisfaction with food quality, or similar grounds.

The first series of mandatory meals cases centered upon the argument that the charge for meals, because it is a condition of occupancy, constituted rent and therefore resulted in a rental charge in excess of the 30 percent of income rent cap specified for Section 8 subsidized facilities. This argument, and a related argument to the effect that mandatory meal programs contravened congressional intent by establishing an impermissible barrier to receipt of subsidized housing, generally have been rejected as a matter of law by the federal courts.[147] However, at least one court has refused to follow the trend and has held that whether meal charges constitute rent presents an issue of fact that can be decided only by a trial.[148]

A second approach has been taken in at least one federal case in New York, in which plaintiffs argued that requiring the purchase of meals as a condition of renting housing constitutes a tying arrangement that violates antitrust law.[149] One response to this argument is that the program of the facility as a whole, including housing, meals, housekeeping, and other services, is a single product rather than several separate products unlawfully tied together. Plaintiffs' antitrust arguments have withstood attempts by defendants to summarily dismiss them, and the district court ruled that the meal program, although approved by HUD, was not exempt from antitrust scrutiny, and certified that question to the Court of Appeals and the question whether, on a stipulated set of facts, the meal program is an illegal tying arrangement.[150] The tying arrangement argument, if successful, can pose a threat to all retirement facilities, whether or not HUD-financed, that offer substantial service programs as a mandatory condition of residence.[151]

A third approach in the challenge to mandatory meals has been to attack HUD guidelines as having been developed without compliance with the public notice and hearing requirements of the federal Administrative Procedure

---

[147] See *Aujero v. CDA Todco, Inc.*, 756 F.2d 1374 (9th Cir. 1985); *Mayoral v. Jeffco American Baptist Residences, Inc.*, 726 F.2d 1361 (10th Cir. 1984), *cert. den.* 469 U.S. 884, 105 S. Ct. 255, 83 L. Ed. 2d 192 (1984).

[148] *Gonzalez v. St. Margaret's House*, 620 F. Supp. 806 (S.D.N.Y. 1985).

[149] See *Johnson v. Soundview Apartments*, 585 F. Supp. 559; 588 F. Supp. 1381 (S.D.N.Y. 1984) and order filed Nov. 17, 1986, reported at 1986-2 Trade Cases, CCH *Trade Regulation Reporter*, ¶ 67,349. The case has since settled.

[150] *Id.*

[151] See discussion concerning condominiums with services, § 7.1(c)(2), above.

Act. It was this attack that brought the most immediate results for complainants. In *Birkland v. Rotary Plaza,*[152] a case involving a HUD Section 236 project, the federal district court for the Northern District of California found the HUD guidelines to be improperly promulgated, and ordered HUD to adopt final rules governing mandatory meals by February 1987.

In response to this federal court order, HUD issued a final rule regarding mandatory meals in March 1987.[153] The final rule permits current HUD-approved mandatory meals programs to continue, but prohibits any new programs in existing or future projects after April 1, 1987.[154] The regulations affect projects with Section 202 direct loans, Sections 221(d)(3) and 221(d)(5) below-market interest rates, Section 236 interest reduction payments, and Section 8 or Section 101 rent subsidy projects.[155] The rules should not apply to Section 231, 232, or 221(d)(4) programs that involve only mortgage insurance by HUD and where no rental assistance is provided.

The final rule reflects HUD's balancing of competing considerations in the mandatory meals program. Continuation of current programs is permitted because HUD views them as providing nutritional and socialization benefits for facility residents, and because if such programs were required to convert to voluntary participation, project sponsors may not be able to obtain necessary sources of subsidies to fund these programs, and thus might terminate them as financially infeasible. HUD saw this result as frustrating the reasonable expectations of both the project sponsors, tenants, and HUD with regard to these projects.[156]

For future HUD-assisted projects, HUD determined that no such reliance considerations existed. Project sponsors for future HUD-assisted projects who decide to offer their tenants a meal service may either site their projects near a community facility with a suitable meals program or make an informed decision to include a central dining facility in their project and offer only a voluntary meals program.[157]

For existing programs, exemptions from the mandatory meals program must be granted for a special diet required for medical reasons, where the tenant has a paying job requiring absence from the project during the mealtime, for temporary absences from the facility of over one week, and where the tenant is permanently immobile or otherwise incapable of attending the central dining facility. A project owner may also grant any tenant an exemption because of dietary practices, for financial reasons, or for any other reasons. An alternative menu that does not conflict with a tenant's religious dietary practices must be offered, or an exemption from the program must

---

[152]No. C84-2026 SW (N.D. Cal. Jan. 10, 1986).

[153]52 Fed. Reg. 6300 (issued March 2, 1987) (to be codified at 24 CFR Pt. 278).

[154]*Id.* at 6300-01.

[155]*Id.* at 6306.

[156]*Id.* at 6301.

[157]*Id.*

be granted. Programs must continue to be offered at cost and with the approval of HUD.[158] All prospective project tenants must also be given notice that participation in the meals program is a condition of occupancy in the project. The regulations also add the requirement that the mandatory meals program must comply with state or local nutritional statutory standards and, where no such standards exist, the project must submit a nutritional statement to HUD on an annual basis.[159]

§ 23   DISCRIMINATION IN ADMISSIONS

Developers and project sponsors must be careful to comply with applicable federal as well as state laws regarding discrimination in housing. Compliance with federal law is a prerequisite for obtaining approval from HUD for either mortgage insurance or direct loans. The principal areas covered by federal law of interest to retirement facilities are statutes concerning discrimination on the basis of age, handicap, religion, and national origin. These provisions are discussed in the sections below. State laws typically cover these areas as well as additional bases of discrimination (such as marital status or gender), and may in some instances be more restrictive than federal law.[160]

§ 23.1   AGE

(a)   Federal Law

The Age Discrimination Act of 1975 provides that no person shall, on the basis of age, be excluded from participation in, denied the benefits of, or be subjected to discrimination under any program or activity receiving federal financial assistance.[161] There are, however, a number of statutory exceptions to this basic provision, which are outlined in detail in the HUD regulations implementing the statute for that department.[162] There has been very little action in the courts under this statute as it relates to housing issues.

It is important to note at the outset that the HUD regulations implementing the Act interpret the phrase "receiving federal financial assistance" to include *either* HUD assistance in the form of funds *or* the services of federal personnel.[163] This interpretation is consistent with that made by other

[158]*Id.* at 6307.

[159]*Id.* at 6306.

[160]Attention should also be paid to local antidiscrimination laws, which may involve emerging areas of concern not covered by federal or state provisions (such as sexual preference).

[161]42 U.S.C. §§ 6101–6107; P.L. 94-135.

[162]*See* 51 Fed. Reg. 45,264 (to be codified at 24 C.F.R. Part 146) (issued December 17, 1986).

[163]*Id.* at 45,266.

federal agencies.[164] This means that *all* projects that proceed under HUD, involving both mortgage insurance and direct loans, must comply with the provisions of the Act. Facilities constructed solely with private monies, but that receive Medicare or Medicaid funds, may also be subject to the provisions of the Act.[165]

The statute sets up two major exceptions to the operation of the Act's discrimination provisions. First, the Act does not apply to age distinctions established under the authority of any law that provides benefits or establishes criteria for participation on the basis of age or in age-related terms.[166] "Any law" is defined to mean age distinctions that are contained in a federal statute, a state statute, or a local statute or ordinance adopted by an elected, general purpose legislative body. For example, Medicare is a program where benefits begin at a certain age by virtue of federal statute enacted by Congress; such age distinctions do not violate the Act. It is important to note that this provision does not provide an automatic exemption to age distinctions that are contained in regulations or in ordinances that are enacted by bodies that are not elected or are special purpose even though elected, such as commissioners or housing authority boards.[167]

Second, a recipient of federal financial assistance is also permitted to make age distinctions if that action reasonably takes into account age as a factor necessary to the normal operation or the achievement of any statutory objective of a program or activity. "Statutory objective" is defined as above.[168] HUD has set up a strict four-part test to determine when age is such a factor:

1. Age must be used as a measure or approximation of one or more other characteristics.
2. The other characteristics must be measured or approximated in order for the normal operation of the program to continue, or to achieve any statutory objective of the program.
3. The other characteristics can reasonably be measured or approximated by the use of age.
4. The other characteristics are impractical to measure directly on an individual basis.[169]

The regulations indicate that the four-part test is designed to weed out age distinctions that are neither directly related to an essential characteristic of

---

[164] *See, e.g.,* the general regulation regarding the Act published by the Department of Health and Human Services (HHS) 45 C.F.R. § 90.4 (1985).

[165] *See* discussion at § 23.2, below.

[166] 42 U.S.C. § 6103(b)(2); 51 Fed. Reg. at 45,270.

[167] 51 Fed. Reg. at 45,270.

[168] 42 U.S.C. § 6103(b)(1); 51 Fed. Reg. at 45,267.

[169] *See* 51 Fed. Reg. at 45,264-5, 45,267, 45,270-71.

a program nor are based on explicitly stated objectives of the law.[170] In order to qualify for this exemption the age distinction must meet *all* four parts of the test, and the burden of proof that the age distinction falls within the exception is on the recipient of federal financial assistance.[171]

As there has been some confusion regarding the application of this four-part test, HUD provided a sample situation in the preamble to the final regulations.[172] In the example, a project providing housing for the elderly or handicapped under Section 202 refuses to accept as tenants persons over 66 years of age. Section 202 housing was generally designed to provide housing for those elderly or handicapped individuals capable of "independent living," and the project in question does not provide services for those unable to live independently.

HUD's analysis of the hypothetical project's action under the four-part test, to determine whether the age distinction is a "factor necessary to the normal operation of a program or activity," reveals that:

1. Age is being used as a measure or approximation of prospective tenants' ability to live independently.
2. The nonage characteristic (the ability to live independently) must be measured for the normal operation of the program or activity to continue.
3. The nonage characteristic cannot reasonably be measured or approximated by the use of age, since there are many people well over the age of 66 who are capable of independent living.
4. It is not impractical to measure the ability to live independently on an individual basis.

   Thus, while the project's action satisfies the first two parts of the test, it fails the second two, and as such violates the Age Discrimination Act.[173]

(b)   State Laws

Retirement facilities are also subject to state statutes and case law regarding discrimination in the provision of housing or services, and developers

---

[170]*Id.* at 45,271.

[171]*Id.* at 45,265, 45,267.

[172]*Id.* at 45,261–62.

[173]An interesting question arises with regard to the application of the Age Discrimination Act to the Sections 221(d)(4) and 223(f) Retirement Service Center programs; *see* § 22.1, above. The HUD guidelines to the program indicate that ReSCs are intended to serve the frail elderly of age 70 or over (Notice H83-58 (HUD) at 3). This age restriction, however, is not contained in any statutory language, as the ReSC program is one initiated by HUD on the basis of the general Sections 221(d)(4) and 223(f) statutes and regulations (*Id.* at 1). Nor would the age limitation appear to meet the four-part test for "necessary to the normal operation of a program," as there are many elderly under the age of 70 who are frail and in need of the services offered by ReSCs. If HUD establishes the age 70 limitation for ReSCs as a firm cutoff without any basis in statute, a conflict with the Age Discrimination Act may arise.

should be sure to check for all applicable state provisions. In one case, for example, the California Supreme Court interpreted the state's general civil rights act to prohibit discrimination on the basis of age in all business establishments, and held that a landlord's "no-children" policy violated the law.[174] While the language of the Act on its face limits its application to discrimination based on "sex, race, color, religion, ancestry, or national origin,"[175] the Court held that the statute barred all types of arbitrary discrimination, and that the reference to particular bases of discrimination was illustrative rather than restrictive.[176]

The California court did, however, recognize the validity of age-limited admission policies for retirement communities or housing complexes reserved for older citizens. It found that such policies were a reasonable means of establishing and preserving specialized facilities for those in need of particular services.[177] This view was later incorporated into state law by statutory amendments[178] that permit limited age discrimination "where accommodations are designed to meet the physical and social needs of senior citizens." The amendments set out in some detail the conditions under which age limitations may be implemented in senior housing, and when nonelderly companions of seniors may reside in such housing.

Retirement facilities that offer health care services may argue that they are not subject to such discrimination in housing statutes on the ground that any admissions criteria are health care related and that housing is incidental to the provision of licensed care.[179]

The Florida Courts have taken a more expansive view of age restrictions in housing. In *White Egret Condominiums v. Franklin*,[180] the Florida Supreme Court upheld a restriction against residency by children under the age of 12 in a condominium apartment. The Court found that this policy was a reasonable means of identifying and categorizing varying desires of the population in regard to housing, and did not violate either the 14th Amendment to the U.S. Constitution or Florida statute. The Court did note, however, that age

---

[174]*Marina Point, Ltd. v. Wolfson*, 30 Cal. 3d 721; 180 Cal. Rptr. 496, 640 P.2d 115 (1982).

[175]Cal. Civ. Code § 51.

[176]30 Cal. 3d at 725. In a later case, the Court found that the Act's reference to "business establishments" also included condominium associations, and struck down a limitation on residency to persons over age 18. *O'Connor v. Village Green Owners Assn.*, 33 Cal. 3d 790, 191 Cal. Rptr. 320, 662 P.2d 427 (1983).

[177]30 Cal. 3d at 742–43.

[178]Cal. Civ. Code §§ 51.2, 51.3; Section 2 of 1984 Stats. c. 787.

[179]The California Legislative Counsel has issued an opinion that the provisions of these sections are inapplicable to licensed care facilities such as health, community care, or adult day care health facilities. Senior Housing, Op. Cal. Leg. Counsel 24969 (Jan. 11, 1986).

[180]379 So. 2d 346 (Fla. 1979).

restrictions cannot be used to unreasonably or arbitrarily restrict certain classes of individuals from obtaining desirable housing.[181]

§ 23.2 HANDICAP

The issue of whether retirement facilities may discriminate in admissions on the basis of handicap has arisen most prominently in the context of projects that were constructed with the assistance of Section 202 direct loans.[182] By statute, four groups are intended to be benefited by the Section 202 program: the elderly, and three subgroups of the handicapped, the "mobility impaired," the "chronically mentally ill," and the "developmentally disabled."[183] The issue in the courts has been whether a project must serve individuals from *all* four groups, or may restrict its programs to one or some groups. Specifically, in the two cases that have arisen, developmentally disabled individuals have sued to gain admission to facilities that restricted admissions to the elderly and the mobility-impaired handicapped.

To date, the courts have rejected both grounds on which the plaintiffs sought admission to the facilities. First, the courts found that restricting admission to only two of the four statutory groups did not violate Section 202.[184] In the *Brecker v. Queens B'Nai Brith Housing Development* opinion, the Court found that Congress precisely drafted Section 202 to permit a sponsor to provide housing for the elderly *or* the handicapped if the sponsor so wished; a sponsor need not serve all eligible needy groups.[185] The facility in question was designed for residents who were capable of independent living, and did not offer the substantial range of services that would be required for developmentally disabled residents. As the Section 202 program was designed to provide *both* a housing and a services component, the facility clearly did not meet needs of the developmentally disabled group. The Court found that a sponsor is not required by the Section 202 statute to change its program in order to accommodate all the groups

---

[181] *See also Metro. Dade County Fair v. Sunrise Village*, 485 So. 2d 865 (Fla. App. 1986) (striking down a municipal ordinance prohibiting housing discrimination on the basis of age as exceeding the legitimate bounds of the police power and refusing to require a mobile home park for the elderly to permit a 29-year-old to reside there).

[182] *See Brecker v. Queens B'Nai Brith Housing Development*, 428 F. Supp. 428 (E.D.N.Y. 1985) *aff'd* 798 F.2d 52 (2d Cir. 1986); *Knutzen v. Nelson*, 617 F. Supp. 977 (D. Co. 1985) *aff'd sub nom. Knutzen v. Eben Ezer Lutheran Housing Center*, 815 F.2d 1343 (10th cir. 1987). For a discussion of the Section 202 program, *see* § 22.3(a), above.

[183] 12 U.S.C. §§ 1701q(d)(4)(A)–(C).

[184] The discussion here will focus primarily on the *Brecker* case, *Knutzen* essentially follows the rationale of *Brecker*.

[185] *Brecker*, 798 F.2d at 55–56.

entitled under the statute. Rather, projects may be targeted to a particular group.[186]

A second and more difficult issue, and one that applies not only to Section 202 but to all federally subsidized housing, is whether discrimination in admissions on the basis of handicap violates Section 504 of the Rehabilitation Act of 1973.[187] Even facilities that were constructed solely with private monies may still be subject to the Section 504 requirements. Although the issue has not finally been resolved, some courts have found that receipt of Medicare and Medicaid funds makes a facility a recipient of federal assistance within the meaning of the Rehabilitation Act, and subjects it to the requirements of Section 504.[188] Section 504 provides that no "otherwise qualified" handicapped individual shall be excluded from participation in, or denied the benefits of, any program that receives federal financial assistance.[189] The plaintiffs in both Section 202 discrimination cases argued that the facility's actions violated this provision of the Rehabilitation Act.

The key to the *Brecker* Court's analysis of this claim was whether the handicapped individuals were otherwise qualified for the facility. The Supreme Court has defined an otherwise qualified individual as "one who is able to meet all of a program's requirements in spite of his handicap."[190] The Court had earlier held that these facilities may restrict admissions to the elderly and the mobility impaired. Since the developmentally disabled patients were neither elderly nor mobility impaired, they did not meet the program's requirements and were therefore not otherwise qualified.[191]

The cases have recognized that Section 504 is not an affirmative action program for the handicapped, and does not require a program sponsor to modify the essential purpose of its program or undergo financial burdens to accommodate all handicapped persons.[192] The *Brecker* Court did note, however, that an application for admission by an individual who was both elderly or mobility-impaired *and* developmentally disabled would raise a

---

[186]*Id.; see also Knutzen*, 617 F. Supp. at 981.

[187]29 U.S.C. § 794. This section applies only to projects that receive "federal financial assistance." The regulations implementing Section 504, like those for the Age Discrimination in Employment Act (*see* § 23.1(a), above), define federal financial assistance to include either the receipt of federal funds or the services of federal personnel. 45 C.F.R. § 84.3. Thus, all projects that proceed under HUD, both those involving mortgage assistance and direct loans, must comply with Section 504.

[188]*See U.S. v. Baylor University Medical Center*, 564 F. Supp. 1495 (N.D. Tx. 1983), *modified* 736 F.2d 1039 (5th Cir. 1984); *U.S. v. University Hospital of SUNY at Stony Brook*, 575 F. Supp. 607 (D.C.N.Y. 1983), *aff'd* 729 F.2d 144 (2nd Cir. 1984). By similar reasoning, the Age Discrimination Act may also apply to facilities constructed with private monies but that receive Medicare or Medicaid funds. *See* § 23.1(a), above.

[189]*Id.*

[190]*Southeastern Community College v. Davis*, 442 U.S. 397, 406 (1979).

[191]607 F. Supp. at 435.

[192]*Id.; see also Southeastern Community College*, 442 U.S. at 410–11.

question of violation of Section 504.[193] Still, the Court felt that admission could be denied if the individual applicant's needs would be inconsistent with the program's design and services.

The key in analyzing whether an admissions policy that places restrictions on handicapped persons violates Section 504, then, is whether the individual's handicap is sufficiently program-related, in that it would prevent the individual from adequately participating in the program or interfere with achievement of the program's goals. Thus, for example, a facility with an included health care program that has established admission criteria based on health status may be able to exclude an applicant requiring kidney dialysis that cannot be offered at the facility, but may not be justified in excluding a blind applicant if the handicap does not preclude participation in the program.

§ 23.3   RELIGION

The Fair Housing Chapter of the Civil Rights Act of 1968 is a comprehensive open housing law that makes unlawful discrimination on the grounds of religion in the sale or rental of dwellings.[194] Unlike the statutes regarding age and handicap discrimination, the Fair Housing Act applies whether or not there has been federal financial assistance to a particular housing facility. Religious organizations may, however, limit sales or rentals of property that they operate for a noncommercial purpose to persons of the same religion unless membership in the religion is restricted on account of race, color, or national origin.[195]

In *United States v. Hughes Memorial Home*,[196] the federal District Court outlined the elements of this "carefully limited exception for certain religious organizations":

1. The exception is limited to *religious* organizations.
2. The exemption applies to mere *occupancy*, as well as the sale or rental of dwellings.
3. The dwellings must be owned and operated for *other than a commercial purpose*.
4. The religion must not discriminate in membership on account of race, color, or national origin for the exemption to apply.[197]

Hughes involved an allegation that a children's home had made dwellings unavailable to black children in violation of the Fair Housing Act. The

---

[193]607 F. Supp. at 438.
[194]42 U.S.C. § 3604.
[195]42 U.S.C. § 3607.
[196]396 F. Supp. 544 (W.D. Va. 1975).
[197]*Id*. at 550.

Court found that the home was not a religious organization, so the Section 3607 exemption did not apply. There appear to be no other reported federal cases that involve the application of this statutory exemption.

The courts have also held that giving preference to certain religious groups in federally assisted housing violates the due process, equal protection, and establishment of religion clauses of the United States Constitution. In *Otero v. New York Housing Authority*,[198] the housing authority had given preference to Jewish families in a low income housing project because it was conveniently located near an old and historic synagogue. The Court found that the Housing Authority's intention to preserve cultural and other values by this preferencing could not overcome the constitutional prohibition against government action in aid of religion.[199]

§ 23.4 NATIONAL ORIGIN

The Fair Housing Act also prohibits discrimination in the sale or rental of dwellings on the basis of national origin.[200] As with discrimination on the basis of religion, the Fair Housing Act applies here whether or not a housing facility has received any federal financial assistance. There appear to be no reported cases involving this particular prohibition of the statute. With regard to retirement facilities, this provision would evidently prohibit a project from formally limiting residence to members of any particular ethnic group or groups, although there might be a considerable amount of voluntary self-selection involved among applicants to the facility.

§ 24 SECURITIES REGISTRATION

One of the most often overlooked subjects in the development of full-service retirement facilities is the application of federal or state securities laws to the financial transaction between the resident and facility operator or developer. Even the traditional practice of many nonprofit continuing care facilities of collecting deposits from prospective residents prior to construction of the facility, and then using those monies to build the project, can raise securities issues that have been largely ignored by developers, consumers, and the government. Perhaps the most significant reason for this phenomenon is that continuing care facilities have largely been nonprofit, church-affiliated enterprises, and in states where continuing care has flourished, other forms of regulation have diverted attention from the securities question.[201] With the trend toward refundable entrance fees,

---

[198]344 F. Supp. 737 (S.D.N.Y. 1972).

[199]*Id.* at 746.

[200]42 U.S.C. § 3604.

[201]In states without continuing care regulation, prosecutors have used securities laws to convict certain promoters of fraudulent life care facility offerings. *See* § 5.1, above.

memberships, and similar structures where a resident expects to receive a payment several years after investing money in the facility, and with the growth of profit-motivated developers, even more serious concerns should exist about the application of securities laws.

Federal law defines a security as follows:

> The term 'security' means any note, stock, treasury stock, bond, debenture, *evidence of indebtedness, certificate of interest or participation in any profit-sharing agreement,* collateral-trust certificate, *preorganization certificate or subscription, transferable share, investment contract,* voting-trust certificate, certificate of deposit for a security, fractional undivided interest in oil, gas, or other mineral rights, any put, call, straddle, option, or privilege on any security, certificate of deposit, or group or index of securities (including any interest therein or based on the value thereof), or any put, call, straddle, option, or privilege entered into on a national securities exchange relating to foreign currency, or, in general, any interest or instrument commonly known as a 'security', or any certificate of interest or participation in, temporary or interim certificate for, receipt for, guarantee of, or warrant or right to subscribe to or purchase, any of the foregoing.[202]

Given the extremely broad language of the statutory definition, it is theoretically possible that a refundable entrance fee contract could constitute an evidence of indebtedness, a preconstruction entrance fee deposit might be classified as a preorganization certificate or subscription, a cooperative share, membership, or condominium interest could be considered a transferable share, and any residence agreement in which the purchaser has a risk of financial loss, or the opportunity to profit might be argued to be an investment contract.

The federal courts interpreting the definition of securities have tended to focus upon whether the investment creates an opportunity for profit. In cases of cooperatives, transferable memberships, condominium sales, or limited partnership or stock purchase arrangements entitling a person to admission in a retirement facility, for example, where a resident might be able to sell the interest, after several years, to a new resident at a profit, there is a substantial question as to whether a security is created.

However, the U.S. Supreme Court held, in *United Housing Foundation, Inc. v. Forman,*[203] that the sale of shares in a cooperative real estate development is exempt from the federal Act, where residents could resell shares to the cooperative at the original purchase price upon termination of occupancy. The Court found that, although that type of investment might ordinarily be characterized as a security, it presented no reasonable expectation of profit from the managerial or entrepreneurial efforts of others. The Court also noted that the promoters emphasized housing and did not seek to attract investors by the prospect of profits. Residents were found to have been

[202] 15 U.S.C. § 77b(1); emphasis added.
[203] 421 U.S. 837 (1975).

attracted solely by the prospect of acquiring a place to live, and not by financial returns on investment.

Although the *United Housing Foundation* case may stand for an exemption from federal securities laws for all forms of housing used as a personal residence, its facts precluded any possibility of profit. At least one federal Circuit Court of Appeals reviewed a transaction where cooperative tenants could sell their shares to a new lessee-purchaser at whatever profit (or loss) the market would bear. In addition, tenants could receive periodic distributions and dividends. The court found that despite the profit opportunity, the continuing requirement that tenants pay monthly fees indicated that the transaction was for housing and not investment in a security.[204] The Tenth Circuit has also reiterated that the promotional emphasis of the developer is central in determining whether real estate sales are securities, and that they are not where "purchasers were induced to obtain them primarily for residential purposes" and where "the benefit to the purchasers of the amenities promised . . . was largely in their own use and enjoyment."[205]

The Securities and Exchange Commission (SEC) has likewise ruled that a proposal to offer retirement condominiums need not comply with registration requirements.[206] Finally, at least two federal district courts have found that nontransferable life care contract interests were not securities.[207]

State laws pose particular concerns with respect to securities registration of retirement facility transactions because state statutes and the interpretations of courts and administrative agencies may differ widely from federal standards. For example, in *Silver Hills Country Club v. Sobiesky*,[208] the California Supreme Court found that a registerable security was issued when developers planning to construct a country club solicited membership fees that were used to finance development of the facility. Members later would be able to sell their memberships at a profit, if possible. The Court determined that because the investment of the prospective members was at risk, the transaction fit within the definition of a security under California law, which is almost identical to the definition appearing in the federal statute. Recently enacted life care legislation in California provides an exemption from treatment as securities for transactions subject to regulation as life care contracts.[209] Other states, such as New York, impose extensive registration and disclosure requirements for cooperative housing offerings.[210]

---

[204]*Grenader v. Spitz*, 537 F.2d 612 (2d Cir. 1976).

[205]*Aldrich v. McCulloch Properties, Inc.*, 627 F.2d 1036 (10th Cir. 1980).

[206]*Culverhouse, et al.*, (SEC 1973) '73-'74 CCH dec. ¶ 79,612.

[207]*Waldo v. Central Indiana Lutheran Retirement Home* (S.D. Ind., Nov. 16, 1979) 1980 (CCH) *Fed. Sec. L. Rep.* ¶ 97,680; *Ashenback v. Covenant Living Centers–North* (E.D. Wis., Feb. 4, 1980) 1979–1980 (CCH) *Fed. Sec. L. Rep.* ¶ 97,369.

[208]55 Cal. 2d 811, 361 P.2d 906 (1961).

[209]West's Cal. Health & Safety Code § 1770(d) (1987).

[210]See CCH, *Blue Sky Law Reports*, ¶ 42,523.

As more developers enter the retirement housing field and develop creative and unusual payment structures for their facilities, the risk of application of state or federal securities laws to retirement facility transactions will increase. Although most elderly people seeking to enter a retirement facility are looking primarily for a principal residence and not an investment, they nevertheless may be risking substantial assets in a venture whose success depends on the development and operational abilities of others. If there are inadequate licensing laws and other protections in a particular state, it is likely that government officials, or consumers who have lost their investment in a failed project, may resort to state or federal securities laws for relief.

§ 25   LOCAL LAWS

§ 25.1   ZONING

The most direct local government impact upon developing retirement facilities is through the zoning and permit approval processes. While specific requirements may vary widely from one jurisdiction to another, several common issues often present themselves.

Lack of understanding of the retirement facility concept is often a principal concern when dealing with local governmental bodies. Uninitiated cities or towns may erroneously view retirement facilities as primarily health care institutions and give them the less favored land-use planning status often reserved for hospitals, nursing homes, or psychiatric facilities. It is therefore important to emphasize the primarily residential character of most such facilities. In general, retirement facilities have been considered by most courts to be excluded from zoning ordinances prohibiting hospitals or hotels in a given area, but included in ordinance definitions permitting apartments or multifamily uses.[211]

Municipalities may, of course, restrict the development of retirement facilities in accordance with their zoning ordinances. There are, however, certain limitations on the arbitrary use of the zoning power or ordinances that are not authorized by the state zoning enabling act. For example, some states prohibit local restrictions on the number of unrelated individuals who may live together in a house.[212] Such a regulation might have an impact

---

[211] *See, generally,* the extensive case annotations on zoning for senior citizen communities and elderly housing at 83 ALR 3d 1084 and 83 ALR 3d 1103. *See also,* J. Hancock, ed., *Housing the Elderly,* Center for Urban Policy Research (New Brunswick, NJ, 1987) 49–56, 95–117, regarding public policy arguments for age-segregated housing for the elderly.

[212] California, New Jersey, Pennsylvania, and Michigan, among others, have struck down such restrictions on state constitutional grounds. *City of Santa Barbara v. Adamson,* 27 Cal.3d 123, 153 Cal. Rptr. 507, 610 P.2d 436 (Cal. 1980); *State v. Baker,* 405 A.2d 368 (N.J. 1979); *Children's Home v. City of Easton* 417A.2d 830 (Pa. 1980); *Charter Township v. Denolfo,* 351 N.W.2d 831 (Mich. 1984). However, most states follow the U.S. Supreme Court's lead in *Village of Belle Terre v. Boraas,* 416 U.S. 1 (1974), which held that consideration of family relationships in zoning ordinances is appropriate under the Due Process clause. *See, e.g., Town of Durham v. White Enterprises,* 348 A.2d 706 (N.H. 1975); *Rademan v. City and County of Denver,* 526 P.2d 1325 (Colo. 1974).

on a small board and care home. Municipalities may also not be able to prevent the development of retirement facilities that are compatible with the other uses already permitted in a district.

The recent U.S. Supreme Court decision in *City of Cleburne v. Cleburne Living Center* is instructive in this latter regard.[213] In *Cleburne*, the city denied a conditional use permit for the operation of a group home for the mentally retarded in a zone that allowed such permits for hospitals, nursing homes, and homes for the aged. The Supreme Court, speaking through Justice White, found that mental retardation was not a "quasisuspect class" and did not merit special scrutiny under the Equal Protection Clause. Nonetheless, the Court held that the Texas statute was based solely on unsubstantiated fears of the mentally retarded, and struck down the statute as having no rational basis. The Court in *Cleburne* used a stricter rational basis test than it has employed in past decisions, and found that group homes for the mentally retarded were no different than those uses already permitted in the area.

It is likely that the Court would apply a similar analysis to a case involving a home for the aged. Like mental retardation, age is not a suspect classification under the Equal Protection Clause.[214] Nonetheless, facilities for senior citizens are unlikely to cause unique problems if their use is generally compatible with others in the zone. Thus, special restrictions on retirement facilities are likely to be struck down under the *Cleburne* rationale. A municipality probably could not prohibit a small board and care home in an area zoned for single-family residences, a senior citizen complex in an area zoned for multifamily use, or deny a conditional use permit to a home for the aged where hospitals were permitted, absent a convincing showing of special circumstances.

On the other hand, many municipalities have enacted ordinances specifically designed to enable the development of retirement centers.[215] These may make appropriate distinctions between congregate housing, board and care, and continuing care facilities, prescribing different treatment for each. Issues such as site size and coverage densities, proximity to health services, grocery stores, and other facilities, parking, kitchens, architectural details and amenities, staffing, basic services, and even resident contract terms may be covered.[216]

Zoning ordinances that provide for districts where residency is restricted to senior citizens have been upheld against a variety of legal challenges. Key cases in New York and New Jersey have held that such

---

[213]471 U.S. 1002 (1985); *see also* Note, "City of Cleburne v. Cleburne Living Center: *Rational Basis With a Bite?*" 20 U.S.F.L. Rev. 927 (1986).

[214]*Mass. Bd. of Retirement v. Murgia*, 427 U.S. 307 (1976).

[215]*E.g.*, Niles, Orland Park, and Schaumberg, Illinois.

[216]*See* Ordinance No. 1540, Orland Park, IL, June 17, 1986.

ordinances are authorized by state zoning enabling acts, which permit zoning for the purpose of promoting the general welfare of the community.[217] These courts have found that communities are promoting the general welfare by providing for the specialized needs of the elderly that are not adequately met in the general housing market.

The courts have also rejected constitutional challenges to age restrictive zoning on due process and equal protection grounds. The Supreme Court of New Jersey in the *Weymouth Township* case[218] closely examined and subsequently rejected these contentions. The Court held that housing is not a fundamental right protected by the fourteenth amendment,[219] nor is age a suspect classification,[220] so that strict scrutiny of the ordinance by the Court was inappropriate. Rather, the municipality had only to show that the ordinance had a rational basis related to the public welfare, a fact already established to the Court's satisfaction in its consideration of whether the ordinance was within the scope of the zoning enabling act.

Finally, courts have generally upheld age restrictive zoning against claims that it violated general state statutes prohibiting housing discrimination on the basis of age. Although conceding facial violations of the general terms of the statutes, the courts refused to give effect to such a literal interpretation, citing the fact that favoritism to the elderly was not among the statute's enumerated prohibited practices, and the state's policies of encouraging construction of housing for the aged.[221] Some states have amended their zoning statutes to specifically authorize zoning to promote housing for the elderly, or have amended their antidiscrimination statutes to remove housing for the elderly from their prohibitions.[222]

One limitation on the extent of age-restrictive zoning has been suggested by the Supreme Court's decision in *Moore v. City of East Cleveland*.[223] There, the court held that a municipality cannot, through the enforcement of a single-family residence zoning ordinance, restrict which family members can live together. Thus, an age restrictive zoning ordinance that operated in such a manner as to prevent family members (even extended ones) from living with one another would probably be unconstitutional.

---

[217] *See, Maldini v. Ambro*, 36 N.Y.2d 330; 330 N.E.2d 403; 396 N.Y.S.2d 385 (1985); *Taxpayer's Ass'n., Inc. v. Weymouth Township*, 71 N.J. 249, 364 A.2d 1016 (1976); *Shepard v. Woodland Township Committee and Planning Board*, 71 N.J. 230, 364 A.2d 1005 (1976).

[218] *Taxpayer's Ass'n., Inc. v. Weymouth Township*, 71 N.J. 249, 364 A.2d 1016 (1976).

[219] *Lindsey v. Normet*, 405 U.S. 56 (1972).

[220] *Murgia*, note 214, above.

[221] *Weymouth*, note 217 above, 71 N.J. 285 n. 16; see also discussion of laws regarding age discrimination in housing, § 23.1.

[222] N.J. Stat. Ann. § 40:55D-65g; Cal. Civ. Code §§ 51.2, 51.3.

[223] 431 U.S. 494 (1977).

25.2   ASSESSMENTS, RENT CONTROLS

Retirement projects tend to raise additional special issues not present in conventional projects. A major concern of local governments is that the project, like most health facilities, will not be on the tax rolls (see discussion of state tax exemptions at § 10). On the other hand, retirement facilities tend to have a less severe impact upon local services than many other types of uses. Retirement facilities, even if operated for profit, may therefore have legitimate grounds for asserting exemption from school district assessments or other payments that do not benefit elderly residents.

However, even if a facility is entitled to exemption under state or local law, it may often be necessary to agree to accept local taxation or assessments as a condition of planning approval. These assessments may be levied by a municipality through the subdivision approval process, the issuance of building permits, or where a zoning variance, conditional use, or rezoning is needed from the municipality in order to secure development approval.

The courts have easily upheld requirements that the developer provide internal streets and similar improvements needed by the subdivision or facility.[224] More difficult problems have arisen where dedications or in-lieu fees are required for off-site streets, parks, and schools. The courts have generally sustained such assessments where two conditions are met. First, the assessments must be authorized by the state's zoning enabling act. Such authority has frequently been implied from the statute, but more and more states are enacting specific provisions authorizing contributions for off-site facilities, such as parks.[225] Second, there must be a rational nexus between the burden on the community created by the development and the municipality's assessment. Such a nexus has generally been found where there is a reasonable basis for attributing the increased off-site community needs to the development.[226] Thus, the development of large retirement facilities might support an assessment for parks or public transportation (if authorized by the statute), but not in-lieu fees to support schools.

Rent controls are another form of local regulation often uniquely affecting retirement facility projects. Often, licensure as a care facility may be a basis for exemption from rent controls on the ground that charges are based largely on facility service costs rather than simply for provision of housing (see discussion at § 20.3(b)). In addition, rules attendant to HUD financing may result in preemption of local rent control laws (see discussion at § 22.5(a)). Local rent control ordinances may also by their terms exclude retirement facilities from their ambit, but such exclusions must be explicit, as courts are unlikely to imply an exclusion from the language of the ordinance.[227]

---

[224] *See, e.g., Blevens v. City of Manchester*, 120 A.2d 121 (N.H. 1961).

[225] Cal. Govt. Code § 65970; Colo. Rev. Stat. § 30-28-133(4)(a).

[226] *Jordan v. City of Menomonee Falls*, 137 N.W.2d 442 (Wis. 1965).

[227] *Klarfeld v. Berg*, 29 Cal. 3d 893, 176 Cal. Rptr. 539, 633 P.2d 204 (1981).

Local laws can be among the most vexing with which to deal due to the general absence of binding interpretive precedents and the sometimes apparently whimsical application of local ordinances to specific projects. Local governmental bodies are often among the first encountered in the process of development. Yet it is all too common an occurrence that retirement facilities-in-planning progress far down the road in development of design, legal structure, marketing, and licensure application, but are ultimately stopped at the local government approval level after numerous hearings. Sometimes, when planning approval is a problem, substantial progress in marketing, design, and financial and legal planning can aid in obtaining approval. Sometimes, it simply represents wasted expense.

Site selection should take seriously into consideration the characteristics of the local jurisdiction and its experience with other related facilities or projects. If possible, local planning approvals should be secured at the earliest possible date, before other expenses mount.

Eight

Financing the Delivery of Care

An elderly person embarking on retirement years should be planning for his or her financial future. The fact that a retired person can no longer look to employment income and must rely on the proceeds of pensions, Social Security, and earnings on investments motivates many to seek a living situation that will provide some measure of economic stability over a long period of time. Although factors such as inflation and other changes in the cost of living pose some concern for anyone planning for the future, a more significant concern for an elderly person is that a serious illness may strike and wipe out a lifetime's worth of savings and force the person to become dependent upon subsistence-level government programs, or to become a burden to family or friends.

Many retirement facilities, both nonprofit and, more recently, for profit, are seeking to help residents ensure that they will be able to maintain a level standard of living for the remainder of their lives by investing in a health insurance type of program early in their retirement years. Retirement facility programs may utilize available government benefits and supplement them with private funds pooled in an in-house reserve, or used to purchase an indemnity policy or to enroll in a health plan furnished by a third party service provider.

The funding of care for the elderly is one of the most timely subjects currently facing national policy makers. At present, retirement facility plans are among the few existing methods by which long-term care for the nonpoor elderly is being funded on a group basis. In coming years, we can expect substantial activity to be devoted to expanding retirement facility health financing programs, creating federal and state incentives to encourage development of privately funded insurance and health plans, and redirecting government resources from expensive acute care to less intensive, longer term health needs.

§ 26   GOVERNMENT FUNDING OF HEALTH CARE EXPENSES

§ 26.1   BASIC PROGRAMS AND BENEFITS

(a)   In General

Approximately $425 billion, or 10.7 percent of the gross national product, is spent annually for health care in the United States.[1] While constituting only 12 percent of the population, persons 65 and over were responsible for about a third of all personal health care expenditures.[2] Two principal federal health financing programs, Medicare and Medicaid, account for 49 percent and 13 percent, respectively, of all personal health care expenditures.[3]

Of the total health care expenditures for older Americans, about 45 percent goes for hospital-related charges, 20 percent each for physician and nursing home services, and the rest for other forms of care.[4] Yet, while government pays about $48 billion of the $54 billion spent on hospital care for the elderly, it pays less than half of the $25 billion expended for nursing care.[5] Of the out-of-pocket health care costs paid by the elderly, only six percent is for hospitalizations, whereas 42 percent is spent on nursing home services.[6] The need for long-term nursing care is thus one of the greatest financial risks facing older persons today.

(b)   Hospital Orientation of Medicare

Fundamental differences in eligibility criteria and coverages of the Medicare and Medicaid programs help explain the disparity in government financing for the different levels of care. The Medicare program is available to, among others, all persons entitled to social security benefits as of the first day of the month in which they attain age 65.[7] The widely available

---

[1] *HHS News*, July 29, 1986, U.S. Department of Health and Human Services, citing 1985 figures.

[2] "Aging America: Trends and Projections," 1985–86 ed. U.S. Senate Special Committee on Aging, pp. 107–108; personal health care expenditures include all expenditures except research.

[3] *Id.*, at 103.

[4] *Id.*, at 104.

[5] *Id.*

[6] *Id.*, at 106.

[7] *See*, CCH, *Medicare and Medicaid Guide*, ¶¶ 1101, 1115.

Medicare dollars for the elderly go predominantly for hospital care (69 percent) and physicians (25 percent), while only *one percent* pays for nursing home care.[8]

Although Medicare coverage is extensive, it by no means covers all hospital costs, and is of minimal usefulness for long-term care needs.

(1) Medicare Copayments and Deductibles for Acute Hospitalization

Medicare covers most acute care costs for the elderly population. Medicare Part A, available to Social Security recipients, covers 150 days of inpatient hospital services for a single spell of illness. In general, the first 60 days are fully covered, subject only to the initial deductible amount ($520 for 1987). Each of the next 30 days is subject to a coinsurance payment by the patient of one-fourth of the inpatient hospital deductible ($130). The last 60 days are subject to a *daily* coinsurance payment of half the inpatient deductible ($260). The last 60 days of coverage are also limited to once-in-a-lifetime use.[9]

Although deductibles and copayments rise rapidly over time, as a practical matter, most hospital stays are of short duration,[10] and "Medi-Gap" insurance policies (see § 27.1) can cover the deductibles and coinsurance payments at relatively little expense.

Certain physician, outpatient hospital, and other charges are covered under Medicare Part B, which is generally available to Part A recipients, for a 1987 monthly premium of $17.90. There is an annual deductible of $75 and a 20 percent copayment requirement for patients.[11] Often, however, physicians will accept the 80 percent paid by Medicare as payment in full.

(2) Minimal Medicare Coverage for Long-Term Care

Most long-term nursing care is not covered by Medicare, which covers only short-term periods of recuperation in a nursing facility begun within 30 days after an acute hospital stay of three or more days.[12] The benefits last for 100 days, but after the twentieth day, a patient coinsurance payment of $65 *per day* (1987 figure) is triggered.[13] Except in areas where nursing care is unusually expensive, this effectively eliminates the benefit for many typical long-term care situations.

---

[8]Aging America, note 2, above, at 107.

[9]*See, generally*, note 7 above, ¶ 1251.

[10]Average hospital lengths of stay range from 9.7 days for those 65 and older, to 11.1 days for those 85 and older and are declining. Aging America, note 2, above, at 99.

[11]Note 7, ¶¶ 3057, 3182.

[12]*Id.*, at ¶ 1304.

[13]*Id.*, at ¶¶ 1358, 1369.

(3) Home Health Limited

Home health benefits are available under Medicare Part A or Part B for persons confined to their homes, and in need of intermittent skilled nursing care, or physical or speech therapy.[14] Services can also include social services and home health aide services.[15] There are no patient copayments or deductibles. Only about three percent of Medicare benefits are for home health.[16] (See also § 20.4 for a discussion of Medicare coverage problems for home health needs.)

(c) Medicaid: Long-Term Care for the Poor

Unlike Medicare, which is available without regard to economic status, Medicaid is a federal- and state-funded program designed to benefit only the poor and near-poor.[17] All state Medicaid programs must permit enrollment of certain categorically needy persons, such as recipients of Aid to Families with Dependent Children (AFDC) or of Supplemental Security Income (SSI).[18] In addition, states may elect to cover medically needy persons who have sufficient income and assets to pay for daily living expenses, but not for health care. For the 30 states that have medically needy programs, eligible enrollees are permitted, on the average, to have no greater than about $1800 in resources.[19]

Unlike Medicare, Medicaid covers nursing care without blanket restrictions on lengths of stay or requirements that patients absorb deductible or copayment costs. While 69 percent of Medicaid expenditures for the elderly is for nursing home costs,[20] elderly persons must first become impoverished before they can take advantage of the program.

In 1985, the American Association of Retired Persons conducted a survey of its members and found that nearly 80 percent of those who thought they would spend some time in a nursing facility believed that the federal government's Medicare program would pay for all or part of it.[21] In fact, however, Medicare pays only two percent of the cost of nursing home care in this country, while Medicaid pays 54 percent of nursing facility

---

[14]*Id.*, at ¶ 1401.

[15]*Id.*

[16]*See,* "Home Care Fact Sheet," April 1986, National Association for Home Care, at 2., citing 1985 Medicare Part A and B outlays.

[17]Note 7, above, at ¶ 14,010.

[18]Note 7, above, at ¶ 14,231.

[19]ICF, Inc., "Private Financing of Long Term Care: Current Methods and Resources," Phase I Final Report, U.S. Department of Health and Human Resources, 1985, at 91 (Phase II also published 1985).

[20]*See* Aging America, note 2, above, at 108.

[21]*See* Garland, S., "Nursing-home Time Bomb Threatens an Aging Nation," San Francisco Examiner Nov. 3, 1985, at E-1.

charges.[22] The elderly themselves, or their families, pay 43 percent of the bill, and only the remaining *one percent* is covered by private insurance.[23] (See discussion of private long-term care insurance at § 27.2).

Becoming eligible for the Medicaid program is not a very desirable alternative for many middle or upper income elderly persons. Although the eligibility criteria may vary from one state to another, the program essentially requires that an elderly applicant spend down virtually all of his or her assets and income to pay for nursing care before the Medicaid program will begin to pick up the bill. One study found that 63 percent of elderly persons without a spouse became poor after only 13 weeks in a nursing facility.[24] Within a year, 83 percent had become impoverished.

In addition, because of the limited resources of government, Medicaid programs in the various states tend to pay considerably less for nursing services than facility owners charge patients who are paying their own bills or who are covered by private insurance. In facilities that cater to Medicaid patients in high percentages, this disparity between the government rate of reimbursement and the usual private pay charges can mean that a lower quality of care and amenities is provided in Medicaid-dependent facilities.

(d)   Miscellaneous Federal Programs

Federal programs that were not necessarily designed specifically to provide care for older persons, but that may be contributing to the cost of care, include Supplemental Security Income, Social Services Block Grants, and the Older Americans Act.[25]

(1)   Supplemental Security Income

Supplemental Security Income (SSI)[26] is a federal assistance program available to aged, blind, and disabled persons whose income falls below certain levels. States may supplement federal SSI payments; about 35 states make specific payments to support persons in some form of community-based group living arrangements with nonmedical services such as personal care.[27]

(2)   Older Americans Act

Grants are made to the states under this program for creation of supportive services for the elderly such as in-home services, home health aides, visitation,

---

[22]*Id.*

[23]*Id.*

[24]Massachusetts Blue Cross-Blue Shield Study, 1985, reported in *Congressional Quarterly*, May 31, 1986, at 1228.

[25]*See* O'Shaughnessy, *et al.*, note 50, below, at 31–39.

[26]*See* 42 U.S.C. §§ 1381 *et. seq.*

[27]O'Shaughnessy et al., note 50, below, at 38–39.

adult day care, respite services, congregate meals, home-delivered meals, long-term care ombudsman programs, and senior centers.[28]

Grants are administered by state and area agencies on aging. The appropriation for 1987 is a relatively small $829 million.[29]

(3)   Social Services Block Grants

The Social Services Block Grant program[30] (Title XX of the Social Security Act) provides federal grants to states for, among other things, "preventing or reducing inappropriate institutional care by providing for community based care, home-based care, or other forms of less intensive care."[31] All states provide some form of home care services under the program, but the orientation is predominantly social services and not health care.[32] The program is not designed for the elderly, and there are many competing demands on the comparatively moderate sums available.[33]

§ 26.2   PROPOSALS FOR FEDERAL PROGRAM CHANGES

(a)   Catastrophic Coverage

Recent proposals for federal legislation—one coming, at the direction of the President, from Health and Human Services Secretary Bowen—have focused serious attention on expanding Medicare benefits to cover so-called catastrophic health care problems. From the numerous proposals emerging in the 100th Congress,[34] the bill which finally emrged, H.R. 2470, would eliminate inpatient hospital copayments, eliminate the current 150 day hospitalization limit, extend nursing coverage from 100 to 150 days, and nearly eliminate the nursing care copayment.[35] Although the bill primarily expands hospital coverage, which is financially more "doable" than providing meaningful coverage of long-term care, a presidential veto has been predicted.[36]

---

[28] See 42 U.S.C. §§ 3001 et seq.

[29] O'Shaughnessy, et al., note 50, below, at 35.

[30] 42 U.S.C. §§ 1397 et seq.

[31] 42 U.S.C. § 1397(4).

[32] O'Shaughnessy, et al., note 50, below, at 31–34.

[33] About $2.7 billion. Id.

[34] E.g., H.R. 65, 1245, 1280, 1281 (100th Congress); See "Panel Considers Alternatives to Bowen Plan," Congressional Quarterly, March 7, 1987, at 434.

[35] See Older Americans Report, July 24, 1987, 1–3.

[36] Id., see also "Congress Takes Ball and Runs After State of the Union Punt," Congressional Quarterly, Jan. 31, 1987, at 208.

Critics of proposals to implement changes primarily affecting hospital care have long contended that the true health financing catastrophe for most elderly people is not the occurrence of an acute illness requiring hospitalization, but rather the onset of a chronic condition requiring long-term nursing care.[37] While long-term care,[38] due to the general lack of comprehensive coverage from government or private insurance sources, almost certainly is the greatest unresolved health financing problem for the elderly, the cost is potentially staggering, and there is wide disagreement regarding how the nation should address the problem.[39]

(b) Harvard Medicare Project Proposals

The Harvard Medicare Project used the occasion of the twentieth anniversary of Medicare to study its successes and failures and make suggestions for fundamental areas of change.[40]

In general, the Project recommended less reliance on beneficiary copayments, and advocated increases in premiums to offset the resulting revenue loss. Copayments, they reasoned, are unpredictable, and strike the sickest most severely, whereas premiums are predictable, do not penalize the sick, and can be adjusted to income levels.

For chronic illnesses, the study recommends expanding Medicare coverage for nursing home care from its currently limited, post-hospital rehabilitative approach to one that pays for long-term illnesses. Funding would be accomplished as for other Medicare benefits, but with a residential copayment from beneficiaries equal to 80 percent of Social Security benefits. The copayment would be designed to help reimburse the nonhealth care residential living expenses that make up a large part of the cost of nursing care.

The study also recommends increasing benefits for less cost-intensive outpatient health services, such as home health, establishing physician reimbursement rate schedules, requiring physicians to accept assignment of Medicare benefits as payment in full for their services, establishing target budgets for hospitals, and creating incentives for health maintenance organizations to create more programs specializing in the health needs of the elderly.

---

[37]See "Long Term Care: The True 'Catastrophe'?" *Congressional Quarterly*, May 31, 1986, at 1227; Brickfield, C., "Long Term Care Insurance: One Piece of the Puzzle," *Health Span* (June 1985), 11.

[38]Long-term care refers generically to nursing care for chronic illnesses, and not long-term hospital stays.

[39]See, e.g., *Congressional Quarterly*, May 31, 1986, discussing federal and private sector alternatives.

[40]See, *New England Journal of Medicine*, 314, No. 11 (March 13, 1986), at 722, for a summary of the findings.

(c)   Public Policy Incentives for Retirement Facility Care Plans

Medicare provides substantial coverage for hospitalization costs, but in the more than 20 years of its existence, it has not reduced the percentage of personal income the elderly must spend on health care.[41] Moreover, while Medicare pays for expensive acute health care for elderly persons who might be able to afford to purchase insurance privately, government funding for less expensive nursing care is available only to the virtually poor. Although cost-based Medicare reimbursement has been largely replaced with a less generous prospective payment system, the Medicare program has created, and may still continue to foster, incentives to care for the elderly in the more costly hospital setting, sometimes unnecessarily.

Approaches to containment of the nation's rising health care costs include direct regulatory efforts, such as limits on government reimbursement, and market-oriented strategies, such as incentives for creation of health maintenance organizations and other alternative delivery systems.[42] Retirement facilities that encourage healthy older persons to invest their resources in plans that will cover or help defray future long-term care costs similarly present a market-oriented strategy that can help relieve the government of its health expenditures burden.[43] And retirement facilities, as residential communities, have even greater opportunities for utilization controls, preventive health care, and use of social/psychological support mechanisms than typical health plans.

There have been very few federal incentives to establish retirement facility plans for long-term care coverage.[44] However, added tax benefits for conversion of home equity to purchase of a qualified retirement facility health plan,[45] or a deduction for periodic contributions made into a restricted long-term care account,[46] could encourage older persons to plan for their future long-term health needs rather than spend down to become eligible for Medicaid. Likewise, if Medicare provided *some* funding for chronic long-term care (as opposed to recuperative benefits), on condition that the beneficiary were also enrolled in a qualified private plan paying a substantial share of the costs, the government might help discourage unnecessary Medicare hospitalizations and reduce Medicaid enrollment. Home

---

[41]The elderly continue to spend about 15 percent of their income on health care, as before the enactment of the Medicare program. *See Aging America*, note 2 above, at 106.

[42]*See* Lundy, J. "Issue Brief: Health Care Cost Containment," Congressional Research Service, October 31, 1986.

[43]*See* § 27.3(a), *below*.

[44]Certain homes for the aging may be eligible for tax exemption (*see* § 9.2), and some continuing care facilities are eligible for an imputed interest rule exemption (*see* § 6.2(b)(2)).

[45]Prepaid medical expenses are already eligible for a tax deduction (*see* § 6.1(c)), but only to the extent they exceed 7.5 percent of adjusted gross income. Large lump sum health care prepayments by the elderly could be exempted from the 7.5 percent threshold.

[46]*See* § 27.3(c).

care may also be more efficiently provided in a retirement facility, and therefore a loosening of Medicare's "intermittent" and "home bound" requirements may be economically justified.[47] Any successful plan would likely be dependent on, but at the same time generate, increased consumer awareness of the general absence of long-term care coverage.

§ 27   PRIVATE FUNDING OF HEALTH CARE EXPENSES

§ 27.1   MEDIGAP INSURANCE

The many out-of-pocket copayments and deductibles chargeable to Medicare beneficiaries in connection with their hospital care[48] have led to a proliferation in the marketplace of so-called Medigap insurance policies designed to cover such expenses. A recent General Accounting Office study, reviewing nearly 400 different policies offered by 92 commercial firms and 13 Blue Cross/Blue Shield plans, represented less than half of the estimated $5 billion Medigap market.[49] About two-thirds of the elderly currently have a Medigap policy in force.[50]

Although plentiful, Medigap insurance policies are not at all effective in filling the largest gap in Medicare coverage—the expenses of subacute care. Federal legislation[51] enacted in 1980 establishes minimum benefit coverage standards for Medigap policies on a nationwide basis. For inpatient hospitalizations, Medigap policies must pay the daily Medicare beneficiary copayment from the 61st through 150th day of stay, plus 90 percent of covered charges from the 151st to the 365th day.[52] But there is no requirement whatsoever that any coverage be extended for skilled nursing or home health care, even for copayments required in connection with Medicare covered convalescent nursing care.[53]

§ 27.2   LONG-TERM CARE INSURANCE

(a)   Historical Unavailability

In sharp contrast with the eagerness demonstrated in the Medigap market, the insurance industry has been exceedingly slow (or reluctant) to respond

---

[47]See § 20.4.

[48]See § 26.1.

[49]"Medigap Insurance," GAO Report to House Subcommittee on Health, Committee on Ways and Means, Oct. 1986, at 3.

[50]O'Shaughnessy, Price, & Griffith, "Financing and Delivery of Long-Term Care Services for the Elderly," Congressional Research Service, Feb. 24, 1987, p. 56.

[51]P.L. 96-265 (Baucus Amendment).

[52]GAO Report, note 49, above, at 20.

[53]Id.

to the need for private sector initiatives to help indemnify the costs of long-term nursing care. Although only 12 policies covering a scant 50,000 persons nationwide were estimated to exist as of early 1985, it has been predicted that, over the next 35 years, the market will sustain a $20 billion industry.[54] Several reasons have been offered for the current scarcity of policies:[55] (1) people believe they are already covered by Medicare; (2) the elderly are unwilling to acknowledge the risk of a need for eventual chronic care while they are still young enough to make premiums affordable; (3) insurers fear overutilization of services; (4) consumers realize Medicaid is available in case of dire emergency; (5) demand for group insurance does not exist, and marketing policies on an individual basis is too costly; (6) state regulations are too diverse, requiring that a custom product be tailored for each state; (7) state regulations are overly broad and fail to make distinctions between long-term care and other types of health insurance; and (8) the product would be too expensive for most elderly persons. Very recently, some innovations have taken place that challenge many of these assumptions (see § 27.2(c)).

(b) Confusing Array of Benefits

Even the few policies that had evolved by early 1986 tended to contain a widely divergent range of conditions of eligibility and limitations on coverages. One review of the nine "most comprehensive" policies[56] revealed a bewilderingly broad spectrum of benefits and limitations:

1. Skilled nursing daily benefits ranging from only $12 to as much as $120;
2. Custodial care daily benefits from as little as $10 after 20 days of skilled or intermediate care, to a high of $120 after skilled care of any duration;
3. Home care benefits from zero to $60 per day following 30 days of nursing care;
4. Prior hospitalization requirements of up to three days within 14 days of nursing home admission;
5. Waiting periods of up to 100 days before benefits commence;
6. Limits on total available nursing coverage ranging from 1000 days to five years; and
7. Annual premiums starting at $179 for some 55-year-olds and reaching $4460 for some 75-year-olds.

[54]ICF, Inc., Phase I, note 19, above, at 12, and *Older Americans Reports,* March 20, 1987, 2.

[55]*See, generally,* Meiners & Gollub, "Long-term Care Insurance: The Edge of an Emerging Market," *Healthcare Financial Management* (March 1984), at 58; *New England Journal of Medicine,* note 40, above, at 725; ICF, Inc., note 19, above, at 81–105.

[56]*See,* Topolnicki, "When a Nursing Home Becomes Your Poorhouse," *Money* (March 1986), at 175.

(c) Long-Term Care Insurance Innovations

(1) Development of Standards and Incentives

Some commentators have found that the confusing array of benefits, conditions, and limitations among long-term care insurance products is reminiscent of the status of the Medigap market in its early stages prior to federal legislation, and have called for uniform definitions, minimum coverage standards, and other reforms.[57]

One recent development that may lead to greater uniformity among long-term care insurance policies, and ease of product development on a national scale, is the adoption by the National Association of Insurance Commissioners, in late 1986, of a Model Long Term Care Insurance Act.

The Model Act requires, among other things, (1) no cancelation of coverage on the grounds of age or mental or physical deterioration, (2) no new waiting period in the event of a conversion or replacement of coverage, (3) no coverage exclusion for losses arising from preexisting illnesses, where the loss occurs more than 12 months following the effective date of coverage for those 65 or over, and 24 months thereafter for those under 65, (4) no mandated loss ratios, (5) no prior institutionalization requirement within a period of less than 14 days, and (5) minimum disclosure standards for advertising materials.[58]

The report accompanying the Model Act also makes recommendations to (1) prohibit optionally renewable policies, (2) preserve prior institutionalization options, (3) promote tax credits or deductions for premiums, (4) restrict Medicaid eligibility via asset spenddown, (5) develop long-term care riders on existing insurance products, (6) establish a data base for pricing and loss ratio determination, and (7) educate consumers.

The federal government has also encouraged greater national interest through legislation establishing a Task Force on Long-Term Health Care Policies.[59] The task force, established in 1986 by the Secretary of Health and Human Services, and comprised of representatives of the insurance industry, elderly consumers, long-term care providers, and federal and state agencies, is charged with making recommendations regarding long-term care insurance policies designed:

(1) [T]o limit marketing and agent abuse for those policies,
(2) [T]o assure the dissemination of such information to consumers as is necessary to permit informed choice in purchasing the policies and to reduce the purchase of unnecessary or duplicative coverage,

[57] See remarks of Lawrence Kirsch, "Private Long Term Care Insurance: The Maturing Market," Conference Proceedings, Jan. 1987, San Antonio, TX, at 11.
[58] See "Long Term Care Insurance: An Industry Perspective on Market Development and Consumer Protection," National Association of Insurance Commissioners (undated (Jan. 1987)), App. M.
[59] See P.L. 99-272, 42 U.S.C. 1395b (1986).

(3) [T]o assure that benefits provided under the policies are reasonable in relationship to premiums charged, and

(4) [T]o promote the development and availability of long-term health care policies which meet these recommendations.[60]

After the task force reports in late 1987, the Secretary has 18 months to report to Congress regarding state actions in response to task force recommendations, and an additional 18 months to report on the necessity, if any, of federal legislative or administrative action to respond to issues raised by the task force or to protect consumers.

In November 1986, the Secretary of Health and Human Services also recommended, in his report to the President, that a limited tax credit for long-term care insurance premiums be given to persons over age 55, that long-term care insurance reserves be given favorable tax treatment now available for life insurance, and that restrictions on employer prefunding of employee long-term care benefits be removed.[61]

States have also taken significant steps toward addressing long-term care insurance issues. At least 21 states[62] have proposed or enacted legislation, or developed study commissions, dealing with product development, statewide risk pools, public employee coverages, income tax deductions for premium costs, establishment of minimum standards for policies, mandatory disclosures and consumer education, development of model policy language, and related topics. In addition, several state legislatures have introduced bills to make long-term care insurance coverage mandatory for group policies sold in the state.[63]

The widespread recognition given to long-term care insurance issues by federal and state governments, and national organizations and interest groups, should help to solve the problems of consumer confusion, lack of standards, disparate and overly broad state regulation, and other barriers to product development and acceptance.

(2) Group Coverages: Retirement Facility Plans, Employee Plans, HMOs, SHMOs

The heightened marketing expenses and underwriting risks involved in selling policies on an individual basis have been perceived as an impediment to long-term care insurance policy development.[64] However, different forms of group long-term care insurance coverages are beginning to develop in the marketplace.

[60] 14 U.S.C. § 1395b(c).

[61] See O'Shaughnessy, et al., note 50, above, at 62.

[62] See L. Lane, memorandum to State executives, American Health Care Association, April 25, 1986.

[63] See O'Shaughnessy, et al., note 50, above, at 63.

[64] See § 27.2(a).

One innovative product offers comprehensive long-term care and Medicare supplemental coverage for residents of a continuing care retirement community.[65] All residents must participate in the noncancelable insurance program and pay premiums as a part of the facility's usual monthly charges.

Employee group health plans have occasionally provided some long-term care benefits beyond the recuperative approach taken by Medicare.[66] Other group efforts include the marketing of a long-term care insurance program in development by the American Association of Retired Persons.[67]

Prepaid group health plans[68] have traditionally not ventured far into the long-term care arena.[69] However, some health maintenance organizations (HMOs) have developed plans, specifically catering to elderly enrollees, with some long-term care and home health benefits.[70] In addition, the Health Care Financing Administration is conducting four demonstration projects for Social Health Maintenance Organizations (SHMOs), which offer coverage for a continuum of care including acute and long-term care. These plans are offered on a prepaid, fixed rate basis, with control of services utilization via a case management system.[71]

(3) Advantages of Retirement Facility Long-Term Care Insurance

The advantage to a retirement facility of purchasing a long-term care insurance product in the market place, rather than self-insuring, is that the risk of loss may be spread over a larger population base, and if the insurance carrier is careful to select its clientele, this can result in substantial cost savings when compared with self-insurance. Insurance carriers that offer their product only to selected retirement facilities rather than the general public, and that pay preferred benefits for health care or custodial care received at selected facilities where there is an incentive to control costs, can significantly reduce the cost of insurance. Of course, the involvement of a well respected insurance company in a retirement facility's health insurance program may also promote consumer confidence and marketing efforts.

From the point of view of many developers, the use of long-term care insurance policies may also be desirable because the developer does not

---

[65]Policy being offered by Provident Life and Accident of Chattanooga, TN, via Johnson & Higgins of Philadelphia, PA.

[66]E.g., Blue Cross of MI, United Auto Workers policy. See ICF, Phase I, note 19, above, at 27.

[67]See remarks of Ronald Hagan, "Private Long Term Care Insurance," note 57, above, at 13–14.

[68]See also the discussion of continuing care, § 27.3(a).

[69]E.g., the Kaiser Health Plan reportedly offers some long term care coverage, but coordinates it closely with Medicare benefits. ICF, Phase I, note 19, above, at 31.

[70]E.g., Blue Cross of Southern California. Id., at 34.

[71]Id., at 33–34.

wish to engage in the business of self-insurance. Instead, by simply arranging for group coverage for the residents of the facility being developed, one can provide many of the benefits of a continuing care type of arrangement, without taking on directly the responsibility of calculating the risks of paying for future health care needs. Shifting the obligation to cover future health care expenses to a licensed insurance company may also have certain regulatory benefits for the retirement facility, depending upon state law. Oftentimes, the laws regulating life care or continuing care facilities exist because of the self-insurance aspect of the transaction. To the extent that state requirements for reserves for continuing care facilities are duplicated by reserve requirements imposed upon the long-term care insurance company, the burden of regulatory compliance may also be passed on to the insurance carrier.

(4) Coordination of Benefits

One problem for new long-term care insurance products will be coordination with other benefits. Unlike Medigap policies, which are designed to build on a uniform base of Medicare benefits, new comprehensive long-term care policies may be providing coverages on top of a potpourri of Medicare benefits, employee health plans, retirement benefits, existing continuing care contracts, Medigap policies, and various other less comprehensive programs of an unpredictable nature. Where an individual has already invested substantial funds in such a program (e.g., a retirement benefits policy), it may be necessary to purchase duplicative base coverage to obtain the desired excess long-term care coverage. Until the market grows and more coverage options become available, it may be difficult to obtain comprehensive long-term care coverage that is supplemental to, but not partially duplicative of, existing coverages already in place.

§ 27.3 SELF-INSURANCE METHODS

In addition to the options of purchasing health care insurance from a third party, or enrolling in a prepaid health plan, consumers may self-insure for their future health care needs by home equity conversion methods such as reverse annuity mortgages, contracting with a continuing care provider,[72] or funding earmarked reserves similar to individual retirement accounts (IRAs).

---

[72]Although similar to a prepaid health plan, continuing care arrangements are treated here as a self-insurance method because enrollment is usually restricted to residents of a given facility, whereas insurance is generally available on a more widespread basis. However, such distinctions are fading as insurers attempt to control care delivery systems and larger continuing care providers spread their risks among multiple facilities.

(a)   Continuing Care

Continuing care facilities were probably the first form of retirement facility to respond in a significant way to the absence of governmental insurance for the costs of long-term health care. Many continuing care facilities that offer nursing care as part of the overall program will not increase substantially the charges to the resident when he or she moves from independent living in an apartment unit to continuous care in the nursing facility. This is made possible by a self-insurance program whereby the facility, using actuarial tables and drawing on experience in the provision of health care, predicts the lifetime cost of caring for the residents in its community and uses a combination of entrance fees and adjustable monthly fees to finance these costs. To the extent that usual monthly fees are insufficient to cover the costs of care, monies may be reserved from entrance fees or other sources.

Continuing care retirement communities (CCRCs),[73] in which residents pay entrance fees and/or monthly fees in return for housing, services, and health care, have been recognized as one of the most important existing methods of privately financing long-term care needs.[74] Absent a strong long-term care insurance market, continuing care communities are, in fact, one of the only material forms of private long-term care financing currently in general use.

CCRCs are often perceived as being primarily for the wealthy,[75] and indeed many such facilities do cater to upper income elderly. However, entrance fees average $35,000 for one person, and may range as low as $11,000.[76] Given the growing need for, and public awareness of, long-term care financing vehicles, CCRC development for middle income groups should expand more rapidly once the higher income market has been saturated.

As with other products, CCRCs may vary considerably in terms of the scope of benefits and the varying costs and means of payment.[77] Some may charge a higher monthly rate for residence in the nursing unit than for apartment living, or may provide a limited number of days of care without any increase in normal periodic fees. Others may have a full indemnity type of plan in which all needed care is provided at a price charged uniformly to all residents. Various combinations of entrance fees and monthly fees, and of refund, unit resale, or fee credit policies further complicate the field.

---

[73] See, generally, §§ 2.3(d), 21.

[74] See, e.g., MacKenzie, "Catastrophic Illness: Private Financing of Health Care for the Elderly," Compensation & Benefits Management (Winter 1987), at 5. ICF, Phase I, note 19, above, at 36–43; O'Shaughnessy, et al., note 50, above, at 64–69.

[75] See, e.g., O'Shaughnessy, et al., note 50, above.

[76] Id. See also discussion at §§ 2.3(d) and 21.

[77] See, e.g., sample contract provisions in Part IX.

Facilities that promise future care or priority access to facilities, but do not offer any significant form of risk-pooled prepayment mechanism or other insurance component, may lead to consumer confusion of the type that led the federal government to regulate Medigap policies. In fact, there is a good deal of disagreement in the industry itself regarding the precise bounds of the continuing care or life care concept.[78]

The self-insurance aspect of continuing care facilities has been viewed by many as the most risky facet of the retirement home business. However, failures of facilities have not resulted as much from a failure to predict the cost of future health care for the resident population as from excessive optimism in one's ability to market the project, or from creation of a fee mechanism that does not allow adjustment to meet rising expenses. (see § 5). Usually, by careful analysis of residents' finances, statistical need for nursing home care, actuarial life expectancies of the specific resident mix, careful enumeration of the health services that are and are not covered by the arrangement, control of health care delivery costs, use of reserve funds, and ability to adjust fees, most continuing care facilities are able to operate on a financially sound basis and continue to offer substantial health care benefits at stable, predictable rates.

At present, there is no federal legislation creating minimum standards for CCRC benefits,[79] and even states that regulate the business most comprehensively do not prescribe minimum health benefits or coverages, loss ratios, eligibility criteria, or permitted levels of fees.[80] Due to the larger risk pools and greater degree of regulation inherent in the commercial insurance industry, long-term care insurance presents an arguably more secure risk than individually self-insured facilities. However, the residential community character of a CCRC introduces lifestyle and utilization controls not present in most health insurance situations. Thus, long-term care insurance may be best used to enhance, rather than supplant, continuing care facility programs.[81]

(b) Home Equity Conversion

Continuing care facilities, discussed above, often rely upon resident home sales to fund the entrance fees required upon admission. However, senior citizens still in their homes may be able to utilize existing equity to purchase a plan that can fund health care needs in the future, before and after moving into a retirement facility.

---

[78]See § 2.3(d).

[79]There is, however, a definition for purposes of qualifying for exemption from imputed interest rules. See § 6.2(b)(2).

[80]See § 21. However, reserves, refunds, and other financial protections do exist in some states.

[81]See generally, MacKenzie, note 74, above, and § 27.2(c)(2).

Home equity conversion may take the form of a reverse annuity mortgage (RAM), in which the homeowner retains title to the property but uses the equity to secure a loan, the proceeds of which are paid out in monthly installments. At the end of the loan term, the principal and interest are due, and may be recovered by sale of the house.[82]

A second form of home equity conversion is a sale-leaseback, in which the homeowner sells the residence to an investor, retains a lifetime tenancy, and receives the purchase price in the form of monthly payments.[83]

In either case, payments could fund present expenses such as home health care, or theoretically could be deferred, with accumulation of interest, to fund future costs of care in a retirement facility setting.

Recent estimates conclude that use of home equity conversion contracts is extremely limited.[84] The kinds of programs described above typically provide small payments over long periods of time, whereas long-term care often requires larger payments over more concentrated timespans.[85] It has been observed that lines of credit, secured by home equity, may be more suitable for funding long-term care than these traditional equity conversion programs.[86] Since the passage of the Tax Reform Act of 1986, which removed personal interest deductions except for certain home loans, banks have begun to offer such home equity lines of credit more regularly.

(c) Individual Medical Accounts

A concept still in the formative stages is that of the Individual Medical Account (IMA). Like an Individual Retirement Account (IRA), the IMA would permit a person to defer taxes on a portion of income deposited each year in a restricted account, the assets of which could be used only for specified kinds of medical expenses. The idea received special public attention when endorsed, in late 1985, by Otis Bowen shortly before his confirmation as Secretary of the U.S. Department of Health and Human Services.[87]

Concerns with this approach include: (1) that people may not be inclined to participate in the plan at an early enough age because they do not believe they will need long-term care, or because they believe Medicare will pay for it, and (2) Congress may not pass such a measure due to concerns about its effect on federal revenues.[88] In fact, the Tax Reform

[82] See ICF, Phase II, note 19, above, at 17.

[83] Id., at 21.

[84] O'Shaughnessy, et al., note 50, above, reports only 300 to 400 contracts nationwide.

[85] See ICF, Phase II, note 19, above, at 25.

[86] Id., at 25–28.

[87] See Congressional Quarterly, May 31, 1986, at 1230.

[88] See ICF, Phase I, note 19, above, at 48–49.

Act of 1986 has greatly restricted the option of depositing funds, tax free, into IRA accounts.[89]

Nevertheless, the Department of Health and Human Services' Task Force on Long Term Health Policies is expected to recommend to Congress in late 1987 that it take steps to institute IMAs or to authorize IRA fund transfers to long-term care insurance programs.[90]

(d)   Use of Transferable Memberships, Refunds, Equity Loans as a Health Care Reserve

Many facilities are now developing creative methods of helping residents to, in effect, self-insure their own health care costs at the retirement facility. The traditional continuing care facility would customarily pool entrance fees and monthly fees on a facilitywide basis and use the funds for operating expenses as well as general reserves for costs of health care and other contingencies. Usually these fees would be nonrefundable, so pooling made sense.

Recently, with the advent of refundable entrance fees, some facilities are keeping separate account of entrance fee refunds or other resident resources that may be drawn upon by the individual to pay for the costs of health care in the facility. Where there are refundable entrance fees, memberships that have resale value, or ownership structures in which a resident may have equity,[91] facilities may be able to draw upon an individual resident's assets or receivables in the event he or she runs out of funds to pay nursing charges, usual monthly fees, or health insurance premiums. While this method of financing health care is probably not a complete substitute for an actuarially planned, pooled insurance program, it can serve as an emergency fund upon which an individual in the facility may rely as a last resort before becoming dependent on government programs.

[89] See I.R.C., § 219.

[90] See remarks of D. DeWitt, "Private Long Term Care Insurance," note 57, above, at 10.

[91] See, generally, Part III for a discussion of different resident payment and ownership structures.

Nine

Resident Agreements

§ 28 RESIDENT AGREEMENT DRAFTING CONSIDERATIONS

§ 28.1 OVERVIEW

Agreements that set forth the rights and obligations of facility residents and owners or operators of retirement communities can be the most important of the many legal documents that are prepared in the course of a project's development. Whether the resident's status is that of property owner or lessee, or whether the facility is congregate housing or continuing care services, the Resident Agreement should articulate comprehensively the services offered, services excluded, payment mechanisms, conditions upon sale of the residential unit or transfer to another unit, termination provisions, rules of occupancy, and the like. The agreements may take such forms as leases, deed covenants or restrictions, real property purchase agreements, continuing care agreements, cooperative association bylaws and contracts, or monthly rental agreements. In every kind of facility, the Resident Agreement should define the parameters of the entire program offered to consumers by the developer or operator.

The forms used in this section are examples of provisions from proposed or actual agreements, and are included for illustrative purposes and not necessarily as models of proper form or content. Often, more complex or extensive provisions are presented than may be required to accomplish a purpose, in order to demonstrate the possibilities and stimulate thinking. The forms generally come from rental, lease, life care, or membership types of contracts, and do not represent real estate sales (e.g., deeds) or corporate ownership documentation (e.g., bylaws). However, much of the language should be useful in service contracts between owners and residents' associations. Readers are encouraged to develop, with advice of legal counsel, custom legal documents to suit their specific programs.

§ 28.2   THE CONTRACT AS A MARKETING DOCUMENT

Retirement facility developers cannot afford to forget that the Resident Agreement is as much a marketing tool as it is a legal document. While every Resident Agreement has its share of legal boilerplate, it also constitutes the prospective resident's definitive opportunity to examine the explicit details of the service program offered, together with the financial provisions associated with such matters as initial occupancy, receipt of optional services, and sale or termination of residence. The Resident Agreement will be scrutinized by the prospective resident, and very possibly the resident's lawyer or financial advisor, particularly in long-term or endowment types of arrangements.

(a)   Naming the Product

The title of the agreement between the facility and resident and description of the product should be given careful consideration, as they characterize the relationship between the parties, and the kind and quality of program offered, and may have legal and marketing implications.

Some providers wish to avoid use of the word *lease* in the agreement because of the possible application of state or local landlord-tenant laws relating to security deposits, fee increases, eviction procedures, or other matters. In facilities where much of the contract may deal with the purchase of services, or occupancy of health or personal care facilities, landlord-tenant laws may be inappropriate or undesirable.

Residence Agreement is a commonly used and generic term, but it refers only to the housing element and does not impart the service oriented character of many facilities. *Care and Residence Agreement* covers both elements, but *care* may have a specific meaning under state license laws, and it is therefore important to limit use of the word to situations where the facility is prepared to offer such services and be appropriately licensed. Similarly, *Congregate Care Agreements* should have provisions covering the resident's personal care needs (e.g., bathing or dressing) and not simply meals or housekeeping. If there is no *care*, as the term may be defined by law, *Congregate Housing* is the more apt term.

Life Care or *Continuing Care* have different connotations, depending on state laws or local custom. Often, *life care* describes the archaic method whereby a person gave all his or her assets to a facility in return for complete care for life. To some, it may also falsely imply that the contract cannot be terminated for the life of the resident, even if there is cause. Usually, however, *life care* and *continuing care* are used interchangeably to describe more modern long-term care arrangements where residents move from independent housing through various levels of care, often in return for an entrance fee and a monthly fee, which does not change substantially when care is needed. On the other hand, for example, California law uses the term *life care* to cover virtually all promises to provide care for more than a year, irrespective of the form of payment or level of care. (For a discussion of terminologies applied to various facility types, see § 2.3, above.)

The title of the agreement can be used to help distinguish a product from the local competition. A developer using a membership structure, for example, may want to present a Membership Agreement, rather than a Residence Agreement, to emphasize that special feature of the project. Conversely, in a locale where a life care facility failure is fresh in the public mind, a more generic term, such as Care and Residence Agreement, rather than Life Care Contract, may help sell the project on its own merit. Some terms may be associated with a low income level, with physical dependence, or even with a low quality of care or service. Consequently, euphemisms such as *independent living, retirement center, assisted living,* and *congregate services,* are often preferred over *elderly housing, rest home, sheltered care,* or *board and care.* This shift in terminology is not necessarily just a marketer's ploy. It reflects as well the increased independence and affluence of the consumer, the decline of retirement facilities as places of last resort, and the need for developers to produce a more attractive product in order to compete in the marketplace.

(b)   You, the Resident

In an effort to make Resident Agreements more readable, some providers have decided to employ a more personal approach to draftsmanship that minimizes the use of legalese and formalistic writing style. For example, rather than continually referring to the consumer as the *resident* or *tenant,* the agreement may address the resident or residents as *you.* In addition, use of such terms as *hereinabove, notwithstanding,* and *wherein* are avoided. Restrictive language or protective boilerplate is minimized, or at least separated from contract provisions that point out the positive benefits of the project.

This colloquial and more personal format can be particularly effective in making the reader aware of the advantages of the service program offered by the facility. (For an example with respect to service descriptions, see Form 28.3A.) In addition, especially difficult passages may be made more comprehendible with the use of plainer language and less jargon. Use of the second person pronoun may also be helpful in clarifying more complicated passages (see, e.g., Form 28.3B). An informal style is not an excuse for sloppiness or imprecision. Careful drafting and the advice of legal counsel are of equal or even enhanced importance. However, marketing professionals should be a part of the team that produces the contract. Rest assured that insurance carriers and others who have employed a consumer-oriented writing style in their contracts have not broadened coverages, made exclusions less effective, or sacrificed legal review.

(c) Positive Phraseology

A corollary of the marketing approach to drafting is to phrase restrictive provisions positively rather than negatively.[1] For example, rather than state that "pets are not allowed unless approved by the manager," the contract may advise that "a pet may be kept in your residence, provided the manager determines that its presence will not interfere with facility operations or disturb other persons." The latter version, while setting more detailed standards, also presents a more optimistic outlook for the prospective resident.

Special sensitivity also should be given to treatment of unpleasant subjects, such as death. Facility names should not convey the impression that they are the final stop before the grave. Cynical observations about retirement homes with names such as "Granite Acres" or "Ebbtide Estates" are not much of an exaggeration upon names occasionally encountered in reality. Similarly, contracts should be carefully drafted to deal artfully with matters of possible mental incompetence, illness, or death. One contract reviewed for this book titled a paragraph simply "Burial"; coincidentally, but ominously, it was paragraph 13. Another specified what happens to your right to remain in your apartment if you "become a mental case." Need we say more?

(d) Selling Services and Amenities

It is important, especially for facilities with significant service programs, to make the opening pages of the agreement serve as an inducement to move into the facility. All of the attractive features of the facility, including furnishings provided, common area amenities, recreational and social activities, parking and transportation services, dining facilities and meal programs, health services, emergency call systems, and other services and amenities should appear immediately after the opening paragraphs of the agreement (see, e.g., Form 28.3C for a simple listing). Some providers may wish to explain the services in more of a narrative form, with a bit of salesmanship (Form 28.3D), or with restrictions intermingled with the description of benefits (Form 28.3E).

In addition, financial or resident property rights provisions that make the project unique or especially attractive, such as refundable fees, transferable memberships, or insurance programs, can be more effective if they are summarized near the beginning of the contract (see, e.g., Form 28.3F). Even though provisions relating to such matters as health care benefits, refundable entrance fees, or other complex matters eventually must be spelled out in great detail and with full explication of all conditions and restrictions, opening paragraphs can present the basic outlines of such provisions. Such general statements should be qualified by reference to the limiting provisions that can follow later on in the document.

---

[1]This is a concept advanced by Ann Hambrook, Hamlyn Associates, Philadelphia, PA.

(e)   Contract Length

The length of the contract may also have a bearing on marketability. While shorter contracts may be easier to read, they may not necessarily be easier to comprehend. Attempts at brevity can lead to vagueness, omission of important points, and unwarranted assumptions and expectations.

A longer contract can be equally or more effective, provided it is written clearly and with an emphasis on the positive features of the facility and its program. Some of the best contracts for programs with substantial services can easily reach 30 or 40 double-spaced typed pages in length. However, when converted to print, the number of pages can be reduced substantially, and the attractiveness of the document increased, without sacrificing readability. Most applicants to retirement facilities are making serious lifetime decisions and will be willing to take the time to scrutinize and digest a longer document. For ease of reference, contracts of 10 or more pages should have a table of contents.

§ 28.3   THE CONTRACT AS A MARKETING DOCUMENT: SAMPLE FORMS

FORM 28.3A: PERSONALIZED AMENITIES

YOUR RESIDENCE AND THE COMMON FACILITIES

You have selected residence no. _____ to be your home. (Retirement Facility) agrees that you shall have a personal and nonassignable right to live in that residence until your death or earlier termination of this agreement, or until a transfer in accordance with other parts of this agreement. You may move into your residence on _____, 19_____. Your residence will be furnished with carpeting, window coverings, appliances, emergency call systems, and smoke alarms. All other furnishings are your responsibility and you are at liberty to place and use your furniture and small appliances without interference, provided retirement facility's safety standards are met. (Retirement Facility) shall be responsible for maintaining the buildings, grounds, utilities, and appliances furnished by it as needed. You shall be responsible for all other internal repairs to your residence.

MEALS AND PERSONAL SERVICES

Nutritionally balanced meals will be provided daily in the dining room or other designated common area. One meal per day of your choosing is included in the regular monthly fee. You may choose a two-meal or three-meal plan at an additional charge, which will be added to your monthly fee. Meal charges may be revised from time to time. You may change your choice of meal plan, provided your change is made in advance, and is for one or more calendar months. You may purchase additional meals for yourself and your guests at the guest meal rates then in effect.

FORM 28.3B: TECHNICAL RULE PERSONALIZED

ACCRUED RESERVE DAYS

When you initially occupy your residence at (Retirement Facility), you will receive an immediate reserve of 10 days of basic services in the health center. As long as you continue to live in your residence, you will receive an additional 10 days to be added to your basic services reserve upon each anniversary of your residence at retirement facility, up to a maximum lifetime reserve of 60 days.

In the event that you need to use the services of the health care center, and such services are not otherwise covered by Medicare, supplemental insurance, or other third party payments, you may use your accrued basic services reserve days.

FORM 28.3C: SERVICE LIST

INCLUDED SERVICES

The following services are included in your Monthly Fee:

1. Dinner served in the dining room each day. During a temporary illness, when authorized by the Director of Nursing, tray service in your residence will be provided.
2. Weekly housekeeping service.
3. Weekly bath and bedroom linen service.
4. An activity program—social, cultural and recreational—for those who wish to participate.
5. Scheduled local transportation.
6. Use of all recreational facilities.
7. If you own an automobile, one (1) covered parking space will be available per residence.
8. Water, sewer, garbage, and common area utilities.
9. Maintenance of building and grounds, including routine maintenance of your residence.
10. Emergency nursing service in your residence.
11. Emergency calls at Retirement Facility by the Medical Director or a physician designated by the Medical Director, whenever summoned by Retirement Facility nursing staff.
12. A comprehensive group health care insurance program, described in Section _____, which has been obtained for you by Retirement Facility.
13. Administration of your medical benefits, including the completion and filing of any necessary forms.

FORM 28.3D: SERVICE AND AMENITIES DESCRIPTION

COMMUNITY FACILITIES

You will be entitled to share with all other residents the use of the grounds and common facilities, and to reserve areas for special occasions in accordance with the Resident Policies and Procedures of Retirement Facility. Common facilities will initially include dining facilities (including private dining rooms, which may be reserved), a physical fitness center, which includes a swimming pool and exercise rooms, a garden center, meeting rooms, lounges, a library, and a postal facility. Retirement Facility may, in consultation with its residents, adapt or change common areas to best meet the needs of the community.

For your convenience, there will be covered walkways throughout the community, and all multistory buildings will contain elevators. You will also be provided with a "smart card," which will be used to ensure security, and which may also be used by you to make purchases in any of Retirement Facility's shops and will contain your medical records. In addition, Retirement Facility will make available to you guest accommodations, space permitting, at an additional charge.

TRANSPORTATION

In order to control pollution and noise, to promote safety, and to enhance the aesthetic quality of the community, Retirement Facility has eliminated individual garages, and all cars will be parked underground. Your basic Monthly Service Fee includes free valet parking at the community building, for one car per resident. A limited amount of self parking will also be available. No long-term on-street parking is permitted. For your convenience, Retirement Facility will provide, at no extra charge, regularly scheduled tram service throughout the community, regularly scheduled minibus service throughout _____ County and transportation as needed to local health care providers.

ACTIVITIES/SERVICES COORDINATION

Retirement Facility will provide at least one full time person to coordinate community trips, social events, group activities, and personal services.

HEALTH SERVICE COORDINATOR

Retirement Facility will provide a Health Services Coordinator. The Health Services Coordinator will be available to schedule doctor or other medical appointments and services and coordinate transportation; maintain current medical records; maintain current medication records and assist with maintenance of prescribed drug regimen; coordinate home health delivery, as necessary; and assist with medical insurance billing.

FORM 28.3E: SERVICES AND RESTRICTIONS (LONG FORM)

ARTICLE I: RESIDENCE ACCOMMODATIONS AND FACILITIES

1. *Your Residence.* You have selected Unit _____ to be your residence (this Unit will be referred to in this Agreement as your "residence"). You shall have a personal and nonassignable right to reside in the residence, subject to the terms of this Agreement and Community rules and regulations, as long as you are capable of independent living. Your residence will be furnished with a modern kitchen, carpeting, individual washer and dryer units, an emergency call system and smoke alarms. All other furnishings are your responsibility, and you may furnish and decorate your residence in accordance with your own individual tastes and preferences. You may place and use your furniture and small appliances as you please as long as this does not interfere with the Community's safety standards.

2. *Parking.* If requested, a parking space will be assigned to you, at no additional charge, for a single motor vehicle used by you. Additional parking space may be available on a separate charge basis. A free parking area for guests will be provided.

3. *Modifications to your Residence.* You will not make any structural or physical change to your residence without the Executive Director's written consent. At your request, for an additional fee, and in compliance with Community policy in effect at the time, Retirement Facility will modify your residence in accordance with the terms of a separate agreement between you and Retirement Facility. Subject to Retirement Facility's approval, you may perform the modification work.

4. *Community Facilities.* You will be entitled to share with all residents in the use of the common grounds and facilities, and to reserve certain areas for special occasions in accordance with Community rules and regulations. The Community will feature facilities for a wide range of social and recreational activities. The Community will include a community center, reception area, library, mail boxes, a barber/beauty shop, auditorium, and a high quality dining room with additional provisions for private dining. The Community, in cooperation with the residents' council, will offer a wide range and balance of social and recreational activities.

5. *Property Protection.* You agree to keep your residence clean and orderly and agree not to permit misuse of or damage to your residence.

ARTICLE II: SERVICES

1. *Meals.* Retirement Facility will make available morning, noon, and evening meals at designated hours with nutritionally well balanced and varied menus. The Monthly Fee entitles you to one meal each day, lunch or dinner, in the Community dining room. Other meals may be obtained in the dining room or coffee shop at an additional charge.

(a) *Tray Service.* Tray service will be provided in your residence if such service is requested by the physician who has been named by Retirement Facility as the Medical Director ("Medical Director").

(b) *Special Meals.* Special diet meals will be provided at no extra charge when approved by the Medical Director.

(c) *Guest Meals.* You may invite guests to any meal, although Retirement Facility requests that you give prior notice so that proper accommodation can be made. Guest meals will be billed to you as an additional charge.

2. *Housekeeping.* At least weekly, Retirement Facility will provide light cleaning services for your residence. Retirement Facility will provide window washing, oven cleaning, and carpet shampooing once a year, or more frequently if necessary, as determined by the Executive Director. Additional housekeeping service may be contracted for with Retirement Facility on an additional charge basis.

3. *Maintenance and Repair.* Retirement Facility will provide necessary repairs, maintenance, and replacement of Community property and equipment. Except in an emergency, such services will be provided during normal working hours, Monday through Friday. Retirement Facility shall have the right to charge you for any repairs, maintenance, or replacement required as a result of the negligence or intentional acts of you or your guests. You are responsible for maintaining, repairing, and replacing your property.

4. *Security.* Your residence will be equipped with an emergency call system by which you can contact personnel who will be available to provide assistance 24 hours a day, seven days a week. Retirement Facility will employ security personnel to supervise the Community buildings and grounds during certain hours, as it deems necessary.

5. *Buildings and Grounds.* Retirement Facility will maintain all Community buildings, common areas and grounds, including lawns, walkways, and driveways. Landscaping and decorative plantings will be provided and maintained by Retirement Facility as it deems appropriate.

6. *Insurance and Responsibility for Resident's Property.* You will be responsible for providing all personal property and liability insurance for you, your property, and your guests. Retirement Facility shall not be responsible for and Retirement Facility insurance will not protect you against any loss or damage to your personal property from theft, fire, or other cause that is not the fault of Retirement Facility, nor does Retirement Facility agree to indemnify you against personal liability for injury to guests or other persons in your residence.

7. *Utilities.* Your residence will be provided with water, heat, air conditioning, and electricity. Water, sewer, and garbage collection fees are included in your Monthly Fee (as described in Article IV, Section E). Electric power for your residence will be individually metered, and you will be entitled to a monthly allowance for electric power. You will be billed monthly for any usage in excess of the monthly allowance. Telephone service to each residence will be available; however, installation of telephones and service costs will be your responsibility.

8. *Transportation.* Retirement Facility will provide scheduled local transportation to shopping centers and other points of common interest.

9. *Personal Assistance.* When approved by the Medical Director, Retirement Facility will provide limited personal assistance to you in your residence, including limited assistance in daily living, consistent with your health, safety, and grooming needs.

FORM 28.3F: MEMBERSHIP FEATURES SUMMARY

I.   MEMBERSHIP IN RETIREMENT FACILITY

A.   Residential and Assisted Status Membership in General

There are two forms of membership at Retirement Facility: Residential Membership and Assisted Status Membership. You initially shall purchase a Residential Membership in Retirement Facility, which together with payment of a Monthly Fee, shall entitle you to residence, services, and use of common areas at Retirement Facility for as long as you are capable of independent living, subject to the terms and conditions of this Agreement and the policies and procedures set forth by Retirement Facility. If you are no longer capable of independent living and require assistance with the routines of daily living or require skilled nursing care, appropriate arrangements for your care will be made available in accordance with this Agreement. If you require such assistance or care on a permanent basis, you will become an Assisted Status Member, as more fully described in Section _____ of this Agreement. As an Assisted Status Member, you will have the option of retaining or selling your Residential Membership.

Your Residential Membership or Assisted Status Membership entitles you to participation in Retirement Facility's health care program and the comprehensive group health care insurance policy obtained on your behalf by Retirement Facility.

Your Residential Membership is intangible personal property and may be sold by you or your estate to a Qualified Buyer, subject to a Transfer Fee, as described later in this Agreement. Your Residential Membership will be evidenced by a Residential Membership Certificate substantially in the form of Exhibit A to this Agreement, and will be signed and delivered upon close of Escrow.

The Assisted Status Membership is intangible personal property, and may be redeemed, as described in Section _____ of this Agreement.

Neither Residential Membership nor Assisted Status Membership gives you any estate, leasehold, or ownership interest in the real or personal property of Retirement Facility or Owner, nor any voting rights in Owner.

You can live in your residence for as long as you (or either of you) live unless you (or both of you) are not capable of maintaining yourself independently in your residence as described in Section _____, unless you breach this Agreement, or if this Agreement is terminated by you or by Retirement Facility, for cause as described in Section _____ of this Agreement.

---

§ 28.4   LIMITING PROVIDER OBLIGATIONS

(a)   Service Exclusions, Restrictions, and Conditions

It is probably as important to list services not provided by the facility as it is to enumerate those that are supplied. Of course, it is impossible literally to list all those services or amenities that are not supplied, but a list of services that are unavailable, or available only for an extra charge, may be called for when the facility does offer many services that could be grouped in the same general classification as those offered, such as health care or meals (see Form 28.5A). For example, where a facility promises to provide or make available, in return for a fixed monthly fee, substantial nursing or personal care services as required by the resident, contracts commonly contain a list of services not provided, such as dental care, cosmetic surgery, organ transplants, eyeglasses, treatment for drug addiction or alcoholism, or treatment for mental illnesses (see, e.g., Form 28.5B for a simple list; Form 28.5C for a comprehensive narrative).

Another important ingredient in limiting the provider's service obligations is avoidance of the unwitting use of language that might be construed to create an obligation to provide a service never intended to be offered. It is easier to make this mistake than it may seem. For example, many facilities, whether congregate housing or continuing care, have emergency call systems, permitting a resident in his or her apartment to summon assistance in the event of a fall or other incident. However, a poorly drafted contract may state that an emergency response system is in place so that the facility can "provide emergency care as needed by the resident." Such a broadly worded statement could have implications far beyond that of monitoring and responding to resident call signals. It could be misconstrued to mean, for example, that the facility will have a trained emergency room physician or nurse on hand at all times, that emergencies occurring off the premises will be covered, or even that the expenses of emergency hospital care or other treatment will be paid for by the facility. Instead, the contract should simply describe the system (Form 28.5D) or state precisely what kind of emergency personnel are available (Form 28.3C).

An innocent oversight in drafting the service provisions of a Resident Agreement can lead to serious misunderstandings, and facility liability. Ambiguities in any contract, and especially those between a business and an elderly person, are usually construed by courts against the business enterprise that drafted the document.[2] Often, such agreements are challenged by relatives of deceased or incompetent residents, who may have few loyalties to the retirement home and little understanding of the parties' intentions. It is, therefore, important to approach each phrase of the agreement that sets forth the benefits and services to be offered with a critical examination of how it might be misconstrued or broadened by another person reviewing it out of context. It is particularly important to approach with caution words and phrases that may have different meanings or implications in common usage than they may have in a particular profession or discipline, or according to statutory or regulatory definitions. Examples are such words as *emergency, medical, personal assistance, supervision,* and *care,* which may have very specific legal or trade usages of which a casual drafter may be unaware.

Contracts describing service programs should also carefully circumscribe such things as the time, place, and manner in which services will be provided.

[2] *See, Restatement of Contracts,* 2d ed., §§ 206, 207.

For example, with respect to meals, the agreement should state whether meals may be taken only in the facility's common dining area, or whether, and under what circumstances, meals may be taken in the resident's room, or taken on outings. Dining policies should also discuss the circumstances under which residents may invite guests or have meals specially prepared for medical or other reasons and for what charge (see Forms 28.5E, 28.5F). In general, the facility may want to specify that it is not responsible to render any services off the premises (Form 28.5G).

Provisions dealing with personal care or health care likewise should specify whether the home covers the costs of services rendered by other institutions, and if so, identify them by name or region (see Forms 28.5H, 28.5I, 28.5C). Agreements also generally specify the extent to which the facility expects the resident to obtain insurance or apply for government benefits such as Medicare or Medicaid prior to receiving benefits from the home (Form 28.5J) and, perhaps, the consequences of a resident's failure to comply (Form 28.5K).

If the facility provides nursing care as part of the regular monthly or other fee, the contract should state the scope and extent to which private duty nursing or other care by staff not regularly employed by the facility will be reimbursed. Similarly, although Medicare pays for most physician services, the agreement should state whether the facility will pay for physician services not covered by Medicare (see Forms 28.5L, 28.5M).

To the extent that a resident is required to submit to a preadmission medical examination, the agreement should state whether preexisting illnesses are covered under any health insurance type benefits of the program, and the effect of failure to disclose such preexisting conditions (see Form 28.5N).

(b) Defining the Parameters of Resident Rights

In addition to the basic program of services and physical features, most retirement facility agreements contain, or may imply, numerous other resident interests and benefits. Contracts may give rise to resident property or tenancy rights, due process obligations upon transfer or discharge, fiduciary duties respecting resident monies, or other rights and remedies that derive from the operation of common law principles or statutory enactments. Often, duties that might be implied from a general review of the relationships between residents and retirement community operators can be limited by careful contract drafting.

(1) Eligibility for Admission

Resident contracts generally do not set forth in great detail the facility operator's criteria for admission to the community. In retirement homes with health services or long-term commitments to residence and services, criteria for admission may encompass such topics as the applicant's financial condition and health status and history. Often, subjective judgments must be made about admissions based on these or other factors, and the contract should not attempt to enumerate such criteria. However, all application forms should be specifically identified in the contract text, attached as exhibits, incorporated by reference, and their accuracy made a condition of performance by the facility operator.

In addition, waiting list policies, or the existence of applicants with a special relationship to the facility (the developer's/benefactor's/bishop's mother) may have a bearing on admissions. In general, waiting list policies, if written, should be separate from the Resident Agreement and should reserve to the facility the discretion on occasion to accept persons not on the list and to admit persons on the list out of order. In addition, there can be technical provisions, such as one describing the remaining priority status, if any, of a person on the list who is called for admission and declines, but wishes to remain on the list for future eligibility.

Resident contracts usually do contain general provisions dealing with age criteria (Form 28.5O) or specifying different benefits for younger residents who are not Medicare eligible (Form 28.5P). However, homes should be careful not to violate state or federal antidiscrimination laws, which, of course, prohibit as an admissions criteria such classifications as race, but may also raise concerns about admissions based on age, handicap, or affiliation with the religious or ethnic group that sponsors the facility (see § 23, above, and Form 28.5Q). Most religiously sponsored retirement facilities do not limit admissions to adherents of the denomination, although such limitations may be permitted. Some sponsors may make it clear, however, that the home will have an atmosphere designed to appeal principally to members of the particular faith (see, for example, Form 28.5R). Others may contractually limit admission to persons of a particular ancestry, or to members of a union, fraternal, or professional group.

(2)   Property Rights

In all retirement facility transactions, some form of property interest or license is given to the resident. It may consist of a fee simple ownership, as in the sale of a residence or condominium unit, a monthly, annual, or lifetime leasehold, as may be encountered in congregate housing facilities or continuing care projects, or a license arrangement that may accompany a membership sale.

Continuing care or life care projects can present one of the more conceptually challenging property problems insofar as their legal status may transcend common law notions of estates and leasehold interests. Most continuing care agreements specify expressly that the resident's right is simply to occupy the premises for the duration of the agreement, and that no interest in real property is conveyed by the agreement (see Forms 28.5S, 28.5DD, 28.3F). This provision is important because a continuing care or life care agreement, which is intended essentially to operate as a long-term lease, could be misconstrued to convey to the resident a life estate in the real property of the retirement facility. Under the common law, life estates in property carry with them certain privileges that retirement facility operators do not wish to make available to their residents. Chief among them is the right to alienate (convey) the property and receive rents and profits from it,[3] until possession reverts back to the grantor upon death of the life tenant. Many of these common law rights of life tenants in real property have been incorporated into the earliest provisions of many state statutes. It is, therefore, important to be assured that continuing care agreements do not inadvertently grant a life estate and, by incorporation of statutory rights as a matter of law, give residents additional rights to use the property, sublet it, or convey it in manners not expressly authorized by the Resident Agreement. Life care contracts are better characterized as leases or licenses permitting possession indefinitely, subject to termination for cause. Avoidance of terms such as *life interest, life estate, life lease,* or *life tenant,* together with a limiting provision, should suffice.

Where appropriate, agreements should specify whether the resident may sublease the premises. Because most retirement facilities cater to a select group of residents, and make promises to provide special services and care based on residents' age, physical condition, and financial status, such contracts are not readily assignable. However, in some circumstances, it may be reasonable to sublease the premises to an approved person, without transfer of any right to services (see Form 28.5T).

(3) Duration of Residence

The term of the Resident Agreement is a relatively straightforward matter except insofar as contracts offer, or border on offering, life care or licensable continuing care (terms greater than one year). While many facilities are designed to offer services for the remainder of the resident's lifetime, contracts often do not expressly state that the resident may remain in the facility for life. Often, agreements are drafted to read that services will be provided so long as the resident performs his or her obligations under the agreement, or some variation of that concept (see Forms 28.5U, 28.5V, 28.5W, 28.5X). The agreement will then be fashioned to be terminable by the facility only for good cause (see Forms 28.11E and 28.11F). Exceptions may exist during initial probationary or cooling-off periods, during which a facility may be entitled to terminate the contract at will, that is, without a showing of good cause.[4]

Other facilities intending to offer continuing care with entrance fees have structured their agreements to be effective for a specific term of years

---

[3] *See,* 31 *Corpus Juris Secundum,* Estates, §§ 30 *et seq.* Other rights include such arcane interests as "estovers" or "botes" (timber) and "emblements" (crops), not suitable to most retirement facility circumstances.

[4] Residents are also entitled to terminate residency during such probationary periods without substantial penalty. *See* § 21, regarding state regulation of continuing care.

that is long enough to cover any reasonably predictable life span of the resident (e.g., 50 years). In such a circumstance, should the resident die prior to the end of the lease term, the contract may allow for the resident's estate to assign to the remainder of the lease term for value to another person who qualifies for residence (Form 28.5Y). The agreement may further provide that any consideration received by the first resident's estate be shared in some calculable fashion with the facility owner (Form 28.5Y). Or, the facility may exercise an option to repurchase the unit (Form 28.5Z).

The manner of expressing the duration of the rights transferred under an agreement may have significant licensing implications. For example, in states where continuing care is defined as a promise to provide care for a period greater than one year, contracts with open ended terms of duration, or options to terminate or renew, can raise questions about the need for licensure. There is often confusion in the minds of many facility developers and operators concerning the legal meaning of a promise for more than one year. Of course, an agreement that has a specified term greater than one year (e.g., a 10 year contract) normally would fit within such a state's continuing care definition. However, if such a contract permits termination without cause by the facility upon 30 days notice, the contract really operates as a month-to-month agreement, and language reciting a 10 year term might well have no significance for continuing care licensing purposes.

Similarly, if the contract were for one year and provided that an extension for another year could be triggered "by mutual agreement of the parties," that clearly should not be considered a contract for more than one year for licensure purposes, because the provider of services is making no commitment to make the services available during the second year. On the other hand, if renewal for a second year could be triggered at the sole option of the resident, the agreement would more properly be considered to be for more than one year because the retirement facility operator is promising that more than a year of services will be available to the resident if the resident so desires.

Agreements that would permit the facility operator to terminate the contract without good cause during the first few days or months after execution might technically be considered inconsistent with the standard definition of a continuing care agreement. However, most states that provide for an initial probationary or cooling off period by definition consider such contracts to be continuing care agreements, provided that there is no opportunity for the provider to terminate at will after the initial period of adjustment. It may be argued, however, that during this initial probationary period, when the provider may terminate the agreement without cause, there has been no commitment to provide life care, and in the event of a death during this probationary period, the provider should not be entitled to retain entrance fees paid in consideration of receiving a life care contract.[5]

---

[5] *See Howe v. American Baptist Homes of the West, Inc.*, 112 Cal. App. 3d 622, 169 Cal. Rptr. 418 (1980).

(4) Miscellaneous Resident Rights

Retirement facility agreements typically provide that the rights of residents are personal to them and may not be transferred to any other person (Form 28.5AA). Similarly, it is often specified that residents have no right to object to the terms and conditions of admission of any other resident (Forms 28.5BB, 28.5CC). Drafters of Resident Agreements should be careful to avoid any inadvertent implication in the agreement that the facility is holding entrance fees or other payments in trust for the particular resident.[6] It should be clear in the agreement that payments made to the facility operator become the exclusive property of the operator and can be used in whatever fashion the operator sees fit (see Forms 28.5DD, 28.5S, 28.3F). Residents of retirement facilities have been known to complain, and even sue operators, on the basis that monies paid as fees were being used to care for other residents, or to fund community service programs, construction of new facilities, or for other purposes.[7] Contracts that require any substantial payment from the resident will often give the resident certain rights to review the facility's financial condition (Form 28.5EE). Sometimes, this is required by state laws (see § 21.6(a)).

Residents may be advised in the contract of their right to organize into a resident's association that may consult with management and raise suggestions or grievances about matters relating to facility operations (see Form 28.5FF). In some states, such a right of organization is mandated by law.[8] Contracts may also specify that residents have the right to elect Board of Directors representatives, although there is widespread opinion that this is inadvisable from a management perspective.[9]

A few contracts provide that a supermajority of the entire resident population of a given facility may vote to change the terms and conditions of residence at the facility (Form 28.5GG). While such provisions may be of comfort to some prospective residents and serve as a marketing incentive, their use should be approached with caution, and the facility operator should retain a power of veto. Residents should not be permitted to make basic changes in the operation of the facility that could lead to a triumph of shortsighted self-interest over management's concerns for the long-term success of the project and the ability to remarket the facility many years in the future, when the entire resident population may have changed. In addition, a tyranny of the majority can result in adverse action taken by the group against the few who are in need of more extensive and expensive personal care, health care, or other services. The prospect of such circumstances could be destructive

---

[6] There are some situations where an express trust may be desirable for tax purposes. *See* § 6.1(b)(4)–(5).

[7] *See, Onderdonk v. Presbyterian Homes of NJ*, 85 N.J. 171, 425 A.2d 1057 (1981), and §§ 21.5 and 21.6(a), above.

[8] *See* § 21.8, above.

[9] *Id.*

to any program designed to provide residents with a long-term sense of security.

Contracts may also cover such matters as the residents' right to keep pets (Form 28.5HH). In certain HUD financed facilities, federal regulations prohibit facility owners from excluding pets (see § 22.5(c)). In general, residents should agree to abide by all rules of the facility, and a copy of printed policies should be provided to them (Form 28.5II).

§ 28.5 LIMITING PROVIDER OBLIGATIONS: SAMPLE FORMS

FORM 28.5A: À LA CARTE EXTRAS

AVAILABLE SERVICES NOT INCLUDED IN MONTHLY FEES

1. Each residence will be individually metered for electricity. You will be responsible to pay for your own electricity, cable television, telephone service, and other services not expressly included in this Agreement.

2. Retirement Facility will make available, upon your request, guest accommodations, additional meals, special diets, additional housekeeping, special transportation, and other special services, upon arrangement for an extra charge. There may be occasions when services such as guest accommodations will be fully reserved and in such cases these services may not be available to everyone who desires them. A list of charges for these additional services will be made available to you periodically.

FORM 28.5B: EXCLUDED HEALTH CARE (SHORT FORM)

HEALTH AND NURSING SERVICES AND SUPPLIES NOT INCLUDED

1. *Services Not Provided.* Retirement Facility will not provide or pay for or indemnify you for medical, surgical, or hospital services or physical examinations, medical consultations, drugs, medications, disposable and nondisposable supplies, x-rays, medical tests, eyeglasses or refractions, hearing aids, dentistry, dentures, inlays, prescriptions, orthopedic appliances, private duty nursing care, podiatric services, physical therapy, treatment for psychiatric disorders, alcoholism, or similar items or services. In addition, Retirement Facility will not be responsible for the costs of furnishing you with services for which reimbursement is available from Medicare or private insurance.

FORM 28.5C: EXCLUDED HEALTH CARE (LONG FORM)

SERVICES NOT PROVIDED

(a) *Schedule of Exclusions.* Retirement Facility will not provide nor arrange for the provision of the following:

(1) Services or supplies that are not medically necessary;

(2) Hospital or other residential care when Resident may receive safe and adequate care as an outpatient;

(3) The services of Christian Science practitioners, faith healers, clinics, or practitioners promoting or featuring the use of medications or medical technique not approved by the American Medical Association;

(4) Dental care or treatment, except for oral surgery when prescribed by a physician;

(5) Cosmetic surgery or related cosmetic services or products relating to the concealment of natural aging processes, as opposed to the alleviation of disfigurement due to accident or illness;

(6) Any nonlegend or proprietary medicine or medication not requiring a prescription, except insulin, and any drug labeled "Caution: Limited by Federal Law to Investigational Use," or experimental drugs;

(7) Experimental treatment and organ transplantation;

(8) Orthopedic care, eyeglasses, and hearing aids;

(9) Treatment for alcoholism, drug addiction, and other chronic substance abuse problems;

(10) Treatment for mental illness, functional nervous disorder, or psychiatric services, including institutional care related thereto, except as provided above;

(11) All services, benefits, or supplies for, or incident to chronic renal dialysis and resulting medical complications;

(12) All services, benefits, or supplies for, or incident to intersex surgery or sex transformation, and resulting medical complications;

(13) All services required while Resident is outside of the fifty (50) states or the District of Columbia of the United States of America;

(14) All services required while Resident is within any of the fifty (50) states or the District of Columbia of the United States of America but is more than ten (10) miles from Retirement Facility; except for acute hospitalization and related physician and emergency care services occasioned by a sudden, serious, and unexpected illness or injury requiring immediate medical attention, but only for so long as it is medically inadvisble for Resident to return to the immediate geographic area of Retirement Facility; and

(15) Any services or benefits for which no charge is made to Resident in the absence of this Agreement.

FORM 28.5D: EMERGENCY CALL

Your residence will include the following:

. . . .

—An emergency call system connecting your residence with personnel who are available 24 hours a day.

FORM 28.5E: CHARGE FOR SPECIAL MEALS

MEALS

1. Three nutritionally balanced meals will be provided daily in the dining room or other designated common area. One meal per day of your choosing is included in the regular Monthly Fee, except for Cottage residents, who shall be entitled to 20 meals per month. You may choose a two-meal or three-meal plan at an additional charge, which will be added to your Monthly Fee. Meal charges may be revised from time to time. You may change your choice of meal plan, provided your change is made in advance, and is for one or more calendar months. You may purchase additional meals for yourself and your guests at the guest meal rates then in effect.

2. The dining room or another appropriate dining area ordinarily will be open for all meals.

3. It is anticipated that from time to time you will travel, dine out, or otherwise be absent from Retirement Facility. Credit is not given when you do not use the services of Retirement Facility.

4. With the approval of the Retirement Facility Medical Director or his designee:

a. Tray service will be available to you in your residence during temporary or extended illnesses at an additional charge.

b. Special diets will be available. A charge may be made if special diets require custom preparation.

FORM 28.5F: SPECIAL MEALS INCLUDED

DINING SERVICES

1. Three nutritionally balanced meals will be prepared daily. One meal per day, lunch or dinner at your daily option, is included in your regular Monthly Service Fee. You may purchase additional meals for yourself and your guests.

2. Special dietary needs will be accommodated at no extra charge.

3. Home meal delivery will be provided at no additional charge, if determined to be medically necessary by the Health Services Coordinator. In addition, tray service to your residence will be available even if not medically necessary, at an additional charge.

4. A registered dietician will be available on a regular basis to provide nutrition consultation at no additional charge.

FORM 28.5G: NO BENEFITS WHILE ABSENT

Personal Obligations of Residents. Retirement Facility shall not be liable or responsible for any expenses, debts, or obligations incurred by you on your own account, nor shall it be obligated to furnish, supply, or give you any support, maintenance, board, or lodging while you are absent from the Community.

FORM 28.5H: HEALTH CARE WHILE ABSENT

Services Away from Community. You will pay all costs of nursing and other medical services incurred away from the Community, whether by reason of illness or accident, unless you are temporarily transferred to an outside facility by Retirement Facility as provided in Section _____.

FORM 28.5I: MEDICAL EXPENSES ABROAD

COVERED MEDICAL EXPENSES OUTSIDE THE UNITED STATES

If at any time you suffer an illness or injury while traveling outside the United States, the group insurance policy provides a benefit of ninety percent (90%) of usual and customary charges.

FORM 28.5J: MEDICARE ENROLLMENT

A. MEDICARE AND SUPPLEMENTAL INSURANCES. If you have not already enrolled, you agree to:
1. Apply for and secure your enrollment in the Hospital Insurance Benefits Program under Part A of Medicare or any successor program; and
2. During the next enrollment period following the effective date of this Agreement, apply, pay the premiums for, secure, and maintain your enrollment in the Supplemental Medical Insurance Benefits program under Part B of Medicare or any successor program.

You agree to obtain and maintain a supplemental insurance policy acceptable to Retirement Facility, to pay Medicare coinsurance and deductible amounts, and to provide major medical coverage in an amount required by Retirement Facility. Should you fail or neglect to arrange for such coverage, you hereby authorize Retirement Facility to make application on your behalf, to pay the premiums, and to bill the costs of obtaining and maintaining the coverage to you on your monthly statement.

If you are not eligible for the above Programs, you agree to obtain equivalent insurance coverage acceptable to Retirement Facility.

FORM 28.5K: FAILURE TO SEEK BENEFITS

YOUR OBLIGATION FOR REIMBURSEMENT

If you fail or refuse to apply for the maximum benefits available under Medicare or other government health and welfare benefit programs for which you may be eligible, now or hereafter enacted, you shall reimburse to Retirement Facility the amount Retirement Facility would have been reimbursed had you so applied or, if Retirement Facility gives written notice to you to apply for benefits and you refuse to so apply, without good cause, within thirty (30) days of receipt of notice, such refusal shall constitute grounds for termination of this Agreement by Retirement Facility.

COOPERATION IN OBTAINING BENEFITS

In order to make certain that the health care program is administered properly, you shall, from time to time as appropriate, take such action and execute such forms as are necessary to secure the payment to any hospital, skilled nursing facility, or other provider of services, or to any physician (including reimbursement to Retirement Facility for services rendered by it) of any and all amounts payable for goods or services provided to you and for which benefits, such as Medicare or insurance, are available, or may be available in the future.

POWER OF ATTORNEY

You hereby appoint Retirement Facility as your attorney in fact for the purpose only of applying for benefits or otherwise handling those matters relating to any of the benefits described in Section _____ from federal, state, or other sources.

FORM 28.5L: SPECIAL MEDICAL PERSONNEL

PERSONAL PHYSICIAN. You shall have the right to consult with or be treated by any physician of your choosing. You shall be fully responsible for payment of any charges for such consultation or treatment.

PRIVATE DUTY CARE. You may employ private duty nurses and sitters at your own expense upon approval of the Director of Health Services or the Retirement Facility administrator. Private duty nurses and sitters will be subject to the rules and regulations of the Retirement Facility Director of Nursing.

FORM 28.5M: PRIVATE CARE GIVER/LIABILITY

Resident is obligated to engage the services of any physician, surgeon, nurses, or other care givers as needed, and the Retirement Facility is not responsible for, or obligated to pay for, services rendered by such persons or by any persons other than those regularly employed or retained by the Retirement Facility. Any adverse conditions resulting from any care administered by persons employed by the Resident are the full responsibility of the Resident.

FORM 28.5N: EXISTING ILLNESSES

Preexisting Conditions. If you move into the Health Center due to a preexisting physical or mental condition within the time periods described in Exhibit A attached to this Agreement, you will pay the per diem rate applicable to nonresidents staying in the Health Center (referred to in this Agreement as the "per diem rate"), as established from time to time by the Executive Director. Determination of a pre-existing condition and the time period shall be made by the Executive Director based on your preadmission physician's report, other medical reports or findings, and after consulting with the Medical Director.

FORM 28.5O: AGE LIMIT

RECITALS: Retirement Facility is a nonprofit corporation engaged in the operation of a Home for the care of persons over 65 years of age, in accordance with the policies and directives of the Department of _____ of the State of _____.

FORM 28.5P: UNDERAGE BENEFITS

Persons under Sixty-Five. If you were less than sixty-five (65) years of age on the date you moved into the Community, you shall not be entitled to Health Center use or services except upon payment of the per diem rate as provided in Article _____. Upon attaining age sixty-five (65) you may apply to the Executive Director and be entitled to Health Center use and services upon agreeing to the terms and policies then in effect.

FORM 28.5Q: NO DISCRIMINATION

Retirement Facility is operated on a nondiscriminatory basis and affords equal treatment and access of services to all persons regardless of race, color, religion, national origin, or ancestry.

FORM 28.5R: SYMPATHY WITH CHURCH

While Retirement Facility is established for members of the _____ Church, applicants from other church constituencies will be considered for admission as space permits, without regard to race, color, gender, national origin, or ancestry.

Since compatibility is the key to happy relationships, applicants for residency must meet certain requirements relating to personal habits, as well as to physical and emotional health. Smoking, for example, is not permitted where the safety, health, and comfort of others are affected, and the use of alcoholic beverages is discouraged. Residency normally does not begin before the age of 62. Sympathy with the religious faith and spiritual concerns of the _____ Church is taken for granted.

FORM 28.5S: LIMITED PROPERTY RIGHTS

You understand and agree that this is an Agreement primarily for services. Your rights as a resident under this Agreement are limited to the rights and privileges expressly granted under it. Though you are granted a right of occupancy, this Agreement is not a lease and you will have no right, title, or interest in any of the real or personal property of Retirement Facility, or any of the rights of a renter, tenant, or lessee. Your rights under this Agreement are personal, and may not be assigned, transferred, inherited, or devised.

FORM 28.5T: SUBLEASING

You may not lease your residence without the express written approval of Retirement Facility. Any approval shall be in accordance with the then current policies adopted by Retirement Facility, which may include, at a minimum, that the lease be only for a short duration to cover a member's temporary absence, that the lessee and the lease agreement be approved by Retirement Facility, that the lease shall expire automatically upon expiration of the lessor's residence agreement, or the lessor's death, or upon lessor's transfer to personal care or skilled nursing, and that no rights to care or services under the residence agreement may be assigned to any lessee.

FORM 28.5U: DURATION UNTIL DEATH OR TERMINATION

From the first day of your residence at Retirement Facility until the time of your death, or until an earlier termination of this Agreement, Retirement Facility will furnish you with the lodging, personal services, medical care, and facilities described in this Agreement.

FORM 28.5V: DURATION UNTIL TERMINATED

For the duration of your residence at Retirement Facility as set forth in this Agreement, Retirement Facility will provide you with the lodging, services, and facilities described in this Agreement.

FORM 28.5W: DURATION UNTIL BREACH

Retirement Facility agrees to furnish the Resident the lodging and services enumerated in this section and in any addenda attached hereto so long as Resident carries out his obligations under this agreement.

FORM 28.5X: DURATION FOR LIFE, CONDITIONAL

Retirement Facility will provide you the services and accommodations described below in this Agreement, for the rest of your life, subject to the terms and conditions specified in this Agreement, including the termination provisions.

FORM 28.5Y: ASSIGNMENT OF LEASE FOR VALUE

In the event Resident dies or this Agreement is terminated prior to the expiration of the term of this Agreement, and Retirement Facility does not exercise its Repurchase Option pursuant to Paragraph _____, the Resident's estate may assign the remaining Contract Rights for a Residency and Care Agreement to a person who meets all of the criteria of Retirement Facility for its residents including, but not limited to, age and physical condition, and any such transferee shall be entitled to an extension of the term of the Agreement for a period that shall expire _____ years from the date of such assignment. Upon such assignment, Resident's estate shall pay to Retirement Facility a transfer fee equal to _____ percent of the consideration received by Resident's estate for such assignment if only one (1) person has been designated as Resident in this Agreement, or _____ percent of the consideration received by Resident's estate for such assignment if two (2) persons have been designated as Residents in this Agreement.

FORM 28.5Z: REPURCHASE OF LEASEHOLD

Repurchase Option. In the event Resident dies or this Agreement is terminated prior to the expiration of the term of this Agreement, Resident hereby grants to Retirement Facility an option (the "Repurchase Option") to repurchase from Resident's estate all residency rights and medical care and treatment rights (the "Contract Rights") created by this Agreement upon the following terms and conditions:

1. The term of this Repurchase Option (the "Option Term") shall commence on the date of Resident's death (or the date of the surviving Resident's death in the event there are two Residents in the Living Unit) and shall continue for a period of _____ days thereafter (but not to expire in any event until _____ days after an executor or administrator is appointed by the Probate Court for Resident's estate).

2. This Repurchase Option may be exercised by Retirement Facility at any time during the Option Term, by giving written notice of exercise to the executor or administrator of Resident's estate.

3. In the event that this Repurchase Option is exercised by Retirement Facility in a timely manner during the Option Term, and if only one person is designated as Resident in this Agreement, the purchase price of the Contract Rights shall be the lesser of:

a. _____ percent of the Entrance Fee for the Living Unit paid by Resident; or

b. _____ percent of the then current Entrance Fee for the Living Unit at Retirement Facility for a _____ year term pursuant to a new Residency and Care Agreement to a person who meets all of the criteria of Retirement Facility for its residents including, but not limited to, age and physical condition.

4. In the event that this Repurchase Option is exercised by Retirement Facility in a timely manner during the Option Term, and if two persons are designated as Residents in this Agreement, the purchase price of the Contract Rights upon the death of the last such Resident shall be the lesser of:

a. _____ percent of the Entrance Fee for the Living Unit paid by such Resident; or

b. _____ percent of the then current Entrance Fee for the Living Unit at Retirement Facility for a _____ year term pursuant to a new Residency and Care Agreement to a person who meets all of the criteria of Retirement Facility for its residents including, but not limited to, age and physical condition.

5. In the event that Retirement Facility exercises this Repurchase Option, the purchase price shall be paid in full in cash subject to a credit for any sums then owing by Resident to Retirement Facility, and such payment shall occur within _____ days of the exercise of the Repurchase Option.

6. In the event the Repurchase Option is not timely exercised or the purchase price is not timely paid as set forth herein, Resident shall be entitled to the transfer rights set forth in Paragraph _____.

FORM 28.5AA: NONASSIGNABLE RIGHTS

Rights and Privileges Are Personal. The rights and privileges of the Resident under this Agreement to living accommodations, facilities, and services are personal to the Resident and cannot be transferred or assigned by the Resident, whether by his own act or by any proceeding of law, or otherwise.

FORM 28.5BB: VARIANCE AMONG AGREEMENTS

You understand that Retirement Facility may enter into Membership Agreements with other persons that may contain terms different from those contained in this Agreement. Despite any such different terms in other Agreements, you understand and agree that this Agreement alone sets forth your rights and obligations with respect to Retirement Facility, and that you are not a third party beneficiary of any other Agreement.

FORM 28.5CC: ADMISSIONS AND DISMISSALS
OF OTHER RESIDENTS

You shall agree that you have no right to determine or appeal the admission, terms of admission, placement, or dismissal of any other resident.

FORM 28.5DD: FEES NOT HELD IN TRUST

All fees paid by Resident to Retirement Facility, including entrance fees, shall become the sole property of Retirement Facility, are deemed payment for residence and services, and are not held in trust for benefit of Resident. Retirement Facility reserves and shall have the right and power, without any objection from the Resident, to apply for and receive all financial and other aid from federal, state, or municipal sources to which it may be legally entitled, and also to apply for or receive financial or other aid or donations by will, deed, or otherwise from any source. The Resident shall have no right, title, or interest in any such fees, property, money, aid, donations, or assistance obtained and received by the Retirement Facility, or any right to demand any accounting therefor.

FORM 28.5EE: FACILITY FINANCIAL CONDITION

The financial condition of the Community is as set forth in the attached financial statement. Upon request, you shall be provided with subsequent annual audited reports, which shall include per capita costs and the status of reserves.

FORM 28.5FF: RESIDENTS' ASSOCIATION

Retirement Facility shall assist the residents in organizing a Residents' Association, which may convene and confer to review budgets, policies, and procedures, help arrange social and recreational programs, and to raise matters of concern among the resident population to the administration of the Retirement Facility. Retirement Facility administration shall meet with the Residents' Association whenever reasonably requested to do so by the Residents' Association. The Residents' Association shall have no legal or contractual right to direct or operate Retirement Facility, or any portion thereof. However, Retirement Facility will consult with the Residents' Association and consider resident concerns and the overall welfare of the Retirement Facility community.

FORM 28.5GG: SUPERMAJORITY AMENDMENT

A. This Agreement is the entire agreement of the parties and may be amended only by a written amendment signed by an authorized representative of Retirement Facility.

B. In addition, with the approval of Retirement Facility and of not less than eighty percent (80%) of the residents of the Retirement Facility, this Agreement may be amended in any respect; provided, however, that no such amendment shall:

1. Reduce the aforesaid percentage of residents that is required to consent to any such amendment; or

2. Permit the preference or priority of any resident over any other resident without the consent of each resident involved.

C. Upon the request of Retirement Facility, accompanied by a copy of a resolution of its Board of Directors certified by the Secretary or an Assistant Secretary of Retirement Facility authorizing the execution of any such amendment, and upon the filing with Retirement Facility of evidence of the consent of not less than eighty percent (80%) of the residents as aforesaid, such amendment shall be effective and any designated residence agreements, which may include this Agreement, shall automatically be amended accordingly.

FORM 28.5HH: PET RULE

Pets. You may maintain a dog, cat, or other pet upon the approval of and on terms prescribed by the Executive Director. No such approval shall be necessary for fish or small birds that are kept in appropriate containers. You will be responsible for ensuring that any pet is properly cared for and that your pet does not create any disturbance or otherwise constitute a nuisance, and agree to comply with any reasonable pet regulations adopted by the Community.

FORM 28.5II: COMMUNITY RULES

For the proper management and operation of the Community and the safety, health, and comfort of the residents, Retirement Facility shall have the right to adopt or amend, either by itself or with or through a residents' association, such reasonable rules and regulations as it deems necessary or desirable. You agree to abide by such rules and regulations.

§ 28.6   FEES AND FINANCIAL PROVISIONS

(a)   In General

All agreements, of course, must set forth all the initial and periodic fees or purchase prices required to be paid in order to gain admission and sustain residence at a retirement facility. The basic fee schedule may be simple (Form 28.7A) or more comprehensive (Form 28.7B), depending on whether the provider chooses to break down component charges, credits, or other variables. Agreements should clearly state which services and amenities are covered by the payment of a regular monthly fee, alone or in combination with an entrance fee, and which services and amenities are available only for an extra charge (see discussion at § 28.4(a)).

In general, agreements should specify when monthly or other periodic payments are due (Form 28.7C), and the consequences of any delinquency in payment, such as late charges or termination of the agreement (Form 28.7D). Agreements should further specify whether any credit toward monthly fees or other regular charges will be given for prolonged absences from the facility, such as vacation travel, for missed meals, or for other absences or less than full utilization of services (see Forms 28.7E, 28.7F).

(b)   Preoccupancy Fees

Many facilities charge an application fee or processing fee to applicants for admission (see Form 28.7B). Even if the facility has refundable entrance fees, the processing fee is usually nonrefundable. The ostensible purpose of the fee is to cover the costs of application procedures, which may involve health screening, financial screening, and other processing that will not necessarily lead to the resident's acceptance at the facility. It may also be used to establish priority on a waiting list.

Facilities with real property purchase or entrance fee structures will usually collect deposits from prospective residents prior to and during construction of the facility. These may be required as evidence of the applicant's bona fide interest, or as a means of financing some development costs. The provisions with respect to such deposits are normally found in deposit agreements. Deposit agreements are separate from the Resident Agreement, which is not signed until the facility is opened for occupancy. (See Form 28.7G for a sample deposit agreement.)

Deposit agreements usually provide for escrow of the deposited monies and will specify the terms and conditions under which deposits may be released from escrow (see also Form 28.7H (Escrow Agreement)). Often, escrow requirements and conditions upon the release of residents' escrowed funds will be mandated by state law (see § 21.3).

Because retirement facility developers may rely heavily on the commitment represented by the resident's deposit on a particular unit, and may intend to use deposits for construction financing once they are released from escrow, many developers will prohibit any refund of a deposit pending construction, or unless the particular unit reserved by the resident has been resold to another prospective resident (Form 28.7G). The deposit agreement should also state whether interest will be paid to the resident or retained by the developer, and the conditions under which the agreement may be terminated and fees refunded. It should be clear that there is no guarantee the project will be completed as planned, and there is no obligation for the developer to enter into the proposed Residence Agreement if insufficient enrollments or other factors make the facility infeasible.

(c) Entrance Fees

In continuing care facilities, the lump sum payment that may be required as a condition of initial admission is often called an *accommodation fee*. Usually, the amount of the fee is related to the capital cost of constructing the project, prorated over the number of units in the building. However, many continuing care facilities are structured so that portions of these initial fees are reserved for the cost of future medical care or other contingencies. To the extent that such fees are to be used to establish medical care reserves, they may be tax deductible by the resident as a prepaid medical expense in the year of admission (see § 6.1(c)(1)). In such cases, use of the term *entrance fee*, rather than *accommodation fee*, will more properly characterize the fee as a payment that is not limited to the costs of the physical accommodations, but is also a prepayment for services that may include future medical care.

Provisions concerning entrance fees should specify the amounts paid (Form 28.7B), but need not specify that the payment is for any particular aspect of the retirement facility program, such as "for occupancy of unit 205," as opposed to payment for services. It should also be clear in the agreement that the payment, once made to the facility, is the facility's unrestricted property, and that while there may be a right to refunds, the fee is not held in trust for the resident's benefit (see § 28.4(b)(4)). Most contracts that contain any sort of entrance fee structure may also contain a clause notifying the resident that whatever rights the resident may have under the contract are subordinate to the rights of lenders who may have mortgage liens or other encumbrances against the retirement community's building or other assets (Form 28.7I).

The most difficult problem for entrance fee transactions concerns provisions for refund in the event of death or withdrawal from the facility (see § 28.10(b) for a detailed discussion).

(d) Membership Structures

Entrance fees or ownership mechanisms, such as condominiums and coops, have been used by developers as a means of obtaining large initial cash payments from residents. A few facilities have begun to employ a membership structure as an alternative to such devices. Like country clubs and health clubs, membership retirement communities sell an intangible personal property interest (the membership) for a fixed charge, payable upon admission, plus payment of a monthly or other periodic fee. Membership gives the resident an opportunity to recover the initial entrance payment and possibly to enjoy appreciation in value in the same manner as a real property owner. However, the developer retains the ongoing control characteristic of entrance fee systems, plus the tax advantages of real estate ownership (see § 7.3).

Unlike entrance fee contracts, membership agreements are cast in the language of a sale rather than a rental or service transaction. Therefore, for example, the payment made by the resident is characterized as the *purchase price*, rather than the *fee* (Form 28.7J). The membership contract must carefully point out that the member is receiving no interest in real property of the facility, but that the membership is personal property that belongs to the resident and may be sold at any time, provided that the buyer meets all of the qualifications for admission to the facility, and the selling resident complies with the terms of the membership agreement (see Forms 28.3F, 28.7K).

Membership agreements should place controls on the resident's resale rights without taking away from the resident the rights and characteristics of true ownership of the membership (see Form 28.7K). It is likely that the facility owner or operator will want to receive some share in any appreciation in value that may be realized by the resident upon resale of the membership (see Form 28.7L). This makes economic sense because increases in value are probably due largely to success of the project concept and design, coupled with competent management over a period of years. It also gives the developer an incentive to stay with the project and ensure its continued success. In order to give the resident a financial incentive to sell the membership at the highest possible price, and to retain for the resident some of the benefits of ownership, the resident also should be entitled to receive a share of any appreciation in value.

While the facility may assist the resident in resale of the membership, it should not guarantee the repurchase of the membership, or else the transaction will appear more like a loan than a sale and possibly lead to imputed interest income for the resident (see § 7.3(c)(1)). Without taking away completely the member's rights of ownership, however, the facility may want to ensure that the resident acts reasonably in effecting a sale (Form 28.7M).

(e) Health Credits

Traditional facilities offering continuing care furnish nearly all necessary personal and health care in return for the entrance fee plus a fixed monthly fee, subject to adjustment. (See Form 28.7N for a comprehensive prepaid care description.) A recent trend has been to limit the scope of care available in return for the entrance fee or a regular monthly fee or to sell health services strictly on a fee for service basis. Some facilities are offering health care reserve days plans, or some similar structure by which a resident is given a fixed annual (Form 28.7O) or lifetime (Form 28.7P) number of days of nursing care, which may be utilized at the facility's health center without any surcharge beyond regular monthly fees. Or, rather than have a fixed lifetime fund that may be drawn down, facilities may establish an account to which days are added, for example, for each year of residence, and are carried over from one year to the next and accumulated (see Form 28.7Q). Others include temporary care as part of the regular fee, but charge extra for extended care (Form 28.7R).

A resident might be able to use accumulated free care days for temporary illnesses during the course of his or her occupancy of the residential unit, or they may be drawn upon at the start of a permanent transfer to nursing or personal care. Individual reserve days may or may not be transferable between spouses. Upon permanent transfer, proceeds from the sale of a residential unit also may be used for paying the costs of care (see Form 28.7S). In addition, a portion of entrance fees may be reserved for use in paying health care costs that are billed on a fee for service basis (Form 28.7T).

Health reserve plans are a matter of individual provider choice, and may be influenced by consumer focus group preferences. Though not available at many facilities, health care prepayment plans are an attractive feature in facilities catering to the expanding older segment of the senior market.

(f) Fee Changes

To the extent monthly fees or charges for optional services are specified in the contract, it should be expressly provided that such fees are subject to adjustment by the facility, together with an indication of the basis, if any, for such adjustment, and the extent of any notice to be given to the resident prior to the effective date of a fee change. Note that many states require that continuing care facilities base increases in monthly fees upon specific criteria articulated in statute or regulation. For example, California specifies that monthly fees may be increased only on one of six alternative bases, the most comprehensive of which is prior year cash per capita costs, projected costs, and economic indicators.[10] Tax exempt facilities likewise may be constrained to offer services at the lowest feasible cost under Revenue Ruling 72-124 (see § 9.2 and Form 28.7U). The frequency with which fees can be raised may be limited (Form 28.7V). However, it is important to allow sufficient flexibility to adjust fees to cover expenses. (See § 5.1, regarding the Pacific Homes bankruptcy.)

§ 28.7   FEES AND FINANCIAL PROVISIONS: SAMPLE FORMS

FORM 28.7A: CHARGE LIST (Simple)

Fees. Resident hereby agrees to pay to Retirement Facility:

1. The sum of _____ dollars payable upon execution of this contract or in accordance with Entrance Agreement. (Credit for any deposit paid with preliminary application will be allowed against this sum, but not the processing fee of _____ dollars. The processing fee covers clerical and related costs for processing the application and is not refundable, except during the ninety (90) day probationary period.

2. The sum of _____ dollars per month, payable monthly in advance, subject to adjustment as noted in paragraph _____.

FORM 28.7B: CHARGE LIST (Detailed)

SCHEDULE OF FEES

The basic fees associated with your residency at Retirement Facility include an Application Fee, an Accommodation Fee, and Monthly Service Charges.

A. Your Nonrefundable Application Fee is $_____

B. Accommodation Fees are refundable only as set forth in Article _____ of this Agreement.

   1. If one Resident occupies your dwelling unit the agreed amount of the Accommodation Fee is $_____

   2. If a second Resident also occupies your dwelling unit, an additional Accommodation Fee is also required in the amount of $_____

   Total Accommodation Fee(s) $_____

[10]Tit. 22, Cal. Admin. Code, § 89730.

Payment received as of date of this Agreement $_____

Interest earned on deposits $_____

Balance due by closing date $_____

C. Monthly Service Fees

Article _____ of this Agreement explains that the Monthly Service Fees may be changed from time to time to reflect changes in the true cost of services, including operating expenses, interest, and taxes. The basic Monthly Service Fee in effect at the time this Agreement is signed are as follows.

1. First Person Fee $_____

2. Second Person Fee $_____

3. Additional cost per person for

( ) Two meal plan $_____

( ) Three meal plan $_____

Adjusted Monthly Fee $_____

FORM 28.7C: FEE DUE DATE

The Monthly Fees are due and payable in advance on the first business day of each month beginning with your assigned occupancy date, and shall be prorated for any applicable period of less than one month. You agree to pay the Monthly Fee applicable to your residence whether you are residing in your residence, in the Health Care Center, or otherwise absent from Retirement Facility. Retirement Facility will provide you with a monthly invoice for any services and supplies provided or obtained for you that Retirement Facility is not obligated to provide. Such invoices are to be paid within thirty (30) days after receipt.

FORM 28.7D: DELINQUENT FEES

You agree to pay your Monthly Service Fee, payable in advance on or before the first business day of each month, in accordance with the schedule appearing in Section _____, or as such Fee may be revised from time to time as provided below. In the event that your Monthly Service Fee is not received by Retirement Facility within five (5) days of the due date, Retirement Facility reserves the right to assess a late penalty of one and one-half (1.5) percent per month until the amount owing is paid. You agree to pay the Monthly Service Fee applicable to your residence whether you are residing in your residence or are absent from Retirement Facility. You will receive a monthly invoice for any goods or services provided for or obtained by you that Retirement Facility is not obligated to provide under this Agreement. Such invoices shall be paid by you within thirty (30) days of the invoice date. Late payment of such invoices may result in assessment of a late penalty as described above. Late penalties will not be assessed if Retirement Facility determines that payments are late due to circumstances beyond your control.

FORM 28.7E: FEE REFUND FOR ABSENCE

Resident Absence. If you are absent from the Community for more than fourteen (14) consecutive days, you will receive a partial refund of your Monthly Fee as determined by Retirement Facility, provided you first give written notice to the Executive Director of the Community at least five (5) days prior to such absence.

FORM 28.7F: MEAL CREDIT FOR ABSENCE

Credits for Absence. If the Resident should be absent from the retirement residence for reasons other than hospitalization under the conditions set out in subparagraph _____ above, the Retirement Facility shall allow a credit on a daily basis of the raw food cost to the Resident during such absence, said credit to commence on the eighth (8th) day of absence. Advance notice of one week to Retirement Facility is required regarding any absence for which credit is to be given, and the period of absence must be continuous in order to receive credit. If the raw food costs of the residence should so indicate, as determined by the Retirement Facility, the amount of said credit may from time to time be increased or decreased, upon prior written notice to the Resident of not less than thirty (30) days. The Resident hereby agrees to abide by any such change.

FORM 28.7G: DEPOSIT AGREEMENT

DEPOSIT SUBSCRIPTION AGREEMENT

THIS AGREEMENT is entered into on _____, 19_____, between _____ _____ (hereinafter referred to as "Retirement Facility") and _____ _____ (hereinafter referred to as the "Subscriber") (if more than one person enters into this agreement, the term "Subscriber" shall refer to each person).

Retirement Facility is engaged in the establishment of a retirement housing and care facility at _____ (hereinafter referred to as the "Facility"). The Subscriber is desirous of becoming a resident of the Facility and has been accepted preliminarily for residence by Retirement Facility. Retirement Facility contemplates that it will complete the Facility by _____, 19_____, but cannot guarantee this completion date.

IT IS THEREFORE AGREED:

1. The Subscriber shall pay the following amounts to Retirement Facility:

a. A priority deposit of _____ dollars ($_____), of which five hundred dollars ($500.00) is a processing fee to cover the administrative costs of processing the Subscriber's application;

b. The sum of _____ dollars ($_____) as an entry fee for the use of residence style _____, which shall be paid as follows:

(1) The sum of _____ dollars ($_____) (which shall be equal to twenty percent (20%) of the entry fee) upon signing this Deposit Subscription Agreement, to be credited against the total balance due.

(2) The sum of _____ ($_____) (which shall constitute the balance of the entry fee) within thirty (30) days after the Subscriber receives notice that the Facility will be ready for occupancy in approximately forty-five (45) days.

2. The amount of the entry fee in Section 1(b) above is based upon the Subscriber's choice of Payment Option _____ for residence unit number _____, and the Subscriber acknowledges that the Payment Option selected will have an effect upon the amount of the monthly fee and upon the refund provisions, as set forth in Appendix A to this Deposit Subscription Agreement and in the Residence Agreement (attached as Appendix B).

3. Retirement Facility shall make the Subscriber's residence unit available for occupancy upon the signing of the Residence Agreement between Retirement Facility and the Subscriber or of any amended version of the Residence Agreement acceptable to both parties.

4. Retirement Facility has entered into an Escrow Agreement with _____, a form of which is available upon request, which provides for the holding of the Subscriber's payment described in Section 1(b)(1) above. The Subscriber shall make that payment jointly to Retirement Facility and _____.

5. The Subscriber's rights under this Deposit Subscription Agreement are limited to the rights expressly granted in this document and do not include any ownership interest in Retirement Facility or in the Facility. The Subscriber's rights under this Deposit Subscription Agreement are subject to any subordination agreements required by the Residence Agreement.

6. Retirement Facility shall make refunds to the Subscribers of the amounts paid under Section 1 above in accordance with the following rules:

a. In the event that (1) the Subscriber terminates this Deposit Subscription Agreement by written notice under Section 8 below, or (2) Retirement Facility terminates this Deposit Subscription Agreement because of the Subscriber's failure to pay any amount set forth in Section 1 above, then Retirement Facility shall refund the amounts paid under Section 1 above, with the exception of the processing fee, without interest. If the termination occurs prior to the start of construction of the Facility, Retirement Facility shall make the refund within thirty (30) days after receiving notice of the termination. If the termination occurs after the start of construction, Retirement Facility shall make the refund within thirty (30) days after another prospective resident has taken the Subscriber's place on Retirement Facility's priority list for the residence style involved and made the necessary deposit subscription payments. The processing fee portion of the priority deposit under Section 1(a) above shall be nonrefundable.

b. In the event that (1) Subscriber dies prior to signing the Residence Agreement, (2) Retirement Facility does not accept the Subscriber for occupancy at the Facility, (3) Retirement Facility terminates this Agreement for good and sufficient cause (other than failure of the Subscriber to pay the amounts due under Section 1 above), (4) Retirement Facility fails without satisfactory cause to construct the Facility by the date set forth above, or (5) Retirement Facility and the Subscriber do not enter into a Residence Agreement for any other reason other than those set forth in Section 6(a) above, then Retirement Facility shall refund all amounts paid under Section 1 above (except the processing fee as set forth below), with interest at the prevailing passbook rate of _____ percent (_____%) during the term of the deposit. Retirement Facility shall make payment within thirty (30) days after receiving notice of the event causing refund. Notwithstanding the foregoing, the processing fee portion of the priority deposit in Section 1(a) above shall be nonrefundable, except where the Subscriber dies prior to signing the Residence Agreement, or where Retirement Facility does not accept the Subscriber for occupancy at the Facility.

c. Retirement Facility shall make any refunds due after the signing of the Care and Residency Agreement in accordance with that Agreement.

7. The Subscriber shall conform to the rules, policies, and principles that exist now or in the future for the operation of the Facility. Retirement Facility shall provide a copy of the Facility's rules and regulations to the Subscriber when they are available.

8. The Subscriber may terminate this Deposit Subscription Agreement at any time by giving written notice to Retirement Facility.

9. By signing below, the Subscriber certifies that he/she has read and understands this Deposit Subscription Agreement and the attached Residence Agreement.

RETIREMENT FACILITY

By: _____

Title: _____

Date: _____

SUBSCRIBER

_____

Date: _____

_____

Date: _____

FORM 28.7H: ESCROW AGREEMENT

ESCROW AGREEMENT

_____
(Escrow Agent)

Escrow Account No. _____

_____
(Street Address)

Date _____, 19_____

_____
(City, State, and Zip Code)

_____
(Telephone Number)

RECITAL: Retirement Facility, a _____ corporation (hereinafter referred to as the "Trustor") plans to construct and operate a retirement housing and care facility at _____ (hereinafter referred to as the "Facility").

This escrow agreement constitutes an arrangement that is acceptable to the _____ Department of _____ under Section _____ of the _____ Code. The Trustor will transfer certain deposit subscription fees described below to the above-named Escrow Agent to be held in trust as provided below.

PROVISIONS: The following provisions shall apply to this Escrow Agreement:

1. The Trustor shall remit to the Escrow Agent all funds collected from the sale of deposit subscriptions on continuing care agreements (except for the _____ dollars ($_____) application fee, which may be retained by the Trustor to cover administrative costs) within forty-eight (48) hours after receipt from the subscriber, together with a duplicate copy of the signed Deposit Subscription Agreement, a copy of the subscriber's deposit receipt, and a deposit summary showing for each subscriber the name, address, the full value of the subscription, and the amount deposited.

2. The Escrow Agent is willing to hold the above funds in trust for the benefit of the Trustor. The Escrow Agent shall invest the funds in the manner approved for liquid assets in Section _____ of the _____ Code, with interest earned to be retained and disbursed as provided in Section 4 below.

3. Subscribers shall make deposit subscription payments to the Trustor and the Escrow Agent jointly by check, draft, or money order.

4. Funds deposited in the escrow account shall be subject to withdrawal only under the following conditions:

   a. Upon written approval from the _____ Department of _____, the Escrow Agent shall make payment to the Trustor or to any subscriber who has deposited funds in the escrow account; or

   b. Upon certification by an officer of the Trustor that the Deposit Subscription Agreement has been terminated pursuant to its terms, the Escrow Agent shall make payment to any subscriber who has deposited funds in the escrow account. The purpose of the payment will be to repay the subscriber the amounts paid under the Deposit Subscription Agreement. Such repayment shall not include interest, except where the subscriber terminates the Deposit Subscription Agreement by written notice to the Trustor or the subscriber fails to pay an amount due under the Deposit Subscription Agreement. Any interest to be paid shall be at the prevailing passbook interest rate of the Escrow Agent during the term of the deposit, and shall be paid directly to the subscriber.

5. The Escrow Agent shall make regular monthly progress reports showing additions, withdrawals, the current escrow account balance, and any other necessary information to the _____ Department of _____ and to the Trustor.

6. In consideration of the Escrow Agent's duties in regard to the escrow account, the Trustor shall pay to the Escrow Agent an initial fee of _____ dollars ($_____), plus the following amounts: _____. Notwithstanding the foregoing, the Trustor's payment shall be no less than _____ dollars ($_____) per year, plus the initial charge of _____ dollars ($_____).

7. The trust created by this Escrow Agreement shall be irrevocable and may be altered or amended only with the written agreement of the Trustor and the Escrow Agent and the written approval of the _____ Department of _____. The trust shall terminate upon instructions from the _____ Department of _____ to release the funds to the Trustor under Section _____ of the _____ Code. Following termination of the trust, the Escrow Agent shall render an accounting to the Trustor and shall distribute the entire escrow account, less any fees due the Escrow Agent, in accordance with written instructions from the _____ Department of _____.

8. During the term of this Escrow Agreement, the Escrow Agent shall not lend any amount to the Trustor for use at the Facility and shall not have any fiduciary responsibilities to lenders or bond holders for the Facility.

9. The Escrow Agent shall not be required to determine any controversy involving third parties concerning the disposition of the escrow account, but instead may await the resolution of the controversy.

RETIREMENT FACILITY   ESCROW AGENT

By: _____   By: _____

Title: _____   Title: _____

Date: _____   Date: _____

FORM 28.7I: SUBORDINATION CLAUSE

Pursuant to the requirements of a bona fide lender, you agree that your rights under this Agreement shall at all times be subordinate and inferior to the rights of the lender under any deed of trust previously executed by Retirement Facility, or any extension, renewal, or substitute for such deed of trust. You also agree that your rights shall be subordinate under any deed of trust hereafter executed so long as it would not jeopardize Retirement Facility's ability to maintain the reserves required by the State Department of _____ to fulfill its obligations under this Agreement, and so long as Retirement Facility has given ninety (90) days written notice to the State Department of _____ and has included an analysis of the impact of the additional indebtedness on its reserves and an analysis of the sources of funds for repaying such indebtedness. You further agree to execute, acknowledge, and deliver such subordination agreement as such lender may require in order to establish the priority of such deed of trust lien against the property.

FORM 28.7J: MEMBERSHIP AS A SALE

RESIDENTIAL MEMBERSHIP PURCHASE PRICE

You are purchasing your Residential Membership for _____ dollars ($_____) in accordance with the terms of the Deposit Subscription Agreement, which is attached to this Agreement as Exhibit B. Purchase of your Residential Membership will entitle you to live in Residence No. _____, which you have selected, according to the terms of this Agreement.

RIGHTS TO INITIAL MEMBERSHIP PROCEEDS

All monies paid to Retirement Facility shall become the unrestricted property of Retirement Facility. As soon as you have paid the Residential Membership purchase price, the Residential Membership Certificate will be your property and may be transferred by you or your estate to a Qualified Buyer as provided in this Agreement, and you or your estate will be entitled to retain the proceeds of sale less the Transfer Fee as provided in this Agreement from the sale of your Residential Membership. Your Residential Membership shall not be mortgaged, pledged, or assigned by you as security for any obligation or subject to a security interest, except as provided in Section _____.

FORM 28.7K: RESALE OF MEMBERSHIP

SALE OF YOUR RESIDENTIAL MEMBERSHIP

Your Residential Membership in Retirement Facility may be sold to a Qualified Buyer at any time, subject to the terms and conditions of this Agreement. You or your estate may sell your Residential Membership for such price as you or your estate and a Qualified Buyer may agree. Payment of the Monthly Fee, and other applicable fees, will continue to be your responsibility until your Residential Membership is fully transferred to a Qualified Buyer.

QUALIFIED BUYER

A Qualified Buyer is a person (or persons) who purchases a Residential Membership from a selling Resident and who is acceptable to Retirement Facility for residency in accordance with the Membership Agreement and the policies and standards established by Retirement Facility at the time of transfer. Such policies and standards include, but are not limited to, meeting the financial and health requirements of Retirement Facility.

FORM 28.7L: MEMBERSHIP APPRECIATION

TRANSFER FEE

When you, your heirs, or your estate sell your Residential Membership, the purchase price paid by a Qualified Buyer will be determined by the marketplace. Retirement Facility will maintain an ongoing marketing program to assist in the sale of your Membership. Upon sale, a Transfer Fee is to be paid to Retirement Facility as follows:

1. _____ percent (_____%) of your Membership purchase price set forth in Section _____.

2. _____ percent (_____%) of the difference between your Membership purchase price and the price paid for your Membership by the Qualified Buyer.

FORM 28.7M: MEMBERSHIP SALE RESTRICTIONS

SIX MONTH SALE OPPORTUNITY

In the event you or Retirement Facility terminate this Agreement, or in the event of your death (or death of the survivor if there are two of you), you, your executor, or your personal representative will have six months from the date of termination or death in which to effect a transfer of your Membership.

RETIREMENT FACILITY MAY TRANSFER YOUR MEMBERSHIP FOR YOU

If your Membership has not been transferred in the six month period set forth in Section _____, you, your executor, or personal representative shall deliver your Membership certificate to Retirement Facility by the end of the six month period, properly endorsed for transfer. If you wish, you may deliver your endorsed Membership certificate to Retirement Facility at any time prior to the expiration of six months. In either event, Retirement Facility will then use its best efforts to find a purchaser for your Membership on your behalf. You or your estate will be entitled to all amounts paid by the Qualified Buyer for your Membership less any monies due to Retirement Facility. No transfer of your Membership may be made at a price less than the amount of your Membership purchase price unless you or your executor or personal representative consent to and approve such transfer. If, after your Membership certificate has been delivered to Retirement Facility for transfer, Retirement Facility obtains a Qualified Buyer who is ready, able, and willing to pay an amount for your Membership at least equal to your Membership purchase price, you, or your estate or personal representative, shall be obligated to transfer your Membership to such Buyer for such price. Retirement Facility does not guarantee that you will be able to sell your Membership for a price equal to the Membership purchase price you paid.

REQUIREMENTS FOR TRANSFER

A transfer of your Membership shall occur only when all of the following events have occurred:

1. Your Membership certificate has been properly endorsed for transfer to the Qualified Buyer, including your representation that it is free of all liens and encumbrances, and surrendered to Retirement Facility for cancelation.
2. The Qualified Buyer has signed a Residence Agreement for residency in the Retirement Facility.
3. The Qualified Buyer has paid the Membership purchase price and Retirement Facility has been paid all monies due under this contract and under the Escrow Agreement applicable to the transfer.
4. The Qualified Buyer has begun paying the Monthly Service Fee due under his or her Residence Agreement.

5. You have released the residential unit described in this Agreement to Retirement Facility in clean and good condition.

TRANSFERS FOR LESS THAN MARKET VALUE

If you transfer your Membership for less than full and adequate consideration, as by gift or bequest or otherwise, the Fair Market Value of your Membership shall be deemed to have been received by you or your estate and a Transfer Fee will be charged accordingly. The Fair Market Value of a Membership for purposes of this Agreement shall be based upon recent arm's length, bona fide sales of Memberships for comparable residential units at the Retirement Facility, and shall be determined by exercise of the reasonable discretion of Retirement Facility.

FORM 28.7N: COMPREHENSIVE PREPAID CARE

Retirement Facility agrees to furnish the Resident the board, room, lodging, care, and services enumerated in this section, and no others, for the rest of the natural life of Resident, and so long as Resident remains in Retirement Facility and carries out his obligations under this contract.

1. *Personal Assistance.* Retirement Facility will provide personal assistance as needed, in the opinion of Retirement Facility Physician, in bathing, dressing, hair care, shaving, eating, and other such incidental personal services in the living unit. Retirement Facility also will provide assistance with medication as needed that has been authorized by a physician for self medication and does not require the exercise of professional judgment.

2. *Medical and Hospital Care.* Medical care furnished by Retirement Facility will include that care that may be given by a licensed doctor of medicine and by the trained nurses regularly employed by Retirement Facility, and does not include dentistry, ophthalmology, chiropractic, osteopathy, podiatry, or religious sect. The medical care must be authorized or prescribed by the Staff Physician. A Resident is at liberty to engage the services of any accredited physician or surgeon, but Retirement Facility is not responsible for or obligated to defray the charges of any such physician for such services rendered or any charge for services rendered by persons other than those regularly contracted for or retained by Retirement Facility. If special care or treatment on the premises is prescribed by such outside physicians, it must be authorized by Staff Physician.

3. Retirement Facility is not responsible for defraying the cost of drugs, medicines, vitamins, dental work, glasses, hearing aids, orthopedic appliances, treatment of mental illness, or of any ailment existing at the time of entrance as a Resident and listed by the examining physician as an exception in this Agreement, or any undisclosed contagious, infectious, or incurable disease existing prior to the execution of this Agreement.

4. Retirement Facility will furnish all hospitalization determined necessary by the Staff Physician, in its own or suitable outside medical facility. Emergency hospitalization within the USA will be furnished or compensated by Retirement Facility to the extent of that provided under the standard daily rate paid for the

accommodation used. Such may, unless the Staff Physician otherwise recommends, be provided through semiprivate accommodations. If private room accommodations are available and desired by the Resident, when in the judgment of the Staff Physician such private room accommodations are not necessary, the Resident shall be obligated to pay the difference between the cost of semiprivate accommodations and such private accommodations. The term *semiprivate accommodations* as used herein refers to a hospital room accommodating more than one, but not more than six persons.

FORM 28.7O: ANNUAL PREPAID HEALTH RESERVE

1. Resident will pay to Corporation, in advance, a monthly general health care charge for certain health care services provided by the Retirement Facility. This monthly general health care charge shall not include the expenses attributable to the care of residents receiving extended or special care. The monthly general health care charge will entitle Resident during each calendar year to nursing care and a room in the Medical Facility for the first five (5) days of each separately diagnosed illness during such calendar year. For extended care in the Medical Facility beyond the first five (5) days for each separately diagnosed illness during the calendar year, an additional amount will be charged on a daily basis for such nursing care and room based on a pro rata share of the operating expenses of the Medical Facility.

2. The monthly general health care charge to Resident is presently in an amount of _____ dollars ($_____), and shall commence upon the earlier to occur of the first day of apartment occupancy in Retirement Facility or within thirty (30) days from the date of notice to Resident that the apartment is available for occupancy. It is understood by and between the parties that the monthly general health care charge and the daily rates charged for extended care in the Medical Facility are based upon estimated operating costs and may be increased or decreased, as deemed appropriate by Corporation, to reflect changes in those costs. Such daily rates charged for extended care are further established on the basis of whether or not the Resident/Patient in the Medical Facility has released his apartment to Corporation.

FORM 28.7P: PREPAID LIFETIME RESERVE (FIXED)

If, in the opinion of your attending physician or the Medical Director, you need nursing care in Retirement Facility health center, we will provide you services there to the extent authorized by our license from the State of _____ on the following terms:

1. We will provide nursing care in Retirement Facility health center without extra charge beyond your regular monthly charges for ninety (90) cumulative days of care (90 days for each of you if there are two, but the allowances cannot be combined and used by only one of you.) However, you will pay for the meals not covered by your monthly Service Fee at the then current charge for extra meals.

2. If you continue to require nursing care in Retirement Facility health center after you have received ninety (90) cumulative days of care, you will pay for the nursing care.

FORM 28.7Q: PREPAID LIFETIME RESERVE (ACCRUING, WITH CAP)

ACCRUED RESERVE DAYS. When you initially occupy your residence at Retirement Facility, you will receive an immediate Reserve of ten (10) days of Basic Services in the Health Care Center. As long as you continue to live in your residence, you will receive an additional ten (10) days to be added to your Basic Services Reserve upon each anniversary of your residence at Retirement Facility, up to a maximum lifetime reserve of sixty (60) days.

In the event that you need to use the services of the Health Care Center, and such services are not otherwise covered by Medicare, supplemental insurance, or other third party payments, you may use your accrued Basic Services Reserve Days.

When two persons occupy one residence, Basic Services Reserve Days shall accrue to each cooccupant as provided above. Except where a cooccupant is transferred on a nontemporary basis to the Health Care Center, as provided below, cooccupants may choose to apply Basic Service Reserve Days accrued to one cooccupant to cover services rendered to the other cooccupant.

Basic Services in the Health Care Center include those services listed in the published room rate and consist of a semiprivate room, routine nursing services, and meals. All ancillary charges and other services including, without limitation, medications, laboratory and x-ray procedures, and special treatments will be charged to your account.

You will continue to pay your regular Monthly Fee at Retirement Facility during all temporary stays in the Health Care Center.

FORM 28.7R: TEMPORARY CARE PREPAID

1. *Temporary Stay.* If you move from your residence into the Health Center and are there for less than sixty (60) days during any ninety (90) day period (referred to in this Agreement as a "temporary stay"), you will continue to pay only your regular Monthly Fee plus a meal charge for two (2) additional meals per day.

2. *Extended Stay.* If you reside in the Health Center for longer than a temporary stay (referred to in this Agreement as an "extended stay"), the fees shall be as follows:

a. If you are a single resident, you will pay your Monthly Fee plus a fee (referred to in this Agreement as the "Health Center Fee") for each day in the Health Center exceeding a temporary stay, as long as you retain your residence. The Health Center Fee shall be an amount equal to (1) the Monthly Fee for single occupancy of a standard one bedroom residence, as may be adjusted from time to time as provided in this Agreement, divided by thirty (30), plus (2) the charge for two additional meals per day. Upon release of your residence, you will thereafter pay only the Health Center Fee.

FORM 28.7S: UNIT SALE PROCEEDS HELD IN TRUST

If you sell your Residential Membership after you have assumed Assisted Status Membership, you will be required to place into a trust account, which Retirement Facility will maintain, the sale price, less Transfer Fees ("net proceeds") from the sale of your Residential Membership. The Trust Account will be administered by Retirement Facility or a trustee obtained by Retirement Facility, and all net earnings from the monies you deposit in the Trust Account will be paid to you when received, except that the trustee shall pay to Retirement Facility, from interest and principal, the amount of any financial obligation that you are unable to pay to Retirement Facility under this Agreement. Upon payment into the Trust Account of the net proceeds of the sale of your Residential Membership, Retirement Facility will deliver to you a signed Assisted Status Membership Certificate and a Trust Agreement. In the event, (1) of your death (if there are two of you, upon the death of the survivor), or (2) you or Retirement Facility terminates this Membership Agreement, your Certificate may be redeemed, and all monies held for you in the Trust Account will be paid to you within thirty (30) days thereafter less any unpaid or deferred charges owed by you to Retirement Facility (e.g., health care charges). You may not sell or otherwise transfer your Assisted Status Membership.

FORM 28.7T: ENTRANCE FEE HEALTH RESERVE (LONG FORM)

EXTENDED CARE BENEFIT. In the event that you are transferred on a nontemporary basis to the Health Care Center for hospitalization, nursing care or other health related services as set forth in Section _____, you shall be entitled to receive an extended benefit. The extended benefit does not apply to health care services received other than in the Health Care Center.

1. For Individual Residents

a. At such time as you are transferred, an Extended Care Reserve Account will be established for your care in the amount of 50 percent of the Accommodation Fee that was paid when you moved to Retirement Facility. In addition, if at the time you are transferred, you have any unused Basic Services Reserve Days, the value of these unused days, which shall be determined by multiplying the number of unused days by the daily rate for Basic Services in effect in the Health Care Center at the time of transfer, shall be added to your Extended Care Reserve Account.

b. If you become a permanent resident of the Health Care Center, your Monthly Fee will be terminated and your residence will be released. However, you will continue to pay to Retirement Facility, on a monthly basis, an amount equal to the Monthly Fee that would be applicable had you remained in your residence. These payments will be added to your Extended Care Reserve Account.

c. All charges that you incur in the Health Care Center will be billed to you. To the extent not covered by Medicare, supplemental insurance, or other third party payments, funds from the Extended Care Reserve Account will be used to pay for services billed to you.

2. For Cooccupants

a. When two persons occupy a residence, the Extended Care Reserve Account as provided above will be established at the time the first person (Resident I) becomes a resident of the Health Care Center on a nontemporary basis.

b. This Extended Care Reserve Account for Resident I will be in the amount of twenty-five percent (25%) of the Accommodation Fee paid; plus the value of one-half of any unused Basic Services Reserve Days accrued to both cooccupants, calculated as provided in Section _____;

c. The second person (Resident II) who continues to live in the residence will continue to pay the current Monthly Fee for one person that is applicable to the residence. The number of Basic Services Reserve Days accrued to Resident II shall be the number of days accrued to both Resident I and Resident II as of the date of the transfer of Resident I, less the number of unused Basic Services Reserve Days applied to the Extended Care Reserve Account of Resident I.

d. Resident I, who has been transferred to the Health Care Center, will have his or her Monthly Fee terminated, but will continue to pay on a monthly basis an amount equal to the Monthly Fee that would be applicable for a second person in his or her prior residence. These payments will be added on to the Extended Care Reserve Account of Resident I. All charges incurred in the Health Care Center by Resident I will be billed to him or her. To the extent not covered by Medicare, supplemental insurance, or other third party payments, funds from the Extended Care Reserve Account will be used to pay for services billed to Resident I.

e. In the event that Resident II also becomes a resident of the Health Care Center on a nontemporary basis, the residence will be released and a Reserve Account will be established for Resident II in the amount of twenty-five percent (25%) of the total Accommodation Fee paid plus the value of any of Resident II's unused Basic Services Reserve Days, calculated as provided in Section _____. Resident II will have his or her Monthly Fee terminated, but will continue to pay on a monthly basis an amount equal to the Monthly Fee that would be applicable had he or she remained in his or her residence. These payments will be added to the Extended Care Reserve Account of Resident II. All charges incurred in the Health Care Center by Resident II will be billed to him or her. To the extent not covered by Medicare, supplemental insurance, or other third party payments, funds from the Extended Care Reserve Account will be used to pay for services billed to Resident II.

f. If either cooccupant dies without having expended his Basic Services Reserve Days and/or Extended Care Reserve Account, the remaining Basic Services Reserve Days and/or Extended Care Reserve Account benefits will be made available to the surviving cooccupant. The charges thereafter to the survivor will be those applicable to Resident II, as described in Sections _____.

FORM 28.7U: FEES AT LOWEST COST (NONPROFIT)

Retirement Facility agrees to maintain the Service Fee Component at the lowest possible rate consistent with sound financial practices and maintenance of the quality and quantity of services called for within this Agreement. It is agreed that Retirement Facility may adjust service fees upon thirty (30) days advance notice to you. Such adjustments shall be based upon Retirement Facility's projected costs (including reserve requirements), prior year per capita costs, and economic indicators as determined by Retirement Facility. You agree that in the event of such adjustment by Retirement Facility, you shall pay such adjusted fee.

FORM 28.7V: FEE CHANGE FREQUENCY

ADJUSTMENTS OF MONTHLY FEE

1. *Adjustments.* Retirement Facility will have the right to adjust your Monthly Fee at any time commencing twelve (12) months after the official opening date of the Community as designated by Retirement Facility, as follows: adjustments shall not be made more than once in each twelve (12) month period nor without at least sixty (60) days notice to you. Such adjustments shall be based on Retirement Facility's projected costs, prior year cash per capita costs, and economic indicators, as determined by Retirement Facility.

---

§ 28.8   CHANGES OF ACCOMMODATIONS

(a)   Voluntary

Resident Agreements should provide for the circumstances, if any, under which a resident may change accommodations in the event another becomes available (see, e.g., Form 28.9A). The provision should cover changes in monthly fees, and adjustments in any entrance fees, due to a difference in the scope of services or quality of the units (see Form 28.9B). Such a provision may be particularly complicated in continuing care facilities where entrance fees are not fully refundable but amortized over a fixed period (see Form 28.9C).

While such a clause may not be necessary in month-to-month rental agreements, those with annual or longer term leases should consider transfer of accommodations provisions. Often, facilities have waiting lists for particular units that are more spacious or attractive for other reasons. When such a unit becomes available, the facility should have a prescribed system for determining who is eligible to occupy the unit and under what circumstances. This can be particularly important when both a nonresident on a waiting list for admission and a resident express interest in the same vacant unit. These matters probably should be handled by facility policy statements, rather than in contract language.

(b)   Health Reasons

Whether or not the facility itself provides personal care or health care services, the circumstances under which a resident must move from an independent living unit to a personal care or skilled nursing facility should be specified in the Resident Agreement. Contracts should give the facility owner or operator the ultimate authority to determine when a resident is in need of moving from independent living to care facilities. It is often difficult for residents to face the sometimes subtle increases in dependency that may come with old age. In addition, the resident's personal physician may have a tendency to support the resident's view that a transfer is unnecessary, whereas a more objective viewpoint would indicate the need for the transfer. To alleviate possible concerns about arbitrary action by the facility operator, the contract may provide that the administration will not make a decision to transfer until it has at least consulted with the resident, the medical director, and the patient's personal physician (see Form 28.9D).

A distinction should be made between temporary and permanent transfers (see Form 28.9E). In the event of a temporary transfer, after the end of the stay in the care facility, the resident generally will be entitled to move back into the residential unit originally occupied. Temporary transfers for health reasons usually are transfers to the skilled nursing facility, which may occur after a fall or a short-term illness.[11] Transfers to the personal care units, however, tend to be long-term placements due to chronic illness, or degenerative changes that may accompany age, such as feebleness or confusion. The Resident Agreement should reflect this phenomenon.

The Agreement should set forth in detail the consequences of a temporary and a permanent transfer. Facility policies differ widely at this juncture. Some require residents to pay fee-for-service charges, which are usually substantially higher than residential monthly fees, for nursing or personal care (see Form 28.9F). Others may provide skilled nursing or personal care services without any substantial increase in the usual monthly fee charges imposed while the person resided in an independent residential unit (see Form 28.7R).

When a transfer is made that is deemed to be permanent, contracts often require release of the residential unit (Form 28.9G). An adjustment in monthly fees, or in amortization schedules for entrance fees (Form 28.9H), if any, may also accompany a permanent move. Some may permit the resident to retain the right to move back to the original residential unit for an extended period of time, provided that the resident continues to pay a monthly charge for keeping the unit open, in addition to charges for residing in the health care or personal care centers (see Forms 28.9I, 28.9G). For those who can afford to do so, this option may be desirable when a resident is unwilling to accede to the permanence of a transfer for health reasons.

However, facility operators should consider some limitation on how long a person in a care facility can keep the residential unit unoccupied and available for his or her return, because the facility will likely have a financial interest in releasing or reselling the residential unit. Often, there will be no way for a resident paying periodic charges in a health center to

---

[11] Of course, permanent transfers to skilled nursing may also take place.

afford, in addition, a surcharge that would duplicate the financial benefit to the facility operator of a new sale or rental of the residential unit, with steady monthly fees and possibly an entrance fee.

(c) Couples

When more than one resident occupies a particular unit, the death or transfer to a health facility of one resident may call for adjustment in monthly fees. Contracts should specify what fees will be required for the person entering the care facility and what reductions, if any, will be available to the spouse or other person remaining in the residential facility (see Form 28.9J).

Termination provisions should also deal with the situation where one resident of a couple residing in a single residential unit dies or leaves the facility. The contract should specify whether the surviving resident may move to smaller accommodations and, if so, what change will be made to entrance fees or monthly fees. Provisions allocating health care credits, entrance fee credits or refunds, fees, or other rights and obligations among spouses can present the most challenging planning and drafting problems (see Forms 28.9K, 28.7Q, and 28.7T).

§ 28.9   CHANGES OF ACCOMMODATIONS: SAMPLE FORMS

FORM 28.9A: TRANSFER TO ANOTHER UNIT

Conditions. All apartment transfers will require Retirement Facility's prior written consent, which will not be unreasonably withheld. The Resident agrees to pay all moving costs and any necessary redecorating costs required to restore the apartment being vacated to its original condition, reasonable wear excepted. The Resident will enter into an amendment of this Contract with Retirement Facility identifying the new apartment and establishing the Basic Monthly Service Fee and the Entrance Fee for the new apartment as set forth below.

FORM 28.9B: FEE ADJUSTMENT ON TRANSFER

Fees. (1) The Resident will pay the Basic Monthly Service Fee for the new apartment at the rate then in effect for the new apartment, prorated if necessary to cover a partial month (and adjusted to reflect a pro rata portion of the Basic Monthly Service Fee paid for the apartment vacated for the unexpired portion of such month), and the obligation to pay the Basic Monthly Service Fee for the vacated apartment will be discharged, all effective as of the date the Resident first occupies the new apartment. (2) Upon transfer, the Entrance Fee for the vacated apartment will be applied to the new apartment. If the Resident transfers to a smaller apartment, Retirement Facility will refund the excess, if any, of the original Entrance Fee paid by the Resident for the apartment being vacated over the amount of the current Entrance Fee for the new apartment. If the Resident transfers to a larger apartment, the Resident will pay an additional Entrance Fee to Retirement Facility in the amount, if any, by which the current Entrance Fee for the new apartment exceeds the original Entrance Fee paid by the Resident for the apartment being vacated, payable on the date the Resident takes occupancy of the new apartment. The balance of the Entrance Fee originally paid by the Resident and any additional Entrance Fee paid by the Resident at the time of transfer will each be subject to refund in accordance with Section _____ hereof.

FORM 28.9C: INTERFACILITY TRANSFER: ENTRANCE FEE ADJUSTMENT

TRANSFER PRIVILEGE WITHIN THE CORPORATION

1. With the approval of both homes, the Resident may move to another of the residence homes of the Corporation, his fees being transferred from one to another.

2. Upon approval, the Resident may exercise his privileges to transfer to other accommodations within the same facility.

3. A Resident may move from Resident's original accommodation to one within the same or in another Corporation facility with an equal or lesser Accommodation Fee without paying any additional Accommodation Fee. If the move is made within the first three (3) months of his or her residency, the Corporation will refund to the Resident an amount equal to the difference between the unamortized balance of the original Accommodation Fee and the Accommodation Fee for the new accommodation. The amortization program for the new Accommodation Fee balance will continue on the basis of the number of months left in the original amortization program.

If the move is made after the Resident's Care and Residence Agreement has been in effect more than three (3) months, and if the unamortized balance of the Accommodation Fee for the accommodation being vacated is greater than the Accommodation Fee for the new unit, the Accommodation Fee for the new unit will be amortized to the Corporation at the rate of one and one-half percent (1.5%) per month, commencing on the effective date of the transfer.

Any difference between the unamortized balance of the previous Accommodation Fee and the Accommodation Fee for the new accommodation will be credited to the Resident as follows:

a. If the difference is less than $1000 but more than $1, it will be credited against the Resident's monthly service fee (Accounts Receivable) in one lump sum.

b. If the difference is $1000 or more, it will be credited to the Resident's monthly service fee at the rate of one and one-half percent (1.5%) per month.

4. A Resident may move from his original accommodation to one within the same or in another Corporation facility with a larger Accommodation Fee by paying an additional Accommodation Fee equal to the difference between the original Accommodation Fee and the current Accommodation Fee for the new accommodation. The total of

the additional Accommodation Fee plus the unamortized balance of the original Accommodation Fee will be amortized to the Corporation at the rate of one and one half percent (1.5%) per month.

FORM 28.9D: TRANSFER FOR HEALTH REASONS: CONSULTATION

Transfer from Residence. Except in case of emergency, Retirement Facility will not transfer you from your residence for health-related or other reasons until Retirement Facility has consulted with you, your personal physician, a member of your family, or your designated representative and the Medical Director. In cases of emergency transfer, these consultations will be held by Retirement Facility within ten (10) days of transfer.

Retirement Facility shall have full authority and right to transfer you from your residence to the Health Center or elsewhere for hospitalization or other health-related services without having to obtain your further consent if the Medical Director or Executive Director determines, after the consultation called for above:

1. That Retirement Facility does not have adequate facilities or staff to provide the nursing services or medical care needed by you;

2. That your continued occupancy of your residence constitutes a danger or health hazard to you or other residents, or is detrimental to the peace or security of other residents; or

3. That you are no longer able to leave your residence without the assistance of another during an emergency and your residence is not approved by the State Fire Marshal for use by nonambulatory residents. If it is necessary to transfer you to an outside health facility, Retirement Facility will endeavor to arrange for transfer to the facility of your choosing. Should you or your family or guardian fail to choose a facility, the Executive Director may choose such facility. All charges for any outside facility shall be your responsibility.

FORM 28.9E: TEMPORARY CARE ALLOWANCE

If you require *temporary* care in skilled nursing, Retirement Facility will provide you with care, without any increase in your monthly fee, except for a charge for the two additional meals served at the care facility. If, at any time, you receive care for more than sixty (60) consecutive days, Retirement Facility and its Medical Director, in consultation with your personal physician and your immediate family, will review your current health status to determine whether you require permanent care.

FORM 28.9F: À LA CARTE CARE

In the event of a move by the Resident into the Nursing Center or other accommodations under the provisions of Section _____ herein, this Residency Agreement shall remain in full force and effect; provided, however, that the Resident shall be relieved of any further responsibility for payment of Monthly Charges on the Residential Premises if properly vacated and shall pay only the charges required for care at the Nursing Center or other accommodations. Retirement Facility may secure new Residents to occupy the Residential Premises upon such a move.

FORM 28.9G: RELEASE OF RESIDENCE

Any permanent or indefinite transfer under Paragraph _____, as determined by Retirement Facility, shall entitle Retirement Facility to release for other occupancy the living accommodations theretofore provided for the Resident. If, however, Resident should recover and no longer need such care, the Resident shall be entitled, as soon as available, to his or her original living unit accommodation, or if unavailable, to a living unit accommodation equivalent to that previously occupied by the Resident. In either event, the Resident shall continue to pay his or her customary monthly rate during the period that he or she is a patient in the Personal Care Section, or in the Health Unit (or other facility as aforesaid). Any transfer made under Paragraph _____ above shall be deemed a termination of this Agreement on the part of the Retirement Facility, as set forth in Subparagraph _____ of this Agreement.

FORM 28.9H: HEALTH TRANSFER: ENTRANCE FEE ADJUSTMENT

If, in the opinion of a physician retained by the Corporation, the condition requiring change of accommodation is permanent, the living accommodations previously occupied by the Resident shall be released for other occupancy. If the Accommodation Fee is not fully amortized, the remaining portion of the Accommodation Fee will apply to the cost of health care in any Corporation facility that does not require an Accommodation Fee, or in any outside facility when such care is not available in a Corporation facility, at the continuing rate of one percent (1%) per month, until Accommodation Fee is completely amortized. Resident will be responsible for the difference between the actual cost of such care and the amount paid monthly from the unamortized balance of the Accommodation Fee. Prorated credit on monthly service fees shall accrue to a Resident when he or she is removed to another unit or institution. Corporation will not pay for outside care other than that specifically provided in this agreement or attached addenda.

FORM 28.9I: PRESERVATION OF RESIDENCE DESPITE PERMANENT TRANSFER

ASSISTED STATUS MEMBERSHIP

1. In the event you permanently require care outside your residence, you automatically become an Assisted Status Member. As an Assisted Status Member, you have the option of maintaining or selling your Residential Membership. As an Assisted Status Member, you will be charged an "Assisted Status Monthly Fee," which is equivalent to the then current total Monthly Fee for Residential Membership in a one bedroom residence, which includes the adjustable service fee component and the fixed sustaining fee component. If you also maintain your Residential Membership, you will pay both the Assisted Status Monthly Fee and your regular Residential Membership

Monthly Fee. To avoid the obligation of paying two Monthly Fees, you may sell your Residential Membership as provided in Section ———.

FORM 28.9J: TRANSFER OF SPOUSE

If one resident of a double occupant residence is admitted to the Health Center on an extended stay basis and the other resident remains in the residence, the Monthly Fee for the resident remaining in the residence shall be the applicable rate for a single occupant of the residence and the resident in the Health Center shall pay the Health Center Fee.

If both residents of a double occupant residence are living in the Health Center on an extended stay basis, each will pay the Health Center Fee. In addition, they will continue to pay the Monthly Fee applicable to single occupancy of their residence as long as the residence is retained. Upon release of the residence the obligation to pay the Monthly Fee ends.

FORM 28.9K: SPOUSE ALLOCATION OF HEALTH CREDITS

If there are two of you, each of you has a sixty (60) day lifetime care allowance. Care allowances are individual and are nontransferable. If only one of you requires care beyond the sixty (60) day allowance, the Monthly Service Fee for double occupancy in the residence will cease. The total Monthly Service Fee for both of you will then be the single occupancy Monthly Service Fee for your primary residence plus the Monthly Service Fee for a one bedroom residence with one occupant. If both of you require care beyond the sixty (60) day allowance and you both occupy the same room, the total Monthly Service Fee for both of you will be the Monthly Service Fee for your primary residence (single occupancy) plus the Monthly Service Fee for a one bedroom residence with a double occupancy surcharge. If you require separate rooms, you will pay the single occupancy Monthly Service Fee for your primary residence plus you will each pay the single occupancy Monthly Service Fee for a one bedroom residence. Upon determination by the Medical Director that you or, if there are two, both of you, can no longer live independently, you may release your primary residence and convert your Residential Membership to Assisted Status Membership as described in Section ——— at any time you wish. After you, or both of you, have converted to Assisted Status Membership, the most you need pay is the Monthly Service Fee for a one bedroom residence plus the charge for a second person, if you occupy the same room.

A chart attached as Exhibit ——— summarizes these alternatives.

§ 28.10   CONTRACT TERMINATION

(a)   General Conditions of Termination

Termination provisions appear in nearly every form of Residence Agreement, but their significance in planning, marketing, and operating a project depends on the complexity of the fee arrangement and service package offered by the facility. In a simple monthly rental agreement, for example, termination is a relatively straightforward matter, from a drafting point of view, and may consist simply of a 30 day notice provision permitting either party to terminate with or without cause (Form 28.11A).

More complicated agreements dealing with long-term periods, open-ended terms, or care for life, present more wide-ranging problems. Contracts should deal with the opportunities for and conditions upon termination by the resident, by the provider, or by reason of some event such as death of the resident, or the resident's need for a level of care or service not provided by the facility (see, e.g., Form 28.11B). Agreements should include provisions governing the duration and manner of giving notice.

The contract should further set forth precisely under which circumstances and during what periods of time either party will need cause to terminate the agreement, and under what circumstances the agreement may be terminated at will. For example, several states require probationary or adjustment periods during the initial term of a continuing care agreement, during which the resident may terminate the agreement without cause and receive substantial refunds (Form 28.11C. See discussion in § 21.8(b)).

In fact, however, it is rare to see contracts, much less laws or regulations, that ever require a resident to have cause in order to terminate the agreement, even after probationary periods have expired. Unlike typical real estate transactions that involve the provision of housing only, retirement facility contracts generally contain services that must be characterized as personal in nature. It is established in the common law that contracts to render personal services cannot be specifically enforced because of the importance of a relationship of trust and confidence between the parties, difficulty of enforcement, and matters of public policy.[12] Most retirement facility developers and operators have expanded upon this principle and permit a resident to terminate the agreement at any time without cause, but a few may impose some form of penalty for early withdrawal, such as the withholding of an extra percentage of the entrance fee (see Form 28.11D).

In addition, providers of continuing care with nonrefundable entrance fees may restrict the ability of a resident to cancel the contract when the resident is in poor health (see Form 28.11B). The rationale for such a provision is that residents who believe they will die soon might cancel the contract before death in order to obtain a more favorable refund of entrance fees, especially in the early years of residence, before the fee is fully amortized. This resident tactic skews the actuarial assumptions built into the fee structure, which is designed to release all entrance fees to the facility upon death of the resident (see discussion at § 21.6(c)). Refundable fee structures tend to have no such health limitation on the right to terminate the

---

[12] See *Restatement of Contracts*, 2d, § 367.

contract, because the fee amounts retained by the facility and refunded to the resident are the same, whether termination is voluntary or due to the resident's death.

(b)   Cause for Termination

All agreements should provide facility operators with the power to terminate for cause, even life care contracts. Typically, a contract lists examples of cause that entitle the provider to dismiss the resident, such as nonpayment of monthly charges, behavior that is disruptive or dangerous to the health or safety of the resident or others in the facility, misrepresentations in the application forms about health status, financial position, age, or other matters, onset of a mental or physical illness or condition that the facility is not equipped to treat, or that is not covered by a facility health insurance program, or change from ambulatory to nonambulatory status that will create fire safety or licensing problems (see Forms 28.11E, 28.11F). Some contracts contain "change of accommodations" clauses that are, for all practical purposes, statements of cause for termination (see, e.g., Form 28.11G). Contracts should be carefully drafted so that it is clear any listing of grounds for termination are merely examples and not a comprehensive or exclusive list.

Providers may wish to give residents an opportunity to cure correctable defaults in their contract obligations. This may have a positive marketing effect, especially in projects where residents must make a substantial financial or other commitment (see Form 28.11H). However, acquiescence in a resident's breach should not be considered a waiver of the resident's continuing contract obligations (Form 28.11I).

Retirement facilities that qualify for tax exemption under Revenue Ruling 72-124[13] must have a policy that permits residents who run out of funds to remain at the facility. However, this obligation exists only to the extent of the facility's financial ability to enforce it, and nonprofit facilities usually list failure to pay monthly fees when due as a ground for termination with cause. The Revenue Ruling does not require that the facility's policy be contained in the residence agreement, although some developers may find that the inclusion of such a policy, if carefully drafted, may have excellent marketing consequences without increased liability (see Form 28.11J). Even for profit developers, aware of the problems of evicting elderly residents, have declared policies making it possible for those who run out of funds to remain at the facility (Forms 28.11K, 28.11L). Facility operators also may permit residents to draw on entrance fee refunds, membership interests, or other equity interest in the facility as a buffer against insolvency. (See, e.g., Form 28.11M. See also the discussion of health credits at § 28.6(e).)

---

[13] See § 9.2.

Occasionally, a resident able to pay the monthly fee may refuse to pay it because of a dispute with the facility, or even due to increased stubbornness or other changes in mental condition. In these circumstances, a termination provision for failure to pay fees is essential, whether or not the facility has "no eviction" obligations as a prerequisite to tax exemption.

For those facilities offering a health care program, it is important to note that the permissible grounds for dismissal from the facility may be more closely circumscribed by law than dismissals from the residential facility. For example, the patients' rights provisions of the Medicare/Medicaid regulations require nursing facilities to agree to transfer or discharge patients "only for medical reasons, or [the patient's] welfare or that of other patients or for nonpayment of his stay," and to be given "reasonable advance notice to insure orderly transfer or discharge."[14] These provisions have been adopted by states that participate in the Medicare and Medicaid programs, and are usually incorporated into nursing facility licensing laws.[15] It should be noted that the fraud and abuse amendments to the Social Security Act prohibit facilities from terminating a resident eligible under the Medicare or Medicaid programs by reason of the patient's or a relative's failure to make a payment to the facility for covered services that is supplemental or in addition to the amount paid under the Medicare or Medicaid program. (See § 9.2(b)(4) for further discussion of these provisions.)

(c) Refunds

In the event of termination of the agreement, whether by the resident or the facility operator, there is often some provision for refund, especially in entrance fee or membership projects. Even in rental projects, refunds may be required of security deposits, prepaid rent, or other payments made to secure the provider's position in the event the resident leaves the premises in a damaged condition or vacates without giving adequate notice. Most states have provisions regulating the receipt of security deposits by residential landlords. Typically, such statutes provide that current deposits be maintained in a segregated account and not be used by the landlord except in the event of a termination of the tenancy. There may be a requirement that the funds on deposit earn interest and specification of time periods within which the landlord is obligated to refund any unused amounts to the resident.

In entrance fee situations, it is important to be sure that the statutory provisions that apply to tenant security deposits do not inadvertently govern the provisions of a continuing care agreement. While this is less of a problem in states with extensive continuing care regulation, it may be wise in states without regulation to review security deposit statutes and determine their impact upon the transaction. In addition, even in states where

---

[14] 42 C.F.R. § 405.1121(k)(4). *See also* § 20.2(a).

[15] *See, e.g.,* Title 22, Cal. Admin. Code § 72527.

there is regulation of continuing care, if a provider has inadvertently structured an agreement that is not in complete compliance with the continuing care statutes, it is possible for a person seeking a refund of fees to argue that tenants' security deposit statutes should apply and supercede the contractual terms or control the refund policies of the facility. As a precaution, it may be wise to specify that the entrance fee is a payment for services and a condition of occupancy, but not a security deposit or prepayment of rent.

A continuing care agreement should specify the circumstances under which refunds are available and the extent of the refund for each circumstance. These provisions may be largely dictated by state laws (see § 21.6(c)). The amounts of refunds may differ depending on whether termination occurs during a probationary or adjustment period, as a result of a later dismissal by the facility, because of cancelation of the contract by the resident, or by reason of death or some other event. Many of the so-called nonrefundable entrance fees, in fact, are refundable at least in part during an initial occupancy period. Fees may be amortized at a rate typically between one and two percent per month, so that if the resident cancels the agreement during the first several years of the contract, the unamortized portion of the entrance fee will be refunded (see Form 28.11N). For very early voluntary withdrawal by the resident, after any statutory probation period, some facilities may impose a higher entrance fee retention penalty, for example, of 10 percent or more (Forms 28.11D, 28.11N). Statutes may require very liberal refund provisions in the event of the resident's dismissal by the facility.[16]

Many traditional facilities provide, however, that in the event of death, the entire entrance fee, including unamortized portions, will be retained by the facility (see Form 28.11O). There may be exceptions to this policy for initial probationary periods, or some facilities may refund the unamortized portion in the event of an early death, even where not required by state law (see, e.g., Form 28.11P).

A growing number of continuing care facilities are using refundable entrance fee structures. In some cases, residents are given the option to enroll in either a refundable program or in the more traditional nonrefundable type, with different entrance fee amounts or monthly fee amounts specified for each option. Refundable fees seldom are 100 percent refundable. The announced policy of the Marriott Corporation's Life Care Division, for example, provides for a 90 percent refund in the event of termination of the contract, whether by the resident, the facility, death, or any other reason. Other facilities may refund a sliding percentage of the entrance fee depending upon the date of contract termination. For example, a facility may structure refunds so that a declining refund is given over time, but reaches a base percentage so that the refundable amount never declines to

---

[16]*See, e.g.,* Cal. Health & Safety Code § 1780, which requires refund of all fees less the actual cost of care.

zero (see Form 28.11Q). Some developers have at least considered offering increasingly higher refunds over time, so that a resident will have a financial incentive to remain at the facility longer and build a capital reserve for later use, or to benefit a spouse or heirs.

In situations where two or more persons occupy a single residential unit, refunds of entrance fees are generally made available when the last surviving resident dies or leaves the facility. A few facilities, however, apportion the entrance fees equally between spouses and provide a refund on the death or termination of each. Some facilities may also provide a partial refund of fees when the residential unit is released for reoccupancy by another party and the prior occupant has moved to a nursing facility or care center under the control of the facility operator.

In connection with membership structures and other sales of personal or real property interests, the term *refund* is probably not appropriate. Rather, the resident will receive payment as a consequence of transferring the membership or title to real property. That interest may be transferred to a new resident or, possibly, to the facility itself. Some facilities retain a repurchase option so that they will have better control over admissions (Form 28.11R), or be able to give priority to certain applicants for admission, for example, those returning from extended nursing care who have since released their own residential units (see Form 28.11S).

If a facility operator guarantees to the resident that the facility will repurchase the property or membership, in the event the resident cannot find his own buyer, the transaction may be vulnerable to characterization as a loan, which could have adverse interest income tax consequences upon the resident. (See discussion of below market loans in § 6.2(b)).

In general, refund provisions should be incorporated into termination provisions, especially where different amounts may be due depending upon the circumstances of the termination.

(d) Miscellaneous Termination Concerns

Many concerns may arise in the event of termination of a resident contract, and not all of these can or should be covered by the Resident Agreement. For example, should it become necessary to terminate a resident against that person's will, there is a question of what procedures must be followed under state law.

Most states have rather elaborate laws dealing with the respective rights and obligations of landlords and tenants when a landlord seeks to evict a tenant from the premises. These laws may prescribe specific notice periods, may state prohibited grounds for termination, and may give tenants substantial due process rights, including the right to a jury trial, before an eviction may be effectuated. On the other hand, such laws generally have not been applied to transfers of patients from health facilities or care facilities, or from such residential enterprises as hotels and boarding houses.

Many retirement facility operators attempt to avoid characterizing the relationship of provider and resident as a landlord-tenant relationship, and seek to emphasize the service components and analogies to hotels and nursing homes. However, it is often difficult to make such distinctions when attempting to evict an elderly person from a residential unit. A contract may provide that the parties agree that the relationship is not one of landlord and tenant, but such a provision would probably be of little avail in the event of an actual contested eviction situation. Each state law governs, and any contrary contractual provisions would probably be deemed void as against public policy.

A matter that can be dealt with in the contract concerns the circumstances that every facility must face in the event of the death of a resident. Often, there may be delays or difficulties in finding the executor, estate administrator, or other responsible person who is authorized to take possession of the resident's furniture and other personal belongings. The agreement should provide that the facility is entitled to remove such belongings from the unit and store them at the expense of the resident's estate, so that the vacant unit may be refurbished and marketed within a reasonable time (Form 28.11T).

Facilities also should be cautious about delivering property of a deceased resident to relatives or others claiming a right to the property, unless the person has letters of administration or other court approved documents indicating a right to collect the assets of the estate. Some states have statutory protections that enable an heir or beneficiary to receive property of a decedent whose estate does not exceed a specified amount, upon presentation of a declaration that the will is not subject to probate. Such statutory forms, if properly filled out in compliance with the law, can protect a facility operator from liability for misdelivery of a decedent's property[17] (see Form 28.11U).

§ 28.11   CONTRACT TERMINATION: SAMPLE FORMS

FORM 28.11A: TERMINATION OF RENTAL

TERMINATION

Either Retirement Facility or the Resident may terminate this Agreement at any time without cause by giving at least thirty (30) days' written notice to the other party. For mailed notice, the date of receipt will be the date of notice. If the Resident does not give the full thirty (30) days' notice, the Resident will be liable for payment up to the end of the thirty (30) days for which notice was required. Retirement Facility may waive the thirty (30) day notice if it is terminating the Agreement because of behavior of the Resident that, in the sole opinion of Retirement Facility, is a direct and immediate danger to the Resident or to others.

[17] See, e.g., Cal. Prob. Code §§ 630, 631.

FORM 28.11B: TERMINATION BY RESIDENT, FACILITY, DEATH

CANCELATION BY RESIDENT

The Agreement may be canceled by you at any time after the end of the probationary period by ninety (90) days' written notice to Retirement Facility in accordance with regulations of the _____ Department of _____, and a certification by a physician approved by Retirement Facility that you are in reasonably good health. The Agreement shall not terminate until the end of such ninety (90) day period, and until such termination date Retirement Facility shall continue to be entitled to all fees required under this Agreement. Upon such termination, Retirement Facility shall refund any amounts paid as an Accommodation Fee, less the sum of one and one-half percent (1.5%) of the Accommodation Fee per month from the date of the Agreement to the date of termination. The Application Fee is nonrefundable.

CANCELATION BY RETIREMENT FACILITY

Retirement Facility may cancel this Agreement at any time for good and sufficient cause with ninety (90) days' written notice. In the event of such termination, refund of the Accommodation Fee and Monthly Fee shall be made within ten (10) days, except that Retirement Facility may retain the per capita cost of care for the period of your occupancy and remit the balance of any such payments made by you or on your behalf.
Good and sufficient cause shall include the following:

1. Failure to perform your obligations under this Agreement, including your obligations to pay the Monthly Fees and other charges;
2. Failure to abide by the rules and regulations of Retirement Facility, including such reasonable amendments as may be adopted from time to time;
3. Material misstatements or failure to state a material fact in your application, financial statement, or health history statement filed with Retirement Facility.
4. Permanent transfer to another public or private institution as described by Article _____.
5. Any other reason deemed by the Board of Directors to be good and sufficient reason.

CANCELATION AND OTHER NOTICES

All notices required by this Agreement shall be delivered to Retirement Facility at _____ to you at the place designated in writing and placed on file with the administrator of Retirement Facility, and to you at your accommodation at Retirement Facility. All such notices shall be effective when personally delivered or when deposited in the mail properly addressed with postage prepaid.

PAYMENT OF REFUNDS

All monies to be refunded to you pursuant to Section _____ shall be tendered by Retirement Facility within ten (10) days.

TERMINATION BY REASON OF DEATH

Upon your death, whether during the probationary period or afterwards, the entire Accommodation Fee paid to Retirement Facility shall remain the property of Retirement Facility and shall not be transferable by your will or subject to claim by your estate or heirs. All monthly fees and other service fees shall be considered as payment for services rendered; such fees shall not be subject to proration.

FORM 28.11C: PROBATIONARY PERIOD TERMINATION AT WILL

There shall be a probationary period of ninety (90) days from the date you sign this Agreement during which this Agreement may be canceled by Retirement Facility, or by you, with or without cause. The canceling party shall give the other party written notice of cancelation at the place specified in Section _____ of this Agreement. Cancelation shall become immediately effective upon the giving of notice as provided in Section _____. A form "Notice of Cancelation" is attached to this Agreement. In the event of such cancelation, and provided the living unit is returned in substantially as good condition as when received, refund of the Accommodation Fee and any Monthly Fees shall be made in accordance with the laws of the State of _____, which provide in essence that Retirement Facility may retain the reasonable value of services rendered to you after the first seven (7) days, and shall remit the balance of any such fees. The Application Fee is nonrefundable.

FORM 28.11D: EARLY WITHDRAWAL PENALTY

Termination of this Agreement after the period of adjustment by the Resident shall be subject to refunds as follows:

1. The Home shall retain all monthly service charges paid by the Resident;
2. The Home shall retain the nonrefundable registration fee;
3. The Home shall retain an amount equal to the cost of any repairs to the living accommodation or for the replacement of property due to damages by the Resident that go beyond ordinary wear and tear; and
4. The Home shall retain one percent (1%) of the accommodation fee per month from the date of occupancy to the date of termination, provided, however, that the minimum charge for termination after the period of adjustment shall be ten percent (10%) of the accommodation fee.

FORM 28.11E: CAUSE FOR TERMINATION (GENERAL)

Good and sufficient cause for termination shall include but not be limited to the following:

1. Conduct by you that constitutes a danger to yourself or others;
2. Failure to perform your obligations under this Agreement, including failure to pay your Monthly Fee or Health Center Fee when due;

3. Material misstatements or failure to state a material fact in your application, financial statement, or health history statement filed with Retirement Facility;
4. Repeated conduct that interferes with the quiet enjoyment of the Community by other residents; or
5. Persistent refusal to comply with written Community rules and regulations.

FORM 28.11F: CAUSE FOR TERMINATION (SPECIFIC)

Retirement Facility will not terminate this Agreement except for just cause. Just cause includes, but is not limited to, the following:

1. Except as set forth below, failure to pay Retirement Facility any charges due.
2. Creation by you of a disturbance within Retirement Facility that, in the judgment of Retirement Facility, is detrimental to the health, safety, comfort, or peaceful living of any of the other residents or staff.
3. Your refusal of treatment or care or to be transferred to an appropriate facility to receive treatment or care that, in the opinion of Retirement Facility, your attending physician, or Retirement Facility Medical Director, is medically or otherwise required for your physical or mental health or the health or safety of other residents or staff.
4. You materially breach this Agreement or are determined to have made a material misrepresentation in the documentation submitted at the time of your application for membership.

FORM 28.11G: TRANSFER AS POSSIBLE TERMINATION

When the Retirement Facility Medical Director or Administrator determines: that Retirement Facility does not have adequate facilities or staff to provide medical services needed by you; that your continued occupancy of your residence constitutes a danger to other residents or to yourself, or is detrimental to the peace or health of other residents; or that you are no longer able to leave your residence without the assistance of another during an emergency and your residence is not approved by the State Fire Marshal for use by nonambulatory residents, and after the consultation called for above, Retirement Facility shall have the full authority and right to transfer you from your residence to the Health Care Center or elsewhere for hospitalization, nursing care, or other health-related services, without having to obtain your further consent.

FORM 28.11H: CURABLE DEFAULTS

WRITTEN NOTICE OF TERMINATION

Prior to any termination of the Agreement by Retirement Facility as described in this Section, Retirement Facility will give you notice in writing of the cause and you will have ten (10) days thereafter within which the problem may be corrected, except as provided below. If the problem is corrected within such time, this Agreement shall not then be terminated. If the problem is not corrected within such time, this Agreement will be terminated ninety (90) days after the original notice of termination, and you must leave Retirement Facility. Refunds, if any, shall be made as required by law. If the Medical Director or the Retirement Facility Administration determines that either the giving of notice or the lapse of time as above provided might be detrimental to you or other residents or staff of the Retirement Facility, or if Retirement Facility determines that the problem constituting cause for termination cannot be cured, then any notice and/or waiting period prior to termination shall not be required.

FORM 28.11I: WAIVER OF BREACH

The failure of Retirement Facility in any instance or instances to insist upon your strict performance or observance of, or compliance with, any of the terms or provisions of this Agreement, shall not be construed to be a waiver or relinquishment by Retirement Facility of its right to insist upon strict compliance by you with all of the terms and provisions of this Agreement.

FORM 28.11J: DEFERRAL OF CHARGES FOR NEEDY RESIDENT

IF YOU ENCOUNTER FINANCIAL DIFFICULTY

It is and shall continue to be the declared policy of the Retirement Facility to operate as a charitable nonprofit organization and not to terminate this Agreement solely by reason of your financial inability to pay the total monthly charges. If you encounter financial difficulty, making it impossible for you to pay your monthly fee for your residence, you shall be permitted to remain at Retirement Facility at a reduced monthly charge based on your ability to pay for so long as you establish facts to justify deferral of the usual charges, and the deferral of such charges can, in the sole discretion of Retirement Facility, be granted without impairing the ability of Retirement Facility to operate on a sound financial basis. The loss of revenue to the Retirement Facility from any such deferral of charges will be borne by Retirement Facility and not be charged back to other residents in their monthly fees. This provision shall be rendered inoperative if you have impaired your ability to meet your financial obligations by making unapproved gifts or other transfers. You agree that any monthly or other charges deferred pursuant to this section shall be treated as a loan to you from Retirement Facility and, by accepting such a loan, you give Retirement Facility a first security interest in your membership, and the proceeds of any sale thereof. You further agree that all such deferred charges, plus interest at the legal rate, shall be an additional charge, in excess of the transfer fee, against the proceeds of any transfer of your Residential Membership, shall be a first lien against your estate, and shall be credited against any trust agreement distribution due to you from Retirement Facility.

FORM 28.11K: BENEVOLENT FUND

1. Retirement Facility anticipates that certain financial difficulties may arise that are beyond the control of a resident. Therefore, Retirement Facility will establish a Benevolent Fund for the purpose of assisting residents who experience financial distress. In order for this Benevolent Fund to be administered fairly, Retirement Facility reserves the right to use monies in the Benevolent Fund as it deems appropriate. In the event that you seek to obtain financial assistance, you may be asked to do any or all of the following at the request of the Administrator of Retirement Facility:

a. Apply for and diligently seek the benefits of any assistance program for which you might qualify. If you should fail to apply for any such benefits, you hereby permit Retirement Facility to apply on your behalf.

b. Report promptly to the Administrator any material increase in your assets or their value, whether the increase occurs by way of gift, inheritance, appreciation in value, or otherwise.

c. Refrain from transferring any material assets for less than their fair value.

d. Make arrangements for the preservation and management of your property by a third party (or parties) including, but not limited to, the execution and funding of a trust agreement for your benefit.

e. Sign any instruments (including notes, assignments, and deeds of trust) that Retirement Facility deems necessary to evidence or secure its claim for repayment of any financial assistance.

f. Provide Retirement Facility with copies of your federal and state income and gift tax returns for three years prior to the request.

FORM 28.11L: LOAN TO NEEDY RESIDENTS

Inability to Pay. If you are not able to pay the Monthly Fee or other amounts owed under this Agreement, you may apply to Retirement Facility for a loan or loans to meet your obligations. Upon receipt of the application and such other information as Retirement Facility may require, Retirement Facility, without waiving any rights under Article _____, Section _____, and/or Article _____, Section _____, will determine whether you have the financial resources and can furnish the security required for the loan. If Retirement Facility decides to make the loan, it shall be on such terms as you and Retirement Facility shall mutually agree. You agree to execute, acknowledge, and deliver a promissory note and other instruments, including financing statements, as Retirement Facility may reasonably require to perfect its security interest.

FORM 28.11M: DEFERRED CHARGES: DEBIT AGAINST
MEMBERSHIP SALE

Deferral Policy. It is and shall be the declared policy of Retirement Facility to operate as a nonprofit organization and not to terminate the residency of Resident solely by reason of the financial inability of Resident to pay the monthly fee, when Resident establishes facts to justify deferral of such charges to Retirement Facility's reasonable satisfaction; subject, however, to Resident's obligations under Paragraph _____ below. In the event of any such deferral of charges, the full amount of such deferral, together with interest compounded annually on each monthly deferred payment from the date of such deferral at an annual rate equal to one percent (1%) over the then prevailing bank prime rate, such rate to be adjusted on each January 1, shall be credited against the price payable to Resident upon Retirement Facility's exercise of the Repurchase Option or added to the transfer fee payable by Resident or Resident's legal representative pursuant to Paragraph _____ in the event the Repurchase Option is not exercised.

FORM 28.11N: AMORTIZED REFUND ON RESIDENT CANCELLATION

This agreement may be terminated by the Resident, at any time after the introductory period, by serving on the Retirement Facility one hundred twenty (120) days' written notice of his or her desire to do so; but, the agreement shall not terminate until the end of the one hundred twenty (120) days except by mutual written agreement. Until such termination, the Resident will continue to pay his or her normal monthly care fee plus other charges as provided herein. Upon such termination, the Retirement Facility shall refund to the Resident the Entrance Fee, less the sum of one and one-half percent (1.5%) of the same per month, or any portion thereof, from the date of occupancy to the date of termination, and $1000 for the Retirement Facility's liquidated expenses. However, the minimum charge for such termination shall be ten percent (10%) of the Entrance Fee.

FORM 28.11O: NO REFUND ON DEATH

Death. Upon death of resident, whether during the probationary period or thereafter, all payments made by him to Retirement Facility shall remain and be the property of Retirement Facility, and shall not be transferable by will of Resident nor subject to claim by his estate or heirs.

FORM 28.11P: EARLY DEATH REFUND

Death of Resident. Upon the death of the last surviving resident who is a party to this Agreement, the entrance fee paid by the resident/transferor to the Retirement Facility shall remain the property of the Retirement Facility and shall not be transferable by the will of the resident or subject to any claim by his or her estate, except as further provided in this Subparagraph _____:

1. If the last surviving resident dies prior to initial occupancy of the residence, the entrance fee shall be refunded to the extent set forth in Subparagraph _____;

2. If the last surviving resident dies during the first ninety (90) days of occupancy, ninety percent (90%) of the entrance fee shall be refunded;

3. If the last surviving resident dies after ninety (90) days of residence, but during the first year of residence, sixty percent (60%) of the entrance fee shall be refunded;

4. If the last surviving resident dies during the second year of residence, thirty percent (30%) of the entrance fee shall be refunded.

FORM 28.11Q: DECLINING REFUND WITH FLOOR

The following refund schedule below shall apply for termination of your residence under sections _____ or _____ . This refund schedule is based upon the Payment Option selected by you. You have selected Option (3). The first year refund for the Payment Option you have selected is (75) percent. Thereafter, two percent (2%) per year is deducted from the amount refundable for the next nine (9) years. After ten (10) years, the refund amount for the Payment Option you selected is (55) percent.

OCCUPANCY OF UP TO 1 YEAR	(75)% of the Entry Fee
1 year to 2 years	(73)% of the Entry Fee
2 years to 3 years	(71)% of the Entry Fee
3 years to 4 years	(69)% of the Entry Fee
4 years to 5 years	(67)% of the Entry Fee
5 years to 6 years	(65)% of the Entry Fee
6 years to 7 years	(63)% of the Entry Fee
7 years to 8 years	(61)% of the Entry Fee
8 years to 9 years	(59)% of the Entry Fee
9 years to 10 years	(57)% of the Entry Fee
10 years and after	(55)% of the Entry Fee

FORM 28.11R: FACILITY REPURCHASE OPTION

PURCHASE BY RETIREMENT FACILITY

In order to help insure that members of Retirement Facility have priority over the general public to purchase a new Residential Membership and move to a different residence, and in order to provide for other contingencies, before you offer your Residential Membership for sale to any other buyer, you shall offer it to Retirement Facility at the Fair Market Value. If Retirement Facility declines to purchase your Residential Membership, or fails to exercise its purchase option within ten (10) days, you are free to sell to any other Qualified Buyer provided, however, that if you obtain an offer from a prospective Qualified Buyer for a price that is less than that which you offered to Retirement Facility, Retirement Facility shall have ten (10) days to match that offer and purchase your Residential Membership. If your Residential Membership is purchased by Retirement Facility, you shall be responsible for paying the Transfer Fee.

FORM 28.11S: RETURN FROM DEPENDENCE

RETURN TO YOUR RESIDENCE AFTER ASSUMING ASSISTED STATUS MEMBERSHIP

If you have become an Assisted Status Member and have sold your Residential Membership, and it is determined by Retirement Facility, in consultation with its Medical Director, that you are again capable of independent living and can return to independent living in Retirement Facility, Retirement Facility will purchase a Residential Membership of a comparable type as that which you owned previously, as soon as one becomes available. Retirement Facility will then sell the Residential Membership to you, in return for your payment to Retirement Facility of the principal amount that you placed into your Trust Account pursuant to Section _____. In the event a comparable Residential Membership is not available, you may purchase the next available Residential Membership for the principal amount that you placed in your Trust Account, with an appropriate adjustment to reflect the different purchase prices.

FORM 28.11T: STORAGE OF PERSONAL PROPERTY

Within thirty (30) days after (1) you move from your residence on a permanent basis or your death, or (2) termination of the Agreement, whichever first occurs, you or your guardian, conservator, executor, or designee, or if none is qualified, your family, will remove your personal property from your residence. If personal property is not removed within this thirty (30) day period, Retirement Facility shall have the right to remove it and place it in storage for one (1) year at your or your estate's expense, after which it shall be sold, pursuant to the requirements of _____ law, and the proceeds, after deductions for expenses, credited to your account.

FORM 28.11U: RELEASE OF DECEDENT'S PROPERTY

DECLARATION REQUESTING TRANSFER OF DECEDENT'S INTEREST IN PROPERTY TO HEIRS AT LAW OR BENEFICIARIES UNDER WILL

CALIFORNIA PROBATE CODE § 630

The undersigned hereby declare(s):

1. _____ was a resident of the City of _____, County of _____, State of California, and died on or about _____, 19____.

2. Decedent left no real property, nor interest therein, in the State of California that has a gross value in excess of Ten Thousand Dollars ($10,000.00). The total value of decedent's estate does not exceed Sixty Thousand Dollars ($60,000.00) exclusive of (a) any amounts due decedent for service in the armed forces of the

United States, (b) any salary, including compensation for unused vacation, not exceeding Five Thousand Dollars ($5,000.00), owing to decedent from his employment, (c) any motor vehicle, (d) any property held in joint tenancy, and (e) any property that passes to decedent's surviving spouse pursuant to Probate Code § 649.1.

. 3. The decedent left surviving the following heirs at law:

Name	Age	Address	Relationship to Decedent

4. No probate proceedings are now being, or have ever been, held in the decedent's estate.

5. Declarant(s) is/are all of the (beneficiaries of the decedent's last Will, a copy of which is attached,/heirs of decedent) and is/are entitled to collect and receive the entire estate without probating the Will, under California Probate Code Section 630.

6. Declarant(s) hereby request(s) that the following property of the decedent be transferred to declarant(s):

7. The undersigned jointly and severally agree to hold _____ harmless and indemnify it against all liability, claims, demands, loss, damages, costs, and expense whatsoever that it may incur or suffer by reason of the transfer, payment or delivery to (me/us) of any property pursuant hereto.

8. This declaration is made to induce _____ to transfer such property to declarant(s).

I/We declare under penalty of perjury that the above is true and correct and that this declaration was executed on _____, 19_____, at _____, California.

(Print Name)	(Signature)
(Print Name)	(Signature)
(Print Name)	(Signature)
(Print Name)	(Signature)

§ 28.12   PROTECTIVE PROVISIONS

There are many miscellaneous provisions that should appear in Resident Agreements setting forth general limitations upon the liability and obligations of the facility and spelling out essential facility policies that are conducive to the sound management of the retirement community. Many of these are technical matters or legal boilerplate, which are exemplified by clauses such as those in Form 28.13A. They should not be taken lightly, however. For example, entire agreement clauses can be helpful and should make reference to the specific exhibits attached and incorporated. The number and variety of exhibits can be substantial over years of facility operation, and it should be clear that the various brochures, verbal representations, and other statements are not contractual in nature. In addition, it can be important to have the resident confirm in writing precisely what documents have been received and reviewed (Form 28.13B). Providers may also wish to include arbitration and attorneys fees clauses to aid in the resolution of disputes.

(a)   Limitation of Liability

Retirement facility agreements generally contain some provision limiting the liability of the facility owner and operator for damages that may result from activities that are not the fault of the home. Contracts may include, for example, a requirement that residents obtain their own insurance covering damage to their furniture or personal property, and liability to guests or invitees to their residential units (see Form 28.13C). In addition, agreements often require residents to indemnify the facility against any claims made by third parties for injury or damages in connection with the resident's occupancy of the facility, and that are the fault of the resident (see Form 28.13D).

Retirement facilities should be cautious about any references in the agreement to persons or organizations other than the corporation or other entity on behalf of which the contract is being executed. References to other persons or organizations may be construed to imply financial responsibility on the part of such other organization. To the extent other organizations are mentioned, the contract should state whether or not they bear any financial or other responsibility for the obligations of the contract and, if so, the precise extent of such obligations (see Form 28.13D). Representations concerning sponsoring or other organizations may be controlled by state statute, especially in the case of continuing care facilities (see § 21.7).

(b)   Liens in Favor of the Facility/Asset Depletion

Contracts in service oriented facilities typically provide that the facility is granted a lien against the resident's estate for unpaid fees or charges incurred during occupancy (see Form 28.11E), or in the event of acquisition or possession by a subsidized resident of property not disclosed to the facility (see Form 28.13F). In addition, when an injured resident has received care from the facility as part of a prepaid plan, residents are often required to assign a lien to the facility against the proceeds of any cause of action the resident may have against the responsible person (Form 28.13G).

Residents commonly are also required to agree that during their lifetimes they will not make substantial gifts of their property or other transfers for less than fair market value without prior approval of the facility (see Form 28.13H). This kind of provision is especially important in facilities that, by reason of conditions on their tax exemptions, are required to care for those who run out of funds, or those who voluntarily have such a policy (see § 9.2(a)(3)). Even if there is no stated policy to retain those who have run out of funds, eviction under such circumstances can be difficult and bad for public relations. It therefore behooves the facility operator to help ensure the financial stability of residents.

(c) Incompetence of the Resident

It is prudent in retirement facility agreements, especially those designed to be in force for long periods of time, to provide for situations where the resident becomes incompetent or unable to handle his or her financial or other affairs.

While powers of attorney normally are effective only so long as the person giving the power is competent, most states now permit a durable power of attorney to be made while the person is competent, which will permit the attorney in fact to make financial decisions or consent to medical treatment after the resident has become incompetent. This is especially useful in matters of health care when it may be difficult to find a relative with authority to consent, or to go to court for appointment of a conservator before making a medical decision. Some states have adopted durable power of attorney statutes specifically dealing with health care decisions.[18]

Contracts should have appended to them at least a durable power of attorney form for health care and suggest that residents execute the form prior to admission in the facility (see Form 28.13I). Note that some states may prohibit making the execution of such a form a mandatory condition of admission to a health facility.[19] Contracts may also expressly permit the facility to apply to the court for appointment of a conservator (Form 28.13J), although contractual authority may not be necessary to make such an application.

Facility owners and operators should be careful that persons appointed as attorneys in fact for health care matters or financial matters are not principals or employees of the facility. Similarly, facility employees or owners should not agree to serve as executors of a resident's estate. It is also wise

---

[18] See, e.g., 20 Penn. Stat. § 5603(h), Cal. Civil Code §§ 2430 et seq.

[19] See Cal. Civil Code § 2441.

for facility employees to refrain from assisting residents in the preparation of their wills, and at least to be sure that the resident's independent counsel is present whenever such a document is executed in the presence of facility staff. Should the facility or any of its employees be named as beneficiary under the wills or be considered to be benefited by any power of attorney, a dissatisfied heir or other relative may contend that the facility or its employee exercised undue influence in procuring the resident's execution of the power of attorney or will.

§ 28.13   PROTECTIVE PROVISIONS: SAMPLE FORMS

FORM 28.13A: GENERAL BOILERPLATE

Waiver. The failure of Retirement Facility in any one or more instances to insist upon strict compliance by you with any of the terms of this Agreement shall not be construed to be a waiver by Retirement Facility of the right to insist upon strict compliance by you with any of the other terms of this Agreement.

Assignment. Your rights under this Agreement are personal to you and cannot be transferred or assigned by any act of you, or by any proceeding at law, or otherwise.

Entire Agreement. This Agreement incorporates Exhibits _____, _____, and _____, and constitutes the entire agreement between Retirement Facility and you. Retirement Facility is not liable for nor bound in any manner by any statements, representations, or promises made by any person representing or proposing to represent Retirement Facility unless such statements, representations, or promises are set forth in the Agreement. Any modification of the Agreement must be in writing signed by Retirement Facility and you.

Partial Illegality. This Agreement shall be construed in accordance with the laws of the State of _____. If any portion of this Agreement shall be determined to be illegal or not in conformity with applicable laws and regulations, such portion shall be deemed to be modified so as to be in accordance with such laws and regulations, and the validity of the balance of this Agreement shall not be affected; provided, however, if Retirement Facility determines, in its sole discretion, that the portion of this Agreement so changed constitutes a substantial change in this Agreement, Retirement Facility may rescind this Agreement and you shall be entitled to a refund as provided in Article _____ of this Agreement.

Construction. Words used in this Agreement of any gender shall be deemed to include any other gender, and words in the singular shall be deemed to include the plural, when the sense requires.

Joint and Several Liability. If two parties execute this Agreement as residents, the term *resident* or *you* as used in the Agreement shall apply to both and they shall be jointly and severally liable under this Agreement unless otherwise provided.

FORM 28.13B: RECEIPT OF DOCUMENTS

You hereby certify that you have received a printed copy of this Agreement, including Exhibits _____ through _____, a copy of Retirement Facility's current financial statement (Exhibit _____) and a copy of the Retirement Facility Resident's Manual, on or before the date set forth opposite your signature below, and have been permitted to inspect a copy of the group health insurance policy for Retirement Facility, the Articles of Incorporation and Bylaws of Operator, and any amendments thereof, and the Lease Agreement between Operator and Owner.

FORM 28.13C: RESIDENT INSURANCE

Property of Resident. The Retirement Facility shall not be responsible for the loss of any property belonging to the Resident due to theft, fire or any cause beyond the control of Retirement Facility. Resident shall have the responsibility for providing any desired insurance protection covering any such loss (or specify minimum terms and coverages).

FORM 28.13D: SPONSOR NOT LIABLE

HOLD HARMLESS

You agree to indemnify, keep, save, and hold Retirement Facility, its agents, employees, successors, and assigns free from all liability, penalties, losses, damages, costs, expenses, causes of action, claims, and judgments arising by reason of any injury or damage to any person or persons, or property of any kind whatsoever, and to whomsoever belonging, including damage to property of Retirement Facility, arising out of your acts or the acts of your invitees during the term of this Agreement or any occupancy hereunder, excepting those proximately caused by the negligence of Retirement Facility. Without limiting the generality of the foregoing, you shall bear the cost of labor and materials for maintenance and repair necessitated by your willful or negligent acts or those of your invitees, and you shall have responsibility for repair and replacement when necessary of your furniture and furnishings except for damage caused by willful or negligent acts of Retirement Facility. No officer, director, principal, agent, or employee of Retirement Facility shall have any personal liability to you for the performance of this Agreement.

FORM 28.13E: LIEN FOR ASSISTANCE

In the event that you remain at Retirement Facility while paying less than your full regular Monthly Service Fee, you agree that Retirement Facility shall have a lien against your estate for an amount equal to any financial assistance you have received from the Benevolent Fund, plus interest on that difference at a rate to be determined. Any funds received from your estate under this paragraph shall be returned to the Benevolent Fund and accrue to the benefit of the community.

You agree that you will not transfer any material assets for less than their fair value in order to qualify for financial assistance.

FORM 28.13F: LIEN FOR UNDISCLOSED PROPERTY

For any Resident who is subsidized in whole or in part by Retirement Facility, the fees charged by Retirement Facility are based, among other consideration, on the representation made by the Resident at time of application as to Resident's financial position and assets. If upon the death of any subsidized Resident, Resident shall own any property not disclosed in the application forms or, if acquired subsequent to the making of such forms, not disclosed promptly upon its acquisition, Retirement Facility shall be entitled to so much of such property, up to the whole thereof, as may equal in value the difference between total fees due from such Resident for the entire time of residency, and the amount paid by the Resident, and this agreement shall operate as an assignment, transfer, and conveyance to Retirement Facility of so much of such property.

FORM 28.13G: LIEN AGAINST LITIGATION PROCEEDS

1. In case of injury to Resident caused as the result of the fault, negligence, or carelessness of some third party or parties, Retirement Facility shall have a lien on any judgment or recovery for all its expenses incurred by reason of such injuries and to take all steps necessary in the name of Resident or otherwise to enforce the payment of such expenses by those responsible for such injuries.

2. Resident or Resident's legal representative shall have the duty to diligently pursue any claim for compensation due from third parties for injury to Resident and to cooperate with Retirement Facility in collecting such compensation and reimbursing Retirement Facility for the cost of such care furnished to Resident by the Retirement Facility.

3. If, however, Retirement Facility is satisfied that Resident or Resident's legal representative has diligently pursued such claims for compensation and that there shall be no recovery, or that the net amount paid to Retirement Facility shall be insufficient to fully compensate Retirement Facility, then the unpaid balance of such charges shall be canceled.

FORM 28.13H: RESIDENT GIFTS

Resident will not make any gift of real or personal property in contemplation of or subsequent to the execution of this contract, which would diminish Resident's estate to the detriment of Retirement Facility's claim. This provision shall apply whether Resident is actually an occupant at the Retirement Facility at time of death or not.

FORM 28.13I: ESTATE PLANNING

Retirement Facility recommends that, prior to taking occupancy hereunder, you make provisions for the final disposition upon your death of all furniture, possessions, payment of funeral expenses and burial, in a lawful will. It is recommended that you also prepare and execute durable powers of attorney for financial transactions and for medical treatment in the forms attached hereto as Exhibits _____ and _____ .

FORM 28.13J: APPOINTMENT OF CONSERVATOR

In the event you become unable to handle your personal or financial affairs and do not have a duly authorized representative, you authorize Retirement Facility to apply to a court of competent jurisdiction for the appointment of a conservator or guardian of your person and estate. All fees in connection therewith shall be paid from the estate of the conservatee or ward.

Table of Internal Revenue Service Rulings

Revenue Rulings	Section Number
54-430; 1954-2 C.B. 101	9.11
55-37; 1955-1 C.B. 347	6.1(c)(2), 7.3(c)(2)
55-449; 1955-2 C.B. 599	9.10(a)
56-185; 1956-1 C.B. 202	9.5
58-17; 1958-1 C.B. 11	6.2(a)
58-303; 1958-1 C.B. 61	9.11
60-135; 1960-1 C.B. 298	6.1(c)(2)
60-76; 1960-1 C.B. 296	7.2(b)(2)
61-72; 1961-1 C.B. 188	9.3
62-177; 1962-2 C.B. 89	7.2(b)(1)
62-178; 1962-2 C.B. 91	7.2(b)(1)
63-20; 1963-1 C.B. 24	15.6(e)
64-231; 1964-2 C.B. 139	9.2(a)(3), 9.3
64-31; 1964-1 C.B. 300	7.1(d)(1), 7.2(b)(2)
66-347; 1966-2 C.B. 196	6.2(a)
67-185; 1967-1 C.B. 70	6.1(c)(1)
68-17; 1968-1 C.B. 247	9.4(a)
68-525; 1968-2 C.B. 112	6.1(c)(1)
69-267; 1969-1 C.B. 160	9.10(a)
69-268; 1969-1 C.B. 160	9.10(a)
69-269; 1969-1 C.B. 160	9.10(a)
69-463; 1969-2 C.B. 131	12.1(b)(1)
69-76; 1969-1 C.B. 56	7.2(b)(1)
69-464; 1969-2 C.B. 132	12.1(b)(1)
69-545; 1969-2 C.B. 117	9.5
70-535; 1970-2 C.B. 117	9.7, 12.1(d)(1)
70-585; 1970-2 C.B. 585	9.4(a)
72-124, 1972-1 C.B. 145	9.2(a), 9.2(a)(3), 12.1(b)(2)
72-147; 1972-1 C.B. 147	9.4

Revenue Rulings	Section Number
72-209; 1972-1 C.B. 148	9.5
72-506; 1972-2 C.B. 506	9.11
73-549; 1973-2 C.B. 17	6.1(b)(2)
74-197; 1974-1 C.B. 143	12.1(b)(1)
74-607; 1974-2 C.B. 149	6.1(b)(4)
75-198; 1975-1 C.B. 157	9.7
75-302; 1975-2 C.B. 86	6.1(c)(1)
75-385; 1975-2 C.B. 205	9.7
76-244; 1976-1 C.B. 155	9.7
76-408; 1976-2 C.B. 408	9.4(a)
76-481; 1976-2 C.B. 82	6.1(c)(1)
77-3; 1977-1 C.B. 140	9.4(a)
77-246; 1977-2 C.B. 190	9.7
77-260; 1977-2 C.B. 466	6.1(b)(3)
79-18; 1979-1 C.B. 194	9.2(a)(1), (a)(3)
79-222; 1979-2 C.B. 236	12.1(b)(1)
79-300; 1979-2 C.B. 112	19.4
81-28; 1981-1 C.B. 328	9.5
81-61; 1981-1 C.B. 355	9.10(a)
81-62; 1981-1 C.B. 355	9.10(a)
82-14; 1982-1 C.B. 460	15.2
83-153; 1983-2 C.B. 48	9.9
83-157; 1983-2 C.B. 94	9.5
84-43; 1984-1 C.B. 27	7.1(d)(1)
85-132; 1985-2 C.B. 182	7.2(b)(2)

Revenue Procedures	
71-21; 1971-2 C.B. 549	6.1(b)(2)
75-21; 1975-1 C.B. 715	12.3(b)
80-27; 1980-1 C.B. 677	9.6
82-14; 1982-1 C.B. 459	12.1(e)
82-15; 1982-1 C.B. 460	15.2
82-26; 1982-1 C.B. 476	15.6(e)

Private Letter Rulings	
7718008	9.6
7733070	9.10(a)
7820058	12.1(b)(2)
7823072	9.4(b)(2)
7852009	6.1(b)(3)
7916068	9.3

Private Letter Rulings	Section Number
7948104	9.5
8022085	9.2(a)(3)
8025132	9.10(c)
8030105	9.2(b)(1)
8101009	9.4(a), 9.4(b)(2)
8111030	12.1(c)
8116121	12.1(c)
8117221	9.2(b)(7), 9.10(c)
8134021	9.10(a), 12.1(b)(2), 12.1(d)(1), 12.1(d)(2)
8138024	12.1(d)(1)
8201072	9.10(a), 12.1(b)(1), 12.1(b)(2)
8206093	12.1(b)(2)
8221134	6.1(c)(1)
8226146	12.1(b)(2)
8232035	12.1(b)(2), 12.1(d)(1)
8243212	12.1(b)(2)
8301003	9.10(a)
8303019	12.1(c)
8312129	9.10(a)
8326113	6.1(b)(5), 6.2(c)
8405083	9.2(a)(3)
8417054	12.1(b)(2)
8425129	12.1(b)(2), 12.1(e)
8427078	9.5
8427105	9.5
8449070	12.1(b)(2)
8502009	6.1(c)(1)
8506116	9.5, 9.9
8510068	9.5
8534089	9.5
8545063	12.1(b)(2)
8616095	9.5
8630005	6.1(c)(1)

General Counsel Memoranda

33671	9.4(a)
37019	6.1(b)(4)
37852	12.1(b)(2)
38478	9.2(b)(3), 9.4(b)(1), 12.1(e)
39326	12.1(c)

United States Code Citations

Internal Revenue Code	Section Number
§ 42	19.7
§ 42(b)	8.3, 19.7
§ 42(c)	19.7
§ 42(e)-(j), (n)	8.3
§ 103(b)	15.1, 15.4(a)
§ 105(h)	13.3(a)
§ 121	7.1(d)(1), 7.2(b)(3)
§ 125	13.3(a)
§ 141(b)	12.1(e)
§ 142(a)	12.2(b)(1)
§ 142(d)	12.2(b)(1), 15.3
§ 145	12.1(e), 15.2
§ 147(b)	15.4(b)
§ 147(f)	15.4(c)
§ 147(g)	15.4(d)
§ 148	15.4(a)
§ 149	15.4(e)
§ 163	7.1(d)(1)
§ 164	7.1(d)(1)
§ 168(b), (c)	12.2(a)
§ 168(g), (h), (j)	12.2(b)(1)
§ 170	9.9, 9.11
§ 183	19.4
§ 213(a)	6.1(c)(1)
§ 216(a), (b)	7.2(b)(1)
§ 262	7.1(d)(1)
§ 368(c)	12.1(d)(1)
§ 401	13.3(a)
§ 410	13.3(a)
§ 414(c), (m), (n)	13.3(a)
§ 416	13.3(a)
§ 451(a)	6.1(b)(4)
§ 465(a), (b), (c)	8.2(b)
§ 469(c), (h), (i), (j)	8.2(a)
§ 482	12.1(c)
§ 501(c)(2)	12.1(c)
§ 501(c)(3)	9.1
§ 501(c)(25)	12.1(c)
§ 501(m)	9.5
§ 502	12.1(c)

Internal Revenue Code	Section Number
§ 505	13.3(a)
§ 509(a)(1), (2), (3)	9.9
§§ 511–514	9.10(a)
§ 512(b)(1)	9.10(c), 12.1(b)(1)
§ 512(b)(3)	9.10(b), 12.1(c)
§ 512(b)(4)	9.10(c)
§ 512(b)(5)	12.1(d)(1)
§ 512(b)(13)	12.1(c), 12.1(d)(1)
§ 512(c)	12.1(b)(1)
§ 514(a), (b)	9.10(c)
§ 528(b), (c), (d)	7.1(d)(2), 9.8
§ 643	6.1(b)(4)
§ 651	6.1(b)(4)
§ 661	6.1(b)(4)
§§ 673–675	6.1(b)(4)
§ 1034	6.1(c)(2), 7.1(d)(1), 7.2(b)(2), 7.3(c)(2)
§ 1245(a)	12.2(a)
§ 1250	12.2(a)
§ 1274(d)	6.2(b)(1)
§§ 4940 *et seq.*	9.9
§ 6110(j)(3)	12.1(b)(2)
§ 7701(e)(1), (5)	12.2(c)
§ 7872(a), (b), (c), (e), (f)	6.2(b)(1)
§ 7872(g)	6.2(b)(2)

Other Code Sections	
12 U.S.C. § 1451	14.1(e)(4)
12 U.S.C. § 1701	22.4(a)
12 U.S.C. § 1701q	22.3(a)
12 U.S.C. § 1701q(d)(4)(A), (B), (C)	23.2
12 U.S.C. § 1701r-1	22.5(c)
12 U.S.C. § 1705	22.4(b)
12 U.S.C. § 1715w	22.2
12 U.S.C. § 1715y	14.1(d)(6)
12 U.S.C. § 1715z-1	9.2(a)(3)
12 U.S.C. § 1717	14.1(e)(2)
12 U.S.C. § 1721(g)	14.1(e)(3)
15 U.S.C. § 13-13c	13.2
15 U.S.C. § 21a	13.2
15 U.S.C. §§ 77a *et seq.*	19.2
15 U.S.C. § 77b(1)	24
15 U.S.C. §§ 3601-3616	7.1(c)(1)

Table of Cases

Index

Note: References are to section numbers in the text.

ABOUT THE AUTHOR

Paul A. Gordon is a partner in the law firm of Hanson, Bridgett, Marcus, Vlahos & Rudy, in San Francisco, California. The firm has represented retirement facility developers and operators for over 25 years.

Mr. Gordon is counsel to the California Association of Homes for the Aging, as well as numerous nonprofit and for profit facility developers and operators. He is a member of the Legal Committee of the American Association of Homes for the Aging, and of the National Association of Senior Living Industries and has lectured frequently on the legal and business aspects of retirement facility development and operations on a nationwide basis.